MENTAL DISORDER IN CANADA:
AN EPIDEMIOLOGICAL PERSPECTIVE

Canada has long been recognized as a leader in the field of psychiatric epidemiology, the study of the factors affecting mental health in populations. However, there has never been a book dedicated to the study of mental disorder at a population level in Canada. This collection of essays by leading scholars in the discipline uses data from the country's first national survey of mental disorder, the Canadian Community Health Survey of 2005, to fill that gap.

Mental Disorder in Canada explores the history of psychiatric epidemiology, evaluates methodological issues, and analyses the prevalence of several significant mental disorders in the population. The collection also includes essays on stigma, mental disorder and the criminal justice system, and mental health among women, children, workers, and other demographic groups. Focusing on Canadian scholarship, yet wide-reaching in scope, Mental Disorder in Canada is an important contribution to the dissemination and advancement of knowledge on psychiatric epidemiology.

JOHN CAIRNEY is an associate professor in the Departments of Psychiatry and Behavioural Neurosciences and Family Medicine at McMaster University and a senior research scientist at the Centre for Addiction and Mental Health.

DAVID L. STREINER is a professor in the Department of Psychiatry at the University of Toronto.

EDITED BY
JOHN CAIRNEY AND DAVID L. STREINER

Mental Disorder in Canada

An Epidemiological Perspective

UNIVERSITY OF TORONTO PRESS
Toronto   Buffalo   London

© University of Toronto Press Incorporated 2010
Toronto Buffalo London
www.utppublishing.com
Printed in Canada

ISBN 978-0-8020-9202-1 (cloth)
ISBN 978-0-8020-9442-1 (paper)

Printed on acid-free, 100% post-consumer recycled paper with vegetable-based inks

---

Library and Archives Canada Cataloguing in Publication

Mental disorder in Canada : an epidemiological perspective / edited by John Cairney and David L. Streiner.

Includes bibliographical references.
ISBN 978-0-8020-9202-1 (bound). ISBN 978-0-8020-9442-1 (pbk.)

1. Psychiatric epidemiology – Canada.   2. Mental illness – Canada.
3. Mental health – Canada.   4. Mental health services – Canada.
5. Mental health policy – Canada.   I. Cairney, John, 1968–   II. Streiner, David L.

RA790.7.C3M378 2010   362.2'04220971   C2009-906452-9

This book has been published with the help of a grant from the Canadian Federation for the Humanities and Social Sciences, through the Aid to Scholarly Publications Program, using funds provided by the Social Sciences and Humanities Research Council of Canada.

University of Toronto Press acknowledges the financial assistance to its publishing program of the Canada Council for the Arts and the Ontario Arts Council.

 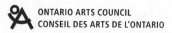

University of Toronto Press acknowledges the financial support for its publishing activities of the Government of Canada through the Book Publishing Industry Development Program (BPIDP).

*This book is dedicated to Alexander Hamilton Leighton, MD
(1908–2007), our teacher, mentor, colleague, guide,
and – most importantly – our friend.
He will be deeply missed.*

Contents

MENTAL DISORDER IN CANADA:
AN EPIDEMIOLOGICAL PERSPECTIVE

Introduction
Psychiatric Epidemiology in Canada:
A Coming of Age

JOHN CAIRNEY AND DAVID L. STREINER

Every year in the fall since 1984, a group of researchers interested in psychiatric epidemiology have gathered on the opening day of the Canadian Psychiatric Association Annual Meetings to spend a day discussing research, and share in good company, good food, and, often more than not, a glass or two of wine. This organization, the Canadian Academy of Psychiatric Epidemiology, or CAPE, was the brainchild of one of the most important figures in psychiatric epidemiology, Alexander Leighton. Although not a Canadian by birth, Alec had a special relationship with this country – especially Atlantic Canada – since his childhood. He would spend summers there as a child and adolescent, absorbing the culture and developing a fondness for and academic curiosity about one of this country's most unusual little inhabitants, the beaver. Indeed, Alec would always maintain a second home in the area, and he would visit there often throughout his life, including one last visit only months before his death.

   This part of the land most surely had gotten under his skin, for, when deciding where to conduct his first community study of mental disorder, he chose this same part of Canada. It was an excellent choice for a psychiatrist who had also trained as a social anthropologist. It had a mix of rural and urban inhabitants, two distinct cultures (French and English), and a host of communities spanning the socioeconomic continuum. It was also a region where many communities were undergoing profound social changes, economic and cultural. These were communities that, from a structural functionalist perspective, were in various states of integration and disintegration. It was just the kind of 'heterogeneity' one would need to address an important, yet understudied, phenomenon – exactly what role did social ecology play in the etiology of mental illness? A detailed review of Leighton's theory in this regard is provided in chapter 3 of this book.

But the Stirling County Study,[1] as it would come to be known, had a much broader impact than just its contribution to social theory and the emerging discipline of social psychiatry. As there were very few community-based studies of psychiatric disorder, and even fewer with a focus on cultural or community impacts on distress and impairment, Leighton and his colleagues had to create what they could not inherit. Unlike contemporary psychiatric epidemiologists, who are able to draw not only upon the Stirling County Study itself, but also on its successors, such as the Epidemiological Catchment Area (ECA)[2] and the National Co-morbidity Studies (NCS[3] and NCS-R[4]), for guidance with issues like sampling, the selection of survey instruments, and the interpretation of results, Leighton and his colleagues had largely to pioneer the modern psychiatric community survey. It is not hyperbole to suggest that they wrote a textbook for doing psychiatric epidemiology as they sought to answer the questions that defined their study. They helped to define the very practice of psychiatric epidemiology, a legacy that continues to this day.

In addition to this work, Alec Leighton and his partner Jane Murphy mentored the next generation of psychiatric epidemiologists. Many of these scientists are contributors to this volume, and several hold an award named in Alec's honour (a lifetime achievement award). Although small with regard to the number of researchers and volume of funding compared, for example, to the United States, Canadian scholarship in psychiatric epidemiology has flourished, building on the legacy of Stirling County. Around the same time the highly influential ECA studies were being conducted, Roger Bland and his colleagues at the University of Alberta provided much-needed community-level data on the epidemiology of disorders.[5] To this day, these data are often cited in relation to our understanding of disorder in the community. Dan (David) Offord, Michael Boyle, and their colleagues at McMaster University made two important contributions to psychiatric epidemiology – the Ontario Child Health Survey (OCHS)[6] and the Ontario Mental Health Supplement.[7] For decades, these studies shaped our understanding of the epidemiology of disorders in children and adults and the major social risk factors associated with them. The OCHS, in particular, has profoundly shaped our approach to the measurement of emotional and behavioural problems in children in community settings – a daunting challenge, given the issues of subjectivity and phenomenology in the reporting of disorder. Researchers from Quebec would continue in this important tradition and again bring scholarly attention to the problem of mental disorders in children through the Quebec Child Mental Health Survey[8] (see chapter 2 in this volume also). Throughout most of the history of the discipline, the focus of study was on specific regions of the country. It was not until early in the twenty-first century that this practice would change, in part through the efforts of a number of scholars, many of whom were involved in the aforementioned studies, and under the leadership of Statistics Canada.

With the release of the Canadian Community Health Survey: Mental Health and Well-Being (CCHS 1.2)[9] in 2005, Canadians now have, for the first time, national estimates of the prevalence of several significant mental disorders. Not surprisingly, important research is currently underway from the newest generation of psychiatric epidemiologists in this country. From Stirling through to the CCHS 1.2, an unbroken line of inquiry into the epidemiology of disorder in Canada is evident. However, although brief commentaries[10–12] and one review of research in psychiatric epidemiology in Canada[13] have been written before, there has never a been a book dedicated to the study of mental disorder at a population level in Canada, nor a book that showcases the important contributions that Canadian researchers have made to the field of psychiatric epidemiology. This book was conceived and completed to fill that gap.

We have divided this book into six sections. The first provides an overview of the history and context of psychiatric epidemiology in Canada, with particular attention to the role that social science has played in the origins of the discipline. The last chapter in this first part describes a shift in the way we have conceptualized and analysed social risk factors and mental disorder in population-based studies. The methodology is addressed in the second section, and in the third section, the epidemiology of major disorders is presented. Although the chapters of part 3 include data from other countries, the focus of these works is on what is known (and sometimes what is not known) about the epidemiology of major psychiatric disorders in Canada. Part 4 we call 'Special Topics' because the focus here is not necessarily on mental disorder per se, but on high-risk groups such as immigrants, persons incarcerated in the prison system, and women, and on topics that continue to be of critical importance to mental health, such as stigma and suicide. The health services and policy section (part 5) reviews the services and interventions aimed at depression, one of the leading causes of disability and diminished quality of life in Canada. But in this section also, we break with tradition a little in order to focus on emerging areas of inquiry and practice – mental health and disorder in the workplace and the role of knowledge translation in mental health policy and practice. In addition to leading epidemiologists in the field of psychiatry, we are also fortunate to have contributions from leading experts in health services and knowledge exchange in this country – evidenced by the high quality of these chapters. Finally, the editors conclude with some thoughts about where the field might head in the future.

The list of contributors represents a mix of senior, mid-career, and junior researchers, all of whom are active recognized scholars in the field of psychiatric epidemiology. We have representation from ten major Canadian universities (representing six provinces east to west), several hospitals, and government and non-governmental research institutes. The disciplinary training of the authors is equally diverse, ranging from psychiatry to infectious disease, nursing, sociology, criminology, psychology, economics, and epidemiology. Given the wide scope of expertise, the importance of the topic area, and the quality of contributions, we hope this book will become an important resource for researchers, professors, and clinicians in the fields of psychiatry, nursing, epidemiology, psychology, sociology, and social work. While it is arguable that Canadian psychiatric epidemiology came of age long before this volume was published, a text such as this one is often the sign of a mature field of inquiry. In any case, we should take the opportunity to both celebrate our achievements and to look enthusiastically to the future, recognizing, as this book highlights, the vibrant and diverse field of study that is psychiatric epidemiology in Canada.

REFERENCES

1 Leighton DC, Harding JS, Macklin DB, Hughes CC, Leighton AH. Psychiatric findings of the Stirling County Study. *Am J Psychiatry* 1963;119:1021–6.

2 Regier DA, Myers JK, Kramer M, et al. The NIMH Epidemiologic Catchment Area Program: Historical context, major objectives, and study population characteristics. *Arch Gen Psychiatry* 1984;41:934–41.

3 Kessler RC, McGonagle KA, Zhao S, et al. Lifetime and 12-month preva-

lence of DSM-III-R psychiatric disorders in the United States: Results from the National Comorbidity Survey. *Arch Gen Psychiatry* 1994; 51:8–19.

4 Kessler RC, Berglund P, Demler O, Jin R, Walters EE. Lifetime prevalence and age-of-onset distributions of DSM-IV disorders in the National Comorbidity Survey Replication. *Arch Gen Psychiatry* 2005;62:593–602.

5 Bland RC, Orn H, Newman SC. Lifetime prevalence of psychiatric disorders in Edmonton. *Acta Psychiatr Scand Suppl* 1988;338:24–32.

6 Boyle MH, Offord DR, Hofmann HG, et al. Ontario Child Health Study. I. Methodology. *Arch Gen Psychiatry* 1987;44:826–31.

7 Boyle MH, Offord DR, Campbell D, et al. Mental health supplement to the Ontario Health Survey: Methodology. *Can J Psychiatry* 1996;41: 549–58.

8 Breton JJ, Bergeron L, Valla JP, et al. Quebec child mental health survey: Prevalence of DSM-III-R mental health disorders. *J Child Psychol Psychiatry* 1999;40:375–84.

9 Gravel R, Béland Y. The Canadian Community Health Survey: Mental Health and Well-Being. *Can J Psychiatry* 2005;50:573–9.

10 Kates N, Munroe-Blum H. Psychiatric epidemiology in Canada. *Can J Psychiatry* 1990;35:383–4.

11 Arboleda-Flórez J. Psychiatric epidemiology in Canada. *Can J Psychiatry* 1997;43:699–700.

12 Streiner DL, Cairney J, Lesage A. Psychiatric epidemiology in Canada and the CCHS Study. *Can J Psychiatry* 2005;50:571–2.

13 Bland RC, Arboleda-Flórez J, Leighton A, Lesage A, Murphy JM, Stuart H. Epidemiology. In: Rae-Grant Q, ed. *Psychiatry in Canada: 50 Years (1951–2001)*. Ottawa: Canadian Psychiatric Association; 2001:211–36.

PART ONE

Context and Theory

1 The Social Science Contribution to Psychiatric Epidemiology

DAVID L. STREINER AND JOHN CAIRNEY

In chapter 2, Bland and Hanson place the recent epidemiological surveys done in Canada in a historical perspective and elaborate on the role that semi- and fully structured interviews have had in making large studies feasible. In this chapter, we briefly review the history of psychiatric epidemiology as a whole and attempt to explain why, for the most part, the field in North America has emphasized psychosocial factors as both causal factors and outcomes, often ignoring genetic and biological ones. We then focus on one of psychiatric epidemiology's most important figures, Alexander Leighton, whose pioneering studies established the modern psychiatric community survey, and whose theoretical works influenced or anticipated many of the ideas that guide research in the field today. His work, rooted as it was in anthropology and social psychology, provides further evidence supporting the important role the social sciences have played in the origins of this field. That this theory was developed and tested in Canada makes it especially significant to this collection.

A Brief History of Psychiatric Epidemiology

The Beginnings

The beginning of epidemiology itself is usually traced back to John Graunt, a haberdasher (not generally considered to be one of the social sciences) in London, who, in 1662, published a book called *Natural and Political Observations Made upon the Bills of Mortality*.[1] 'Bills of Mortality' were death records, which Graunt gathered from parishes in and around London in order to determine factors that affected when people were born and when and why they died. The book was revolutionary, as it was the first time that an attempt was made to discern patterns of morbidity and mortality in the population based on data from individuals.

Psychiatric epidemiology, though, was somewhat of a late starter, and did not emerge until the middle of the nineteenth century. In Europe, psychiatry had taken mainly a biological perspective, abetted in part by the discoveries that 'general paresis of the insane' (tertiary syphilis) and 'pellagra psychosis' were both due to physical causes, the former by a spirochete[2] and the latter by a deficiency of nicotinic acid in the diet.[3] This led to the hope that biological underpinnings could be found for all of the other psychiatric disorders. However, the United States was dominated at the time by a psychosocial paradigm, one that looked at societal and familial factors as the sources of pathology.[4] According to Grob,[5] the majority of nineteenth century psychiatrists in the United States were superintendents of psychiatric hospitals. Many of them believed that by gathering data they could uncover the underlying laws of disease, including mental illness, and that inductive science would validate their Protestant religious beliefs.

Perhaps the most prominent of these psychiatrists (or 'alienists,' as they were then called) was Edward Jarvis (1803–1884), who, before he became the head of a psychiatric hospital in Dorchester, Massachusetts, had aspirations of becoming a preacher, reinforcing Grob's thesis. As superintendent, he conducted a number of studies, finding, for example, that there was an inverse relationship between the distance people lived from psychiatric hospitals and their use of them. He recommended that there should be more small, geographically distributed hospitals rather than a few large, centralized ones.[6] In 1854, he was asked by the Commonwealth of Massachusetts to head up a Commission of Lunacy, charged with determining the number of mentally ill patients in hospitals.

Paradise Lost

Jarvis's report[7] was an amalgam of hard data and conclusions that had less to do with what he found than what he believed. For example, his religious beliefs (and those of others on the commission) led him to view small-town and farm life as bastions of moral virtue, and to see large cities as places marked by immigration, poverty, rapid social change, and anomie. Because of the pace of urbanization at the time, the Commission on Lunacy felt that the incidence of insanity should also be rising rapidly, and, although their data showed no such trend, this is what they concluded.

Srole and Fischer[8] describe this belief as the 'mental Paradise Lost' paradigm. 'One key tenet in this ideology is the pervasive conviction, often accepted as prima facie axiom, that mental health in the population at large has long been deteriorating and at an accelerating tempo during the modern era.'[8(p209)] Phenomena as disparate as situating psychiatric hospitals in rural 'idyllic nature' settings, erroneously concluding that rates of mental illness parallel rates of urbanization, or stating, as did Eric Fromm, that 'schizoid or schizophrenic qualities ... of a chronic low-grade type ... [are] common ... to most of the urban population' (cited in Srole[8(p210)]) can be attributed to this belief that we have left the 'Lost Paradise' of country life.

The American Censuses

This interest in counting the insane in Massachusetts was paralleled on a national level by the U.S. Bureau of the Census. In the sixth census, conducted in 1840, it attempted to count them for the first time. There were columns into which the enumerator could enter, for each household, 'How many idiotic or insane whites' and 'How many idiotic or insane slaves and free blacks.' The results of that census were (and remain) highly controversial and contentious. It stated that the rate of insanity among Blacks was ten times higher in the northern states than in the South, leading proponents of slavery to conclude that it was necessary 'because the African is incapable of self-care and sinks into lunacy under the burden of freedom.'[9] It has been proposed by some[10] that the secretary of state at the time, John C. Calhoun (under whose purview the Bureau of the Census fell), a slave-owning Southerner, staffed the bureau with like-minded political appointees who 'fudged' the data. Indeed, when he took a closer look at the data, Jarvis[11] found that, for example, there were 133 Blacks listed in the census as patients at the Massachusetts Insane Asylum. However, in reality, the asylum accepted only White patients, and Blacks were rarely admitted into other hospitals in the north. Similarly, northern towns that were said to have significant numbers of blind, insane, and idiotic Blacks had no Blacks at all living within their boundaries.

Further jeopardizing the work of the bureau was the lack of any formal nosological schema. There was serious disagreement within psychiatry regarding whether, to use just one example, paranoia was a distinct entity, or should be placed within the schizophrenias,[12] and parallel disagreement about the key features that should define each diagnostic category. Perhaps spurred by his re-examination of the 1840 census, Jarvis became involved with the bureau for the next thirty years. Between 1852 and 1882, he was the president of the American Statistical Association (ASA). He helped plan the seventh census (1850), wrote the section on vital statistics for the eigth census and, during his tenure as ASA president, worked closely with the bureau to improve the accuracy of their data collection. Under the direction of the superintendent of the census, Francis A. Walker, who had succeeded Jarvis as president of the ASA, one of the twenty-five volumes resulting from the 1880 census was on 'dependency,' a term that included the mentally ill, the retarded, and criminals, written by Frederick H. Wines.[13] Not surprisingly, given Jarvis's close involvement with the project, the volume concluded that the increase in 'dependency' was related to urbanization and organized society.

Over the next few decades, two different perspectives vied for supremacy within American psychiatry, initiating a struggle that still exists in various guises. One camp, led by the American Medico-Psychological Association (which later became the American Psychiatric Association), felt that psychiatry could advance only if the haphazard diagnostic criteria, which often varied from one hospital to the next, were made more uniform. They attempted to devise an agreed-upon system of diagnostic categories that would be used in all hospitals, a move that ultimately culminated in the first edition of the *Diagnostic and Statistical Manual (DSM)*.[14] The opposing camp, led by Adolph Meyer, who is often seen as one of the founders of academic psychiatry in the United States, and who was the chair at Johns Hopkins, objected to what he called 'one-word diagnoses' and the attempt of statistics to solve psychiatric and social problems. In what must be seen as an ironic twist of fate, the last resident he trained was Alexander Leighton, who is considered to be the father of psychiatric epidemiology.

The Introduction of the Social Sciences

In the United States, from the time of Jarvis until well into the 1950s, psychiatric epidemiology was dominated by social scientists. For example, the special census in 1910 that focused on the mentally ill was headed by Joseph A. Hill, who was a political economist,[5] and social scientists were prominent in the mental health agencies of New York and Massachusetts. Grob states that 'To social scientists the census was not merely an instrument to collect data. On the contrary, the census represented a radical faith that quantitative research, when merged with administrative rationality, could replace politics.'[5(p231)] During this period, a number of books reinforced the 'biopsychosocial,' as opposed to the medical, conceptualization of the roots of mental disturbances. These included the Lynds' *Middletown*,[15] Landis and Page's *Modern Society and Mental Disease*,[16] and Faris and Dunham's major ecological study, *Mental Disorders in Urban Areas*.[17]

Although there was continued interest within the Bureau of the Census in counting the insane, as reflected in the special censuses in 1904 and 1910, there was growing realization that the counts were of those people who were in institutions, and that a multitude of non-psychiatric factors, such as distance from a hospital, urban/rural residence, social support, the availability of beds, social policy, and so forth, were major determinants of who was or was not hospitalized. Consequently, a different approach was needed: studies that measured psychiatric disorders in the community. These began to be conducted after the Second World War, when psychiatric epidemiology entered what Klerman[4] and Weissman[18] called its second generation and its 'golden age.'

The Later Generations

In Canada, Alexander Leighton and his colleagues began the Stirling County study,[19] which is still being led by Jane Murphy.[20] In order to see if the results could be generalized from a predominantly rural setting to a more urbanized one (and, in part, as a test of the 'Lost Paradise' hypothesis), Leighton collaborated with Rennie, Srole, and Langner in the equally famous Midtown Manhattan Study[21] in New York. Unlike previous studies, these featured larger, more representative samples of the general population, high response rates, and measures of overall impairment, rather than the unreliable, psycho-analytically-informed diagnoses of *DSM-I*.[14] Again, the studies highlighted the causal role of social factors in the genesis of mental disorders.

We will not discuss what Klerman[4] and Weissman[18] call the third- and fourth-generation studies, as they are well covered in the Bland

and Hanson chapter, except to note that they, as did the previous generations, focused primarily on psychosocial factors.

The Contribution of Social Theory

While it may appear as though, at least with regard to methods, there has been a reasonably linear development in psychiatric epidemiology from its inception, the same pattern is difficult to discern when we examine the contribution of social theory in psychiatric epidemiology both in Canada and elsewhere. In fact, the relationship, were we to graph it, would probably look more like a U-shaped curve, where the complexity of theory (depicted on the y-axis) is highest in the 1950s (x-axis), declines throughout the next three or so decades, and shows some evidence today of an upward trend. This is not to say that in specific disciplines such as sociology, theory has not continued to evolve. Psychiatric epidemiology is rooted in psychiatry and is multidisciplinary by definition. Our observations, therefore, are specific to it, and not a comment on other fields of inquiry. Given the early richness of social theory in early psychiatric epidemiology, it is important to review this work (see chapter 3, which picks up the upward trend in our curvilinear model).

Social Theory – Historical Reflections

There is a joke among some academics with regard to their epidemiology colleagues that says, 'Epidemiologists are like accountants, only less interesting.' Epidemiology does often seem like little more than accounting – how many individuals suffer from condition X? And certainly the caricature of someone who engages in this kind of 'accounting' might be reasonably portrayed as a staid, dry individual, hardly the 'life' of the academic party. The joke, however, reflects a more deep-seated concern, shared by many epidemiologists themselves: the sometimes tenuous relationship academic epidemiology has with theory.[22] In fact, theory in epidemiology often takes a backseat to the more matter-of-fact task of ensuring that one gets the numbers right.

In many ways, psychiatric epidemiology is one of the exceptions to this criticism. Almost from the beginning, theory, especially social scientific theory, has occupied an important place in the development of the discipline. Indeed, the field relies almost exclusively on social science, often at the expense of other fields such as genetics and neu-

rology. This is, in part, a matter of practical necessity. Psychiatric epidemiology depends heavily on the science of surveys as the principal
means by which its data are collected, and certain forms of data (e.g.,
demographic) are simply easier to collect than others (e.g., biologic
material), for both technical and ethical reasons. It is also the case,
however, that many of the leading figures in the field, both yesterday
and today, are social scientists or are trained in this tradition (e.g., Alec
Leighton, Jane Murphy, Bruce and Barbara Dohrenwend, Ron Kessler,
Bruce Link, William Eaton, Myrna Weissman). The attraction of social
scientists to the field has almost certainly influenced the development
of the discipline. The impact of this is perhaps most apparent in the
application of psychometrics (meeting the daunting challenge of
measuring psychological disturbances without the use of trained clinical personnel) and social psychological measurement (meeting the
equally daunting challenge of measuring social structural and interpersonal factors that may give rise to these disturbances) to the practice of community psychological surveys. Both of these traditions are
guided by the theoretical frameworks that inform the practitioners of
these disciplines.

Sociology, anthropology, and psychology have been and continue to
be important guiding parent disciplines to the field and its methods,
even if this is not always stated explicitly. Yet there have been times
when theory, social or otherwise, has taken a backseat to 'getting the
numbers right.' This is true in Canadian psychiatric epidemiology as
elsewhere, but we are fortunate to have had several key figures in the
field of mental health who developed and tested major theories
regarding the social etiology of mental disorder. In this part of the
chapter, we will review the theoretical work of Leighton and will end
with a brief discussion of the theoretical linkages of his ideas to theories that continue to shape our theoretical understanding of risk factors
for mental illness to this day – a thread that will be pursued further in
chapter 3.

The Social Theory of Alexander Leighton and
the Stirling County Study

It is difficult to overstate the importance of Alexander Leighton and
the Stirling County Study to the field of psychiatric epidemiology in
Canada, and, indeed, the field elsewhere. More often than not, the
importance of his contribution has been thought to lie in his methods

and findings, rather than in the theory that underlies them. We must remember, however, that the trilogy documenting the initial findings of the Stirling county study included complete works on theory (*My Name is Legion*[19]), method (*The Character of Danger*[23]), and on the results of the exhaustive anthropological fieldwork conducted by Leighton and his team (*People of Cove and Woodlot*[24]). It was clear that theory, as much as method or results, occupied a place of central importance in his work and that of his colleagues. As such, we believe it important to give particular attention to the theoretical work developed in the Stirling County studies, especially inasmuch as it illustrates an important incorporation of social theory into psychiatric epidemiology.

A Lifetime of Reflection: Fundamental Conclusions

Leighton's acceptance speech for the Malinowski award in 1984 provided a unique insight into his views on social theory and cultural anthropology.[25] Others, too,[26] have used this text to summarize his work and our review draws as much on these works as it does on the original text. Essentially, the collective findings of both his early experiences in the military during the Second World War, and his anthropological and epidemiological fieldwork, including but not limited to Stirling County, led him to draw three fundamental conclusions in relation to our understanding of both society and the individual:

1 There is a tremendous amount of intra-cultural variation. On reflecting upon early ethnographic accounts of numerous cultural groups, Leighton concluded that the actual practice of culture (expressed in values, beliefs, and rituals, for example) was far more variable than one might be led to believe from summaries of these accounts. In his words, 'patterns of life (family, child care, response to illness) varied considerably within social groupings and from individual to individual.'[25(p214)] In other words, the stories or narratives of culture, typified in the ethnographic accounts of early and mid-twentieth century anthropology and sociology, tended to homogenize the lived experience of the participants under study, and the varied ways they respond to and, indeed, define the conditions of existence, social and otherwise. The world Leighton encountered was far richer and more diverse than the ethnographic accounts expressed. This observation, apparently reached quite early in his intellectual development, would have a profound

impact on his work in Stirling. This proposition is widely held today in modern ethnography, which suggests Leighton was ahead of his time in reaching this conclusion.[26]

2 There is a common core (or bundle) of strivings that are shared by all people. This was a major theoretical proposition and was central to his theory of psychopathology, as outlined in *My Name Is Legion*.[19] Although we will return to this idea later, in essence the 'bundle of strivings' originally catalogued by Leighton included, among others, the need for physical security, sexual satisfaction, love, security, individual recognition, a sense of belonging to a group, orientation toward oneself and one's place in a social group (society), the expression of spontaneity (creativity), a sense of belonging to a moral order, and a feeling of being 'right in what one does.' It is important to note that the universality of these strivings suggested that these are not products of culture. Rather, they are essential, defining elements of the human condition, and are therefore better conceived of as biological imperatives rather than socially defined or created ones. It is this last point that would likely raise the eyebrows of many contemporary social scientists, especially those who adhere to a social constructivist paradigm.[27] Leighton's interest and early training in evolutionary biology opened up a possibility for explaining fundamental elements of our humanity that likely would not necessarily have been so obvious (or desirable) to a social scientist.[26]

3 The final conclusion concerns inter-individual variability (what Leighton described as 'person-variability') within cultures. This is simply a statement about diversity. Where the first observation deals with cultural homogeneity (e.g. values, ritual practices), this observation is about individual homogeneity. Many ethnographic accounts in Leighton's time disregarded individual variability within cultural groups, thereby disregarding or ignoring individual functioning and personality differences that were, to Leighton, everywhere evident. Quite simply, even within cultures, people vary in attitudes and opinions, but also in temperament, cognitive abilities, and so forth. Again, this point is widely accepted in modern sociology and anthropology, but earlier works from these disciplines, especially those from the post–World War II period in America, tended to emphasize the concept of 'national character' and demonstrate a general interest in the role of culture and social structure in personality formation.[28] Leighton describes his experi-

ences in post–war Japan and southeast Asia and the belief among many of his contemporaries in the service that the isolated pockets of Japanese soldiers, unaware that the war had ended, would be unlikely to surrender when confronted by allied troops, given the authoritarian nature of the 'Japanese personality.'[ψ] It was only by interviewing captured Japanese soldiers and the analysis of diaries found at battle sites, that this homogenized conceptualization of the 'Japanese character' came to be challenged.[25]

Conclusions 1 and 3 speak directly to issues of central concern in the social sciences – the nature of the relationship of the social to the individual (person in society, society in person). They are direct challenges to social or cultural relativity and social/cultural determinism. Rather than being simply products of social forces, determined by culture or society, individuals are shaped as much by internal forces as external ones. Human experience is rich and varied within social settings and specific historical periods. When we also consider the second proposition – that there is a core universal element that binds all of humanity together – we all essentially strive for the same things and this is part of our biological make-up. Together, these conclusions offer a challenge to an overly socialized conception of human beings, and at the same time, champion the idea of the importance of the individual in social experience.

The Role of the Social in Psychopathology

Leighton's second conclusion was fundamental to his conceptualization of psychopathology, and was described in detail in *My Name Is Legion*.[19] We have reproduced some of the original figures used in that text to illustrate these ideas. Figure 1.1 depicts what we have already identified as a central proposition in Leighton's conceptual system – all individuals, represented here as personality, strive to fulfill a set of fundamental human needs (e.g., love, recognition, security) depicted as objects. Leighton labelled the whole act of striving as the essential psychical condition and viewed this as a biological imperative necessary for sustaining life.[19] Psychical balance (psychological health or well-being) is achieved and maintained when the striving produces the desired outcome (e.g., securing meaningful relationships). Failure to acquire, or loss of, these objects results in tension and distress – a disruption of psychic well-being.

Figure 1.1   Leighton's Essical Psychical Condition

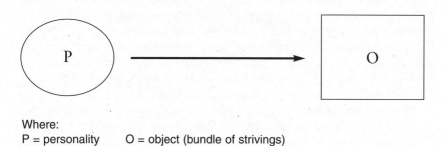

Where:
P = personality   O = object (bundle of strivings)

Figure 1.2   Disrupted Essential Psychical Condition

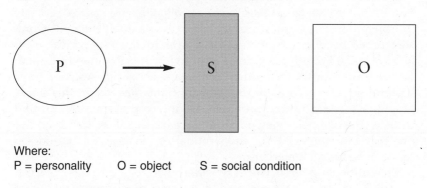

Where:
P = personality   O = object   S = social condition

In figure 1.2, the concept of the social is introduced, and a mechanism linking social factors to mental disorder is offered. Specifically, the social in this system can act as a 'blockage,' interfering with the attainment of desired objects. An example of this can be found in relation to economic activity. Imagine an individual who trains his whole life to obtain and sustain occupancy in a particular occupation, only to lose his job because it becomes redundant or unnecessary due to major, macro-economic changes. The collapse of the fishing industry in eastern Canada, and the current travails of the manufacturing sector in Canada and the United States provide contemporary examples. The salient points here are: (1) the disruption and resultant dislocation of the person through an event such as unemployment blocks one's attempts to satisfy fundamental human needs; and (2) the change is brought about not by the actions of the individual, but by forces (social and cultural) beyond the control of the person(ality). The role of the social, then, is as a force that prevents the satisfaction of fundamental human desires. It is, of course, also true that societies, through the provision of services such as education or universal health care, can also facilitate the acquisition of these necessities. In this conceptualization, we are challenged to look for instances where social forces either block or facilitate our fundamental human strivings.

This particular view of the social is not unique to Leighton, but the characterization of social forces as sources of interference with our humanity is quite different from Freud's theory of civilization as a sublimating force for sexual energy,[29] and Fromm's socialist utopian society.[30] Both of these theorists embrace the idea that the society acts as a force to limit human expression and the fulfillment of needs and desires; but where Freud sees the forces of civilization as necessary to achieve progress, Leighton sees social forces as a double-edged sword, sometimes beneficial, sometimes harmful to one's psychical well-being. Unlike Fromm, Leighton did not view the abolition of capitalism as a necessary precondition for creating a social system free of harmful interferences with fundamental human needs. In this sense, Leighton's contribution provides an interesting middle ground between the two polar viewpoints in the psychoanalytic tradition, and one that rests neither on Freud's model of the unconscious nor on Marxian historical materialism.

An additional point is worth considering in regard to this theory. It is clear that Leighton[19] accepted that psychopathology could arise from other mechanisms, some internal to the individual, and some external, but different from either Fromm's or Freud's the models. In the essential psychical condition, Leighton noted that the failure to secure objects could arise from a defect inherent to the person, or a defect in the object itself. In this sense, social forces are one potential etiological agent, that likely acts in concert with other internal (person) and external (e.g., interactional) forces to shape the psychical well-being.

It is clear that if social forces are etiological agents in mental disorder, then some method of operationalizing these are required. Community, and in particular, community integration and disintegration, become the key concepts through which Leighton and his colleagues could explore the role of social forces as source of interference. People live and identify with communities, and although there is no easy (or singular) way of characterizing them, in Stirling County, hamlets (defined geographically and politically) were the unit of observations. Communities could be characterized as integrated or disintegrated, in a Durkheimian inspired system of classification. Disintegrated communities were those that suffered one or more of the following insults: (1) recent history of disaster, (2) extensive poverty, (3) cultural confusion (conflicting cultural groups), (3) extensive secularization, (4) widespread migration, or (5) rapid social change.[31] The visible signs of disintegration were high rates of crime and 'deviant' behaviour, an absence of strong community leaders, and decaying infrastructure and other observable signs of poverty (decrepit buildings, few or no recreational facilities, etc.).[19]

Social disintegration, then, was the social force that blocked the essential striving conditions required for psychological well-being. Results of the initial survey in Stirling county revealed that the probability of psychiatric disturbance ('caseness') was greater in communities that were disintegrated than in those that were not. At the individual level, within communities, socioeconomic status, gender, age, and religiosity emerged as important risk markers for disorder. Unlike many population surveys of psychiatric disorder undertaken since Stirling (e.g. ECA, NCS, CCHS 1.2), disorder was found to be most common among the elderly. Otherwise, women, those who were poor, and those who scored low on religiosity were at greater risk for disturbance. Similar associations were reported by other studies of the same period (e.g., Midtown Manhattan Study), and have been replicated many times since. Perhaps most importantly, further evidence for the role of community (dis)integration in psychiatric disturbance was obtained after a ten-year follow-up of the original survey.[32] One of the communities had undergone profound social change (economic revitalization) since this original survey, so much so that the community could be reclassified as integrated at the time of the follow-up. A significant decrease in psychiatric disorder compared to the original survey was also observed, leading Leighton and his colleagues to conclude that the community-level change had indeed led to improved mental health among residents. This remains an important and powerful demonstration of the role of the social environment in psychopathology.

So, were we to put these threads together, a unique conceptualization of the person in society, and of the society in person, emerges. According to Leighton's theory, human beings attempt to achieve and

maintain a state of psychological striving. This is a biological imperative, not a social or psychological one. All individuals, regardless of
culture and individual differences, seek to maintain this state. To
Leighton, however, people are biologically, psychologically, and
socially constituted. In other words, while the essential psychical condition is universal, lived experience is determined by a confluence of
different factors, some biological, many others social. It is also clear
from this work that there is a dynamic relationship between personality (self) and society in this system of thought. Social forces can block
or interfere with our fundamental strivings, and these forces are
evident at the multiple levels of social organization (community integration or disintegration, position in the social structure). But social
forces interact with persons across their life course (or what Leighton
termed the 'life-arc'), so people are molded not only by their biology,
but also by their biographies and their place in history. Finally, it is
clear in Leighton's theory that individuals are not simply products of
culture or biology, but also have the capacity to resist social forces and
to adapt positively to their circumstance. Persons, to use the parlance
of our day, may be vulnerable and reactive, but they are also active and
resilient.

To many readers, this may all sound a little familiar. These ideas
summarized resonate with contemporary theory on the determinants
of mental health. Leighton's theory anticipates the biopsychosocial
perspective, for it recognizes the role of each of these factors in shaping
health and disorder. The role of stress – the source of which is social
(e.g., community disintegration) – in Leighton's work recalls the stress
process framework, especially that espoused by Leonard Pearlin and
his colleagues.[33,34] The concept of the life-arc, the notion that the
timing of one's biography influences not only the act of striving, but
also the consequences of its blockage – parallels Life Course theory,
especially the perspectives of Glen Elder[35] and John Clausen.[36] And
finally, the inherent capacities of the individual, in concert with
resources in the social environment, to resist or cope with interference
to the essential psychical condition sounds very much like resiliency –
that magical trait hotly sought after by social scientists seeking to
explain why most individuals, when confronted with adversity and
trauma, do not become psychopathological. What is truly remarkable
about Leighton's theory is not only its comprehensiveness and complexity, but that it is relevant to contemporary theory on the role of
social environment in shaping health and development in individuals.

Conclusions

In many respects, psychiatric epidemiology has come a long way since its first, faltering steps in the middle of the nineteenth century. We now use psychometrically sound instruments and complicated, multi-stage sampling procedures, and rely heavily on computers to store the masses of data that emerge and to run the sophisticated analyses that are required to tease apart the complicated relationships among predisposing, enabling, and protective factors and the outcomes. Edward Jarvis and his colleagues would be amazed at the progress that has been made, and jealous of the tools at our disposal. In other regards, though, they would feel right at home and comfortable with the general approach.

While the underlying social theories governing our choice of variables have increased in complexity and in their list of intra-individual and social factors, the focus has remained relatively unchanged. Jarvis felt that large cities were inherently pathogenic. Leighton's work showed that small towns could also produce pathology; and that healthy communities, both large and small, contributed to the mental well-being of their inhabitants. But the focus on the social milieu as a, if not *the*, causative agent would not be at all foreign to him. By the same token, he would likely not be surprised that other factors, such as biological or 'constitutional' ones, have been largely ignored. Jarvis could be excused to some degree; Galton didn't publish his book on the inheritance of intelligence until 1869.[37] We do not have that excuse, but we are hampered by the invasiveness and costs, as well as the logistical, legal, and ethical challenges required for genetic testing. We will return to this issue in the last chapter, in which we discuss where we think psychiatric epidemiology should be heading in the future.

Despite this relative narrowness in focus, psychiatric epidemiology has accomplished much in the past 150 years, and the Canadian contribution has been considerable, for both its theoretical and methodological insights. In the following chapters, some of the leading figures in Canada outline where we've been, and what we have found.

NOTES AND REFERENCES

ψ   It was believed and practised in many instances by Japanese soldiers that death (by ritual suicide) was preferable to capture. The prevailing belief among psychiatrists and psychologists working for the allies was that this practice could only be explained in a personality that had surrendered personal interests to a collective will/authority – what was described as an authoritarian personality.

1 Graunt J. *Natural and Political Observations Made upon the Bills of Mortality*. Baltimore: Johns Hopkins Press, 1662/1939.
2 Noguchi H, Moore JW. A demonstration of Treponema pallidum in the brain in cases of general paralysis. *J Exp Med* 1913;17:232–8.
3 Goldberger J, Waring CH, Willets DG. The prevention of pellagra. A test of diet among institutional inmates. *Pub Health Rep* 1915;30: 3117–31.
4 Klerman GL. Paradigm shifts in USA psychiatric epidemiology since World War II. *Soc Psychiatry Psychiatr Epidemiol* 1990;25:27–32.
5 Grob GN. The origins of American psychiatric epidemiology. *Am J Pub Health* 1985;75:229–36.
6 Jarvis E. The influence of distance from and proximity to an insane hospital, on its use by any people. *Boston Med Surg J* 1850;42:209–22.
7 Jarvis E. *Insanity and Idiocy in Massachusetts: Report of the Commission on Lunacy, 1855*. Cambridge, MA: Harvard University Press, 1855/1971.
8 Srole L, Fischer AK. The Midtown Manhattan Longitudinal Study vs 'the mental paradise lost' doctrine. *Arch Gen Psychiatry* 1980;37:209–21.
9 Cooper R. *Psychiatry and Philosophy of Science*. Stocksfield, UK: Acumen, 2007.
10 Maultsby MM. Why American Blacks distrust psychiatrists. In: Turner SM, Jones RT, eds. *Behavior Modification in Black Populations: Empirical Findings and Psychological Issues*. New York: Plenum Press, 1982.
11 Jarvis E. Insanity among the colored population of the free states. *Am J Med Sci* 1844;7:71–83.
12 Schanda H. (2000). Paranoia and dysphoria: Historical developments, current concepts. *Psychopathology* 2000;33:204–8.
13 U. S. Bureau of the Census. *Report on the Defective, Dependent, and Delinquent Classes of the Population of the United States*. Washington: Government Printing Office, 1888.
14 American Psychiatric Association. *Diagnostic and Statistical Manual: Mental Disorders*. Washington: Author, 1952.
15 Lynd RS, Lynd HM. *Middletown: A Study in Contemporary American Culture*. New York: Harcourt Brace and Co, 1929.
16 Landis C, Page JD. *Modern Society and Mental Disease*. New York: Farrar and Rinehart, 1938.

17 Faris REL, Dunham HW. *Mental Disorders in Urban Areas: An Ecological Study of Schizophrenia and Other Psychoses.* Chicago: University of Chicago Press, 1939.

18 Weissman MM. The epidemiology of psychiatric disorders: Past, present, and future generations. *Int J Methods Psychiatr Res* 1995;5:69–78.

19 Leighton AH. *My Name Is Legion: The Stirling County Study of Psychiatric Disorder and Sociocultural Environment. Vol. 1.* New York: Basic Books, 1959.

20 Murphy JM, Horton NJ, Laird NM, et al. Anxiety and depression: A 40-year perspective on relationships regarding prevalence, distribution, and comorbidity. *Acta Psychiatr Scand* 2004;109:355–75.

21 Srole L, Langner TS, Michael ST, et al. *Mental Health in the Metropolis: The Midtown Manhattan Study.* New York: McGraw-Hill, 1962.

22 Shy CM. The failure of academic epidemiology: Witness for the prosecution. *Am J Epidemiol* 1997;145:479–84.

23 Leighton DC, Harding JS, Macklin DM, Macmillan AM, Leighton AH. *The Character of Danger: Psychiatric Symptoms in Selected Communities.* New York: Basic Books, 1963.

24 Hughes CC, Tremblay MA, Rapoport RN, et al. *People of Cove and Woodlot.* New York, NY: Basic Books, 1960.

25 Leighton AH. Then and now: Some notes on the interaction of person and social environment. Society for Applied Anthropology, 2002. Retrieved January 2, 2006, from http://www.sfaa.net/malinowski/monograph/chapter 14.htlm.

26 Barkow JH. Alexander Leighton and the evolutionary perspective. *Transcult Psychiatry* 2006;43:45–55.

27 Berger PL, Luckmann T. *The Social Construction of Reality: A Treatise in the Sociology of Knowledge.* Garden City, New York: Anchor Books, 1966.

28 Kohn M. *Class and Conformity: A Study of Values.* Chicago: University of Chicago Press, 1969.

29 Freud S. *Civilization and Its Discontents* (J. Strachey, trans.). New York: W. W. Norton, 1929/1961.

30 Fromm E. *The Sane Society.* New York: Rinehart & Company, 1955.

31 Blazer DG. *The Age of Melancholy: 'Major Depression' and Its Social Origins.* New York: Routledge, 2005.

32 Leighton A. Poverty and social change. *Sci Am* 1965;212:21–7.

33 Pearlin LI. The sociological study of stress. *J Health Behav* 1989;30:241–56.

34 Pearlin LI. The stress process revisited: Reflections on concepts and their

interrelationships. In: Aneshensel CS, Phelan J, eds. *Handbook on the Sociology of Mental Health*. New York: Plenum Press, 1999:395–415.

35 Elder G. *Children of the Great Depression: Social Change in Life Experience* (25th Anniversary Edition). Chicago: University of Chicago Press, 1988.

36 Clausen J. *American Lives: Looking Back at the Children of the Great Depression*. New Jersey: Free Press, 1993.

37 Galton F. *Hereditary Genius: An Inquiry into Its Laws and Consequences*. London: Macmillan, 1869.

2 The History of Psychiatric Epidemiology in Canada: The Development of Community Surveys

ROGER C. BLAND AND TARA HANSON

Community surveys were initially done to determine the prevalence of mental disorders within a specific population. Fifty years ago, large-scale studies were simply not feasible for several reasons. Standardized, structured interviews did not exist, and computers were not available for scoring, handling large data sets, and sophisticated statistics. Physicians or other mental health professionals were needed to conduct individual interviews and confirm diagnoses within a community. These mental disorders were diagnosed before the establishment of standardized diagnostic criteria. Without computers, the volume of data collected had to be limited to what could be analysed manually.

Severe psychiatric disorders have low prevalences, requiring suitable methodologies to sample large numbers in the population to produce accurate estimates. Diagnostic instruments must be reliable and valid enough to be used by non-clinician interviewers in order to keep study costs manageable. In addition, there must be an adequate way to manage the large amounts of data collected on each participant and to make necessary adjustments in the sampling methods. Another consideration, which has become increasingly apparent, is that knowing the number of people with a particular diagnosis does not give a clear indication of the level of disability from which they are suffering nor whether they will need, access, or benefit from treatment services.

Several factors contribute to accurate approximations of the prevalence of mental disorders in a given population. Widely adopted diagnostic schemes ensure that disorders are classified according to common criteria. During the 1960s and 1970s, a major study conducted in the United States and the United Kingdom found that there was a higher frequency of schizophrenia being diagnosed in the United States and a higher prevalence for manic depressive disorder and depression being diagnosed in the United Kingdom.[1] Once a standardized diagnostic tool – the Present State Examination (PSE) – and systematic interviewing techniques were introduced, the reported rates of schizophrenia and manic depression in these countries were similar, an illustration of the need for consistent criteria for diagnosis.

By consistently employing reliable diagnostic instruments, researchers are able to compare study results among countries and populations. Validity, however, is often problematic because external means of confirming diagnosis (e.g., laboratory tests) do not exist. The methodologies involved in conducting prevalence surveys evolved alongside technological advances, gradually expanding community survey research into national and international arenas.

The history of psychiatric epidemiology in Canada is best understood within an international context. Advances in population mental health research approaches have been adopted and shared worldwide. Canadian researchers applied advanced methodologies and fashioned new tools as the need appeared. There are important international pioneers in this field who have contributed to the generation of knowledge in psychiatric epidemiology.

Prior to the 1950s, over sixty psychiatric epidemiological studies were reported from Scandinavia and Central Europe, but few were available in English. At that time, little of the research was focused on social psychiatry or epidemiology. Academics were interested in exploring the relationships between mental illness and genetics. Many studies incorporated small sample sizes, unrepresentative of the whole population, while some simply relied on hospital statistics. Nevertheless, Strömgren[2] was able to conclude that the lifetime risk for schizophrenia was 0.72%, and 0.21% for manic depressive illness. These estimates are reasonably concordant with conclusions from more recent studies.

Several early studies may be regarded as landmarks due to their sampling methods. The Lundby studies initiated by Essen-Möller[3] and the later follow-ups by Hagnell and colleagues[4,5,6] included all inhabitants living in a Swedish community in 1947 (i.e., the sample was the whole population of a geographically limited area). The residents served as a cohort which has been followed up several times since, including those who left the community and others who arrived during the interviewing periods. Follow-up studies with this initial cohort continue to be conducted.

Different sampling methods were used in North American studies including the Eaton and Weil study of Hutterites in Canada and the United States.[7] Medical and non-medical sources identified potential cases and key informants were used to further identify cases. The final diagnosis was determined by physician-review of the interviews and some direct psychiatric interviews. Fremming[8] in Denmark and Helgason[9] in an Icelandic study used birth cohorts as a method for obtaining a representative population sample and were very successful in tracing the subjects (92% for Fremming and 99% for Helgason). The method of studying birth cohorts has become known as Klemperer's method, named after the person who first used this method in Munich in 1933.

In Atlantic Canada, Alexander Leighton and his associates[10] initiated the Stirling County study. This study, along with the Midtown Manhattan study by Srole et al., [11] used written protocols and structured interviews administered by non-medical interviewers that were then reviewed by clinicians. Further information on study participants was gained through hospital medical records and later verified by general practitioners. Both of these studies have been described as second generation epidemiological studies since they introduced major advances in sampling large populations. The New Haven study by Weissman et al.[12–15] was probably the first among the third generation studies that incorporated sophisticated sampling methods plus standardized diagnostic tools, using the Schedule for Affective Disorders and Schizophrenia (SADS-L) based on the Research Diagnostic Criteria (RDC) administered by trained non-medical clinicians.

The results of the Midtown Manhattan study showed that 80% of the sample had current affective or psychophysiological symptoms and 20% were judged to be severely impaired.[16] According to the study results, females with lower socioeconomic status experienced greater social adversity and were at a high risk for exhibiting symptoms of mental illness. From the Stirling County Study, Leighton et al.[10] reported similar conclusions. Streiner et al. elaborate that these studies 'were marked by large representative samples, high response rates, and the use of measures of overall impairment rather than the unreliable psychiatric diagnosis of the day.'[17(p571)] The Stirling County researchers used the Health Opinion Survey and used key informant and participant-observation methods to build community models based on the *Diagnostic and Statistical Manual* (*DSM-I*) criteria.[18] Screening scales were developed for both of these studies and have been adopted and used in several community surveys that explored the correlation between stress and symptoms of mental illness.

The Stirling County study is particularly remarkable. Dr. Jane Murphy was cognizant of the advances made in psychiatry since the start of that study, including the development of the third *Diagnostic and Statistical Manual* (*DSM-III*),[19] and the launching of the Epidemiological Catchment Area Program that used the Diagnostic Interview Schedule (DIS). She was able to review all the psychiatric interview materials from the 1952 Stirling County surveys and concluded that the interview procedures were extremely similar to the *DSM-III*/DIS approach. She then reanalysed psychiatric data collected from the 1952 to 1970 community surveys based on the *DSM-III* criteria.[19,20] In addition to analysing the data based on new methods, she drew a new sample and conducted a complete follow-up of everybody who had been interviewed at earlier dates. Between 1991 and 1996, Murphy went into another phase of active fieldwork and expanded the database to contain over 4000 subjects.[16] The project captured information recorded by physicians pertaining to virtually all the individuals who participated. Dr. Leighton served as a senior consultant for the additional project, and together they have produced 40-year findings from the longitudinal Stirling County Study.

Operationalized criteria for the diagnosis of mental illness according to categories of specific disorders did not appear before the 1970s. Clinician-administered standardized assessments were introduced as a means to systematically diagnose patients presenting symptoms of mental disorders. A significant contribution was made by the World Health Organization's (WHO) 1974 international research program on schizophrenia. The WHO study used the Present State Examination (PSE) as the standard assessment tool for diagnosing schizophrenia in these investigations. The PSE could be reliably applied in different cultures around the world.[21] The PSE identifies symptom patterns that are then matched to give a best fit for diagnoses, thus using a dimensional rather than categorical approach.

Henderson et al.[22] in Australia developed a technique of two-stage sampling, by screening a large population with the General Health Questionnaire (GHQ), determining the level of 'caseness' for each score on the GHQ, and then having clinicians administer the PSE to a stratified sample according to GHQ score. This provided good estimates of current prevalence combining screening large populations with selective clinical interviews.

Major efforts were made to develop standard reliable criteria for diagnosis resulting in the Feighner Criteria[23] (with the accompanying Renard Diagnostic Interview), the Research Diagnostic Criteria[24] (which led to the Schedule for Affective Disorders and Schizophrenia[25]), and eventually the third edition of the *Diagnostic and Statistical Manual*.[19] The development of these instruments and the accompanying interview schedules proved to be of great importance in the evolution of psychiatric epidemiology.

The Research Diagnostic Criteria (RDC)[24] were developed in 1975, enabling research investigators to apply a consistent set of criteria to describe sample participants with functional psychiatric illnesses. Development of the RDC was a collaborative project primarily with regard to depressive disorders, and was sponsored by the Clinical Research Branch of the National Institute of Mental Health (NIMH).The initial work on the RDC focused on modifying and elaborating on the diagnostic criteria developed in 1972 at the Washington University School of Medicine in St. Louis. These criteria are referred to as the 'Feighner Criteria' (named for the senior author of an article summarizing criteria for 15 conditions).[23,24]

The Schedule for Affective Disorders and Schizophrenia[25] (SADS) was developed in conjunction with the RDC. The production of these instruments resulted from the NIMH's aim of improving the reliability and, therefore, the validity of psychiatric diagnostic practice. The SADS was at that time unique among structured diagnostic interviews. It advanced the previous limitations of instruments such as the Present State Examination, which did not collect historical information. Therefore, diagnoses requiring such information, such as bipolar affective disorder or antisocial personality, could not be made.

In 1978, The U.S. *Report of the President's Commission on Mental Health* (PCMH) identified major epidemiological and services research gaps.[26,27] Shortly thereafter, in the early 1980s, the American Psychiatric Association published the third edition of the *Diagnostic and Statistical Manual of Mental Disorders (DSM-III)*.[19] The book dramatically influenced the future of psychiatric epidemiology. It was the first official classification of psychiatric disorders to include operational criteria for all major diagnoses. The Epidemiological Catchment Area (ECA) studies were initiated to provide answers to questions raised by the PCMH about how the mentally ill were being served, the extent of under-servicing, and who were suffering by this under-service.[27] It was recognized that for large-scale community surveys to be feasible, an instrument that could be administered by less highly trained interviewers and that could be computer scored was necessary.

The Diagnostic Interview Schedule (DIS)[28] was created at the request of the National Institute of Mental Health in preparation for the ECA studies. The DIS incorporated the general design and features of the Renard Diagnostic Interview. It also incorporated diagnosis by *DSM-III* criteria, the RDC, and the Feighner criteria. The DIS evolved into a highly structured diagnostic interview that could be administered by non-clinically trained interviewers to determine diagnosis. The DIS combined the strengths of several existing tools created to meet these requirements. This translated into direct benefits; the costs of using mental health professionals in large-scale community surveys were reduced and funds could be invested into other areas of survey methodologies including expanded sample sizes. Training for the interviewers was standardized, and the diagnostic algorithm was computer scored. Tests of reliability and validity were conducted, including test-retest and inter-rater reliability; they also included criterion validation, comparing the results against clinician interviews. Results were considered satisfactory to proceed to large-scale community studies.

The transition to computers provided several new opportunities for the ECA studies. No longer limited to manual calculations, researchers were able to conduct larger studies and incorporate a larger number of variables to achieve greater clarity about the symptoms and diagnosis of specific mental disorders. Over 20,000 respondents were interviewed in New Haven, Connecticut; Baltimore, Maryland; Durham, North Carolina; St. Louis, Missouri; and Los Angeles, California.[29] The ECA study is significant because it marks a new generation of approaches to epidemiological studies in mental health using large random samples of an entire population, standardized interview techniques conducted by trained lay interviewers, and computer scoring for diagnoses and data analysis.

In Ontario, Offord and Boyle[30,31] initiated and conducted the Ontario Child Health Study in response to a request from the Ontario Ministry of Community and Social Services. The project aimed to estimate the prevalence of emotional and behavioural disorders among children aged 4 to 16. Four disorders were selected for the focus of the study: conduct disorder, attention-deficit disorder with hyperactivity, emotional disorder, and somatization. The research team recognized that previously available checklists did not provide thresholds for individual psychiatric disorders based on *DSM-III* criteria.[31] To solve this problem, items were chosen from the Child Behavior Checklist[32] that appeared to operationalize *DSM-III* criteria for specific disorders.[31] For measurement purposes, the team developed scales composed of problem behaviours that were added together to form scores. The augmented Child Behavior Checklist was administered to parents, teachers, and adolescents aged 12 to 16. This was one of the largest and most significant epidemiological studies on children's mental health in North America. The findings have been widely used by many jurisdictions to plan changes to children's mental health programs. High rates of mental health problems in children were revealed, as well as the failure, in most jurisdictions, to provide any form of treatment.

In Edmonton, Alberta, between 1983 and 1986, Bland, Newman, Dyck, Thompson, Orn and their associates conducted long-term outcome studies on a cohort of patients with schizophrenia and affective disorders upon their first admission to medical institutions.[33] They also investigated mortality in large samples of treated patients with schizophrenia and affective disorders. The researchers conducted a series of studies eventually involving over 10,000 community respondents using the DIS and methodology similar to that used in the ECA study.[33,34] Extensive interviews were conducted with family members and spouses of the individuals who participated. Also included were institutionalized samples of the elderly, and a random sample of provincial jail inmates. These investigations yielded prevalence and some incidence data, and also information about health care use.[33] In addition, Thompson investigated the association between the rate of social problems and the prevalence of psychiatric disorders.[33] The data collected were further analysed to provide insight into individual psychiatric disorders within the Edmonton area study sample. Several papers were published on findings related to major depressive disorder, mania, obsessive-compulsive disorder, phobias, panic disorder, drug abuse, and antisocial personality disorder.[35]

The results from these investigations led to the group's invitation to participate in the Cross-National Collaborative Group led by Myrna Weissman. Epidemiological data on mood disorders were compared among 10 countries including Canada, the United States (including Puerto Rico), France, Italy, West Germany, Lebanon, Taiwan, Korea, and New Zealand.[36] The comparison was made possible because investigators in all 10 sites had assessed psychiatric disorders in large population samples with the same instrument, the DIS for the *DSM-III* (or *DSM-III R*).

In 1982, the World Health Organization (WHO) and the United States Alcohol, Drug Abuse and Mental Health Administration (ADAMHA) engaged in a collaborative project to review and assess the diagnosis and classification of alcohol, drug abuse, and mental disorders and formed a Task Force on Diagnostic Instruments. This was charged with developing diagnostic definitions and criteria to be incorporated into the forthcoming tenth revision of the *International Classification of Diseases* (ICD-10), the American Psychiatric Association's *DSM-III*, the Present State Examination (PSE), and others.[37] The project resulted in the creation of the Composite International Diagnostic Interview (CIDI). The CIDI combined questions from the DIS and the PSE. The instrument was designed to enable cross-cultural epidemiologic and comparative studies of psychopathology. Such studies can focus on estimates of the prevalence rates of specific disorders across countries, cultures, and languages and describe patterns of comorbidity, risk factors, and social consequences for specific disorders.[37] The CIDI was developed as a fully structured interview instrument that could be administered by trained non-clinician interviewers. Another advantage of the tool was that computers could manage the scoring of diagnosis.

In 1987, Offord, Boyle and others used the CIDI to conduct the Ontario Health Supplement study, a province-wide prevalence study and needs assessment of 10,000 respondents aged 15 to adult. The aims of the study were to improve the understanding of mental disorder and provide a rational basis for developing programs and policies to prevent and treat mental disorder more effectively.[38] The data from this study were used for the planning and organization of services, but also raised significant questions regarding how services are used and the level of disability occurring in those with psychiatric disorders. Since the Ontario study used instruments and methods similar to those of the U.S. National Comorbidity Study, comparisons can be made, particularly regarding some of the differences in the prevalence rates found between these two investigations.[33]

The 1990–1992 and 2001–2002 National Comorbidity Surveys led by Kessler et al. assessed mental disorders in the United States using a modified CIDI (the UM-CIDI). The introduction of this tool is important for two reasons. The high prevalence of psychosocial symptoms reported by earlier studies was replicated in studies focused on recognizing particular psychiatric disorders.[16] Also, correlates of psychosocial symptoms identified in earlier surveys had been shown to be associated with specific diagnosable disorders.[16] Study results were interesting, wide-ranging, and concluded that psychiatric disorder overall is quite common, and that the major burden of psychiatric disorder is found in those with high comorbidity.[29]

The Canadian Study of Health and Aging was launched in 1991 in response to recommendations from an advisory committee to the Department of National Health and Welfare. The committee requested a nation-wide prevalence study of dementia, including Alzheimer's disease, using standard screening and diagnostic criteria.[39] The committee further suggested analytic studies of risk factors and of caregiving for patients with dementia and that a longitudinal study be conducted. In total, 18 study centres across Canada were divided into five regions. Random samples of people aged 65 and older were drawn from the population including a sample of those living in institutions. Screening was done using the Modified Mini-Mental State Examination (3MS) to identify cognitive impairment. Prevalence results suggested that 8.0% of Canadians aged 65 and over met the criteria for dementia. These rates were found almost equally among the community and institutional samples; the female:male ratio was 2:1. The age-standardized rate ranged from 2.4%, among those aged 65 to 74 years, to 34.5%, among those aged 85 and over.[39] The study predicted that if the prevalence estimates remain constant, the number of Canadians with dementia will more than double by 2021 solely due to the changing demographic structure of the Canadian population.

The Quebec Child Mental Health Survey was conducted in 1992 based on a need to obtain provincially based epidemiological data for planning more effective services for children.[40] The survey included a representative sample of 2400 children and adolescents aged 6 to 14 throughout the province. Children, parents, and teachers participated in the study. The disorders assessed included simple phobia, separation anxiety disorder, overanxious disorder, generalized anxiety disorder, major depressive episode, dysthymia, attention deficit hyperactivity disorder, oppositional defiant disorder, and conduct disorder. A combination of the Diagnostic Interview Schedule for Children, Version 2.25[41] and the Dominic Questionnaire[42] were used for the study.

The results led the authors of the survey to conclude that collaboration between the health and education sectors was to be encouraged by policy makers. Specific recommendations included the need to ensure that health professionals were aware of the needs of elementary school teachers and that teachers needed to be better informed about disruptive disorders of childhood. It was also recommended that clinicians develop new ways of helping elementary school teachers with children with ADHD and the sharing of information with parents was encouraged. In addition, study findings revealed that young boys and adolescent girls were at greater risk of internalizing disorders. This was considered serious by the researchers and they recommended that these results be used by policy makers to improve public education campaigns about the internalization of disorders by children.[36]

In Australia, it was decided that the country required its own estimates regarding the prevalence of mental disorders rather than relying on imported estimates. The Australian National Survey of Mental Health and Well-Being[43] had three specific aims: to estimate the 1-month and 1-year prevalence of mental disorders and of significant psychological symptoms in the Australian population, to estimate the amount of disablement associated with such morbidity, and to estimate the use of health and other services by persons with such conditions. To achieve these aims, the survey developed three complementary parts: surveys of children and young persons, surveys of adults, and a special survey for low prevalence disorders, the psychoses. Before the national survey was launched there was only limited information on the prevalence of dementia and severe cognitive impairment among adults in Australia.

The automated Composite International Diagnostic Interview (CIDI-A) was used in the study. The CIDI-A is a psychiatric interview for research developed in Australia and, since, used internationally. Professional interviewers, but without experience in psychiatry, administered the tool. The interview incorporated diagnostic criteria based on the World Health Organization's tenth edition of the *International Classification of Diseases* (ICD-10) issued in 1993 and the *DSM-IV* published by the American Psychiatric Association in 1994. Questions were added to screen for psychosis, neurasthenia, and eight personality disorders. Goldberg's 12-item General Health Questionnaire was also included. People over the age of 65 were given the Mini-Mental State Examination (MMSE) to assess cognitive impairment.

The Australian Bureau of Statistics (ABS) targeted approximately 13,600 private dwellings and within each dwelling one person aged 18 years or over was randomly selected for an interview The interviewers successfully completed interviews on 78% of the targeted sample . The Australian National Survey was comprehensive and thorough in addressing the intended aims of the research. While several results were consistent with indicators provided from previous studies, the researchers found some unexpected results in regard to anxiety disorders, substance abuse disorders, and depression. For example, there was no evidence to support certain risk factors that had been commonly associated with predicting the development of depression. The exemplary methodology used in the Australian Study showed where mental disorders are distributed in the Australian general population, the disablement they cause, and where the unmet need is most evident.[43] Researchers hope that the conclusions drawn from the national survey can be used by the government to make positive changes that will protect and improve the mental health of Australians.

The recent European Study of the Epidemiology of Mental Disorders (ESEMeD) project was the result of the efforts of investigators from several European countries in collaboration with the World Health Organisation World Mental Health Surveys.[44] Before the ESEMeD, a number of population-based studies addressing specific mental disorders had been carried out in different European countries. This project, by using standardized methods in its cross national investigation, aimed to overcome some of the gaps and apparent differences in prevalence rates and in the burden and care of individuals with mental disorders found in individual studies. Data were collected to gain representative samples of adults, including individuals aged 65 and older, in Belgium, France, Germany, Italy, the Netherlands, and Spain. The ESEMeD is considered the largest comparative study of the epidemiology of mental disorders in Europe with more than 21,400 participants representing a population of about 213 million. The comprehensive study collected data on a range of mental disorders, risk factors, disability and quality of life, and the use of services and medications.

This study is the first European survey to use *DSM-IV* for the classification of mental disorders. Inclusion of the ICD-10 enabled direct comparison between the two diagnostic instruments. The instrument used to assess mental disorders in ESEMeD was the CIDI administered by trained interviewers who were not mental health professionals. The CIDI provides computerized algorithms for lifetime and current diagnoses of mental disorders. The latest version of the CIDI used in

ESEMeD was developed in coordination with the WHO World Mental Health (WMH) surveys investigators and gives an assessment of the clinical severity of the disorders. The use of this research instrument allows for the comparability of ESEMeD data with those of all the other countries included in the WHO World Mental Health surveys initiative. The European Study resulted in the creation of a database from which information will continue to be extracted, studied, and compared to produce sound evidence on the prevalence, disability burden, and unmet needs related to mental disorders. This source of reliable data is intended to inform health policy throughout all of Europe.[44]

The 2002 Canadian Community Health Survey: Mental Health and Well-Being (CCHS 1.2) was the first national mental health survey in Canada. The initiative aimed at several goals beyond determining prevalence rates in relation to major depression, mania, panic disorder, social phobia, and agoraphobia. The study set out to examine links between mental health and social, demographic, geographic, and economic variables; mental health service utilization; and perceived needs and disabilities associated with mental illness.[45] Approximately 48,000 dwellings were selected from the 10 Canadian provinces and one person per household aged 15 years or over was invited to participate in an interview. More than 85% of the interviews were conducted face-to-face and the overall combined response rate for Canada was 77.0%.

Interview questions were based on the WHO World Mental Health 2000 Project's new version of the CIDI (the WMH-CIDI). The national survey only partially coded mental disorders to the *DSM-IV* criteria. The CCHS 1.2 team, claiming the support of its Mental Health Expert Group and the WMH 2000 Project, made modifications to the content of the disorder modules to reduce response burden and clarify concepts.[45] As a result, comparing the results from CCHS 1.2 and the WMH-CIDI modules diagnosis and prevalence rates is a challenging task.[41] The CCHS 1.2 questionnaire was developed in consultation with Statistics Canada's Questionnaire Design Resource Centre. In their opinion, after pilot testing, they decided that the interview was too long, questions were too verbose, and some screening criteria were deemed to be too broad.[45] The survey questionnaire was then revised to be briefer. Due to these modifications, results cannot be directly compared to any other survey.

Statistics Canada trained interviewers to administer the questionnaire using Computer-Assisted Personal Interviewing (CAPI). The

Centre for Addiction and Mental Health in Toronto provided ongoing support for those administering the questionnaires including training in the awareness of and sensitivity to mental health issues. All survey respondents were asked questions on mental health service use, medication, and mental health determinants. Questions pertaining to the impact or cost of mental health problems were not directly addressed. Instead, the survey used the generic terminology for mental health – problems with emotions, drugs, and alcohol – to refer to any mental disorders or problems experienced by the respondent. Other survey content areas included eating troubles and behaviours, gambling problems, suicidal ideation and behaviours, and alcohol or illicit drug use and dependence. Instruments used to measure these mental health issues were based on tools used in Statistics Canada surveys such as the National Population Health Survey, CCHS1.1 and the Health Promotion Survey.[45]

In addition to the questionnaire differences between the CCHS 1.2 and the WMH-CIDI, they also note that there were variations in the way the derived variables for each disorder were computed, representing additional challenges for data comparisons. These derived variables for the selected disorders only partly meet *DSM-IV* classification criteria. However, the algorithms for major depression, mania, panic disorder, social phobia, and agoraphobia were tested by CCHS analysts and by various expert groups.[45]

Twenty studies based on the analysis of the CCHS data were approved for funding in the initial competition (others were approved under other auspices). The question of results cannot simply be put as 'What did they find?' The question of this national study and others is, 'What are they finding?' The data gathered continue to be studied and analysed by researchers across the country and internationally. A few examples of such studies include: Beck and associates reporting on psychotropic medication use in Canada,[46] Thompson's research on the variations in the prevalence of psychiatric disorders and social problems across Canada,[47] and Bergeron et al.'s work on the determinants of service use among youth with mental disorders.[48] Other studies will likely be forthcoming, as access to data can be requested through Statistics Canada.

The Canadian Senate Standing Committee on Social Affairs, Science and Technology, chaired by Senator Michael Kirby, issued a report on mental health and addiction in 2004.[49] The report acknowledged that Canada lacks a national information base to enable accurate identification of the prevalence of either mental illness or addiction to measure the mental health status of Canadians and to assist in the evaluating policies, programs and services in the fields of mental health. This is a major challenge in determining the need for and providing appropriate treatments and services for people with mental health issues. Kirby noted that Statistics Canada's release of the Community Health Survey has helped by providing for the first time a set of data on some mental illnesses, substance use disorders, and gambling. The committee recommended that this survey should be repeated soon and cover a wider range of disorders. The committee also recommended that a national survey should be undertaken to assess the prevalence rates of mental disorders among children and adolescents. The Senate report outlines the epidemiological gaps in knowledge that remain to be addressed regarding mental illness in Canada. The report acknowledges the contributions that the first national survey has made and emphasizes that there still remains much to be done.

Ironically, impediments to the research process include innovation, because, as new interview schedules are developed, studies are conducted using different methods and become less easily comparable, locally and internationally, particularly when translation has to take place and testing of each instrument in each different cultural environment. Nevertheless, the development of survey instruments that can be administered by non-clinically trained individuals and of methods for obtaining large representative samples of whole populations have enabled major studies to be implemented.

Have we lost something by removing clinicians' experience from the process? How many clinically trained researchers remain active participants in research today? Henderson et al.[43] caution and remind us that when 'diagnoses' are made by computer-scored standardized instruments they are only an approximation of what an experienced research clinician would produce. They are not clinicians' diagnoses. The research community must await more information on the validity of these instruments across a range of diagnostic groups and, as Henderson points out, these groups, as defined in ICD-10 and *DSM-IV*, are themselves only an arbitrary nosology.[43]

Critics of community surveys may comment that they are simply tools used to gather information on prevalence. Partially true, but these investigations reveal changes in psychiatric morbidity in the community. They provide evidence-based information to support governments in making policy changes that will have a positive impact on mental health outcomes. Recent surveys have returned to some of the concepts found in the earlier Stirling County and Midtown Manhattan studies by examining the extent of disability, the need for treatment, whether people are accessing services and by identifying the potential barriers to improving mental health. Instruments such as the Health of the Nation Outcome Scales (HoNOS)[50] help generate knowledge in these and other important areas by enabling clinicians to track treatment outcomes.

In 1993, the UK Department of Health commissioned the Royal College of Psychiatrists' Research Unit to develop scales to measure the health and social functioning of people with severe mental illness, with the goal of improving the health and social functioning of people with mental illness. The HoNOS instrument[50] contains 12 items used to measure behaviour, impairment, symptoms, and social functioning. The scales are completed after routine clinical assessments. Ratings are scored, repeated after a course of treatment, and then compared for use as clinical outcomes measures. The scales were developed using stringent testing for acceptability, usability, sensitivity, reliability, and validity. Issues covered in the scale include: psychiatric symptoms, addictions, disability, relationships, housing, and occupational stressors. Several versions of HoNOS are available for working age adults, people over 65 and children, and adolescents. Clinicians can monitor their patients' service-use patterns and responses to interventions. The tool is widely used to monitor mental health services in England.

While it is imperative to study and record this information, it is also important to consider that mental health is associated with a variety of social conditions including poverty, violence, justice, self-determination, family structure, employment, and resilience. Neither the mental health system nor mental health research can conceivably alleviate all of these problems. There is the distinct danger that the mental health system and researchers will be perceived as failing when problems associated with these contributors are not resolved.

The systematic classification of diseases dates back to the nineteenth century. Medical statisticians William Farr (1807–83) and Jacques Bertillon (1851–1922) initiated early groundwork. It has taken a significant amount of time for mental illnesses to gain serious attention and research investment. Much more work is required to reduce the stigma and misunderstandings associated with these diseases. Advancing mental health requires the continued collaborative efforts that have been demonstrated in the area of psychiatric epidemiology for the past fifty years.

REFERENCES

1 Cooper JE, Kendell RE, Gurland BJ, et al. *Psychiatric Diagnosis in New York and London: A Comparative Study of Mental Hospital Admissions*. Maudsley Monograph number 20. London: Oxford University Press, 1972.

2 Strömgren E. Statistical and genetical population studies within psychiatry: Methods and principal results. In: Sjögren T, ed. *Psychiatrie sociale*. Paris: Herrman, 1950:155–88.

3 Essen-Möller E. *Individual Traits and Morbidity in the Swedish Rural Population*. Copenhagen: Munksgaard, 1956.

4 Hagnell O. *A Prospective Study of the Incidence of Mental Disorder*. Stockholm: Svenska Bokförlaget Norstedts-Bonniers, 1956.

5 Hagnell O. The Lundby study on psychiatric morbidity (Sweden). In: Mednick SA, Baert A, eds. *Prospective Longitudinal Research: An Empirical Basis for the Primary Prevention of Psychosocial Disorders*. New York: Oxford University Press, 1981:189–206.

6 Hagnell O, Lanke J, Rorsman B, et al. Current trends in the incidence of senile and multi-infarct dementia: A prospective study of the total population followed over 25 years: The Lundby Study. *Arch Psychiatr Nervenkr* 1983;233:423–38.

7 Eaton JW, Weil RJ. *Culture and Mental Disorders*. Glen Coe, IL: Free Press, 1955.

8 Fremming KH. The expectation of mental infirmity in a sample of the Danish population (based on a biographical investigation of 5500 persons born in the years 1883 -1887). *Occasional Papers on Eugenics*, No. 7. London: The Eugenics Society and Cassel, 1951.

9 Helgason T. Epidemiology of mental disorders in Iceland: A psychiatric and demographic investigation of 5,395 Icelanders. *Acta Psychiatr Scand* 1964;(suppl 173).

10 Leighton DC, Harding JS, Macklin DB, et al. *The Character of Danger*. New York: Basic Books, 1963.

11 Srole L, Langner TS, Michael ST, et al. *Mental Health in the Metropolis*. New York: McGraw-Hill, 1962.

12 Weissman MM, Myers JK. Rates and risks of depressive symptoms in a United States urban community. *Acta Psychiatr Scand* 1978;57:219–31.

13 Weissman MM, Myers JK. Affective disorders in the US urban commu-

nity: The use of the Research Diagnostic Criteria in an epidemiological survey. *Arch Gen Psychiatry* 1978;35:1304–11.

14   Weissman MM, Myers JK, Harding PS. Psychiatric disorders in a US urban community. *Am J Psychiatry* 1978;135:459–62.

15   Weissman MM, Myers JK. Psychiatric disorders in a US urban community: The application of Research Diagnostic Criteria to a resurveyed community sample. *Acta Psychiatr Scand* 1980;62:99–111.

16   Susser E, Schwartz S, Morabia A, et al. *Psychiatric Epidemiology*. Oxford: Oxford University Press, 2006.

17   Streiner DL, Cairney J, Lesage A. Psychiatric epidemiology in Canada and the CCHS study. *Can J Psychiatry* 2005;50:571–2.

18   Tremblay MA. Alexander H. Leighton's and Jane Murphy's scientific contributions to psychiatric epidemiology: A personal appreciation. *Transcult Psychiatry* 2006;43:7–20.

19   American Psychiatric Association. *Diagnostic and Statistical Manual of Mental Disorders* (3rd ed). Washington DC, APA, 1980.

20   Murphy JM. Continuities in community based psychiatric epidemiology. *Arch Gen Psychiatry* 1980;37:1215–23.

21   Wing JK, Cooper JE, Sartorius N. *The Measurement and Classification of Psychiatric Symptoms: An Instruction Manual for the PSE and Catego Program*. London, Cambridge University Press, 1974.

22   Henderson S, Duncan-Jones P, Byrne DG, et al. Psychiatric disorder in Canberra: A standardized study of prevalence. *Acta Psychiatr Scand* 1979;60:355–74.

23   Feigner JP, Robins E, Guze JB, et al. Diagnostic criteria for use in psychiatric research. *Arch Gen Psychiatry* 1972;26:57–73.

24   Spitzer RL, Endicott J, Robins E. *Research Diagnostic Criteria (RDC)*. New York: Biometrics Research, New York State Psychiatric Institute, 1975.

25   Endicott J, Spitzer RL. A diagnostic interview: The Schedule for Affective Disorders and Schizophrenia. *Arch Gen Psychiatry* 1978;35:837–44.

26   Dohrenwend BP, Dohrenwend BS, Gould MS, et al. *Mental Illness in the United States: Epidemiological Estimates*. New York: Praeger, 1980.

27   Eaton W, Kessler L. *Epidemiologic Field Methods in Psychiatry: The NIMH Epidemiologic Catchment Area Program*. Orlando, FLA: Academic Press, 1985.

28   Robins LN, Helzer JE, Croughan J. et al. The National Institute of Mental Health Diagnostic Interview Schedule: Its history, characteristics and validity. *Arch Gen Psychiatry* 1981;38:381–9.

29   Kessler R. The National Comorbidity Survey of the United States. *Int Rev Psychiatry* 1994;6:365–88.

30 Offord DR, Boyle MH, Szatmari P, et al. Ontario Child Health Study. II.
    Six month prevalence of disorders and rates of service utilization. *Arch
    Gen Psychiatry* 1987;44:832–36.

31 Boyle MH, Offord DR, Hofman HG, et al. Ontario Child Health Study. I.
    Methodology. *Arch Gen Psychiatry* 1987;44:826–31.

32 Achenbach TM, Edelbrook C. *Manual for the Child Behavior Checklist and
    Revised Child Behavior Profile*. Burlington, VT: University of Vermont,
    Department of Psychiatry, 1983.

33 Bland R, Arboleda-Flórez J, Leighton AH, et al. Epidemiology. In: Rae-
    Grant Q, ed. *Psychiatry in Canada: 50 years*. Ottawa, Canadian Psychiatric
    Association, 2001:211–36.

34 Bland, R, Newman S, Orn H. Epidemiology of psychiatric disorders in
    Edmonton. *Acta Psychiatr Scand* 1988;77(suppl 338).

35 Bland R, Newman SC, Russell JM, et al. Epidemiology of psychiatric dis-
    orders in Edmonton: Phenomenology and comorbidity. *Acta Psychiatr
    Scand Suppl* 1994;89(suppl 376).

36 Weissman MM, Bland RC , Canino GJ, et al. Cross-national epidemiology
    of major depression and bipolar disorder. *JAMA* 1996;276:293–9.

37 Robins LN, Wing JK, Wittchen HU, et al. The Composite International
    Diagnostic Interview: An epidemiologic instrument suitable for use in
    conjunction with different diagnostic systems and in different cultures.
    Arch Gen Psychiatry 1988;45:1069–77.

38 Boyle MH, Offord DR, Campbell D, et al. Mental Health Supplement to
    the Ontario Health Survey: Methodology. *Can J Psychiatry* 1996;41:549–58

39 McDowell I. Study of Health and Aging: Study methods and prevalence
    of dementia. *Can Med Assoc J* 1994;150:899–913.

40 Breton J-J, Bergeron L, Valla J-P, et al. Quebec Child Mental Health
    Survey: Prevalence of DSM-III-R mental health disorders. *J Child Psychol
    Psychiatry* 1999;40:375–84.

41 Shaffer D, Fischer P, Piacentini J, et al. *Diagnostic Interview Schedule for
    Children (DISC-2.25) – Child Version – Parent Version*. New York: Division
    of Child and Adolescent Psychiatry, New York State Psychiatric Institute,
    1991.

42 Valla JP, Bergeron L, Berube H, et al. A structured pictorial questionnaire
    to assess DSM-III-R-based diagnoses in children (6–11 years): Develop-
    ment, validity and reliability. *J Abnorm Child Psychol* 1994;22:403–23.

43 Henderson S, Andrews G, Hall W. Australia's mental health: An
    overview of the general population survey. *Aust N Z J Psychiatry*
    2000;34:197–205.

44 Alsonso J, Angermeyer MC, Lépine JP. The European Study of the Epi-
    demiology of Mental Disorders (ESEMed) project: An epidemiological

basis for informing mental health policies in Europe. *Acta Psychiatr Scand Suppl* 2004;109(suppl 420):5–7.

45 Gravel R, Béland Y. The Canadian Community Health Survey: Mental Health and Well-Being. *Can J Psychiatry* 2005;50:573–9.

46 Beck C, Williams JVA, Wang J-L, et al. (2005). Psychotropic medication use in Canada. *Can J Psychiatry* 2005;50:605–13.

47 Thompson A. Variations in the prevalence of psychiatric disorders and social problems across Canadian provinces. *Can J Psychiatry* 2005;50:637–42.

48 Bergeron E, Poiriers L-R, Fournier L, et al. Determinants of service use among young Canadians with mental disorders. *Can J Psychiatry* 2005;50:629–36.

49 Kirby MJ. *Mental Health, Mental Illness and Addiction: Issues and Options for Canada.* Interim Report of the Standing Senate Committee on Social Affairs, Science and Technology, 2004.

50 The Royal College of Psychiatrists. What is HoNOS? Retrieved on October 25, 2006. Available at: http://www.rcpsych.ac.uk/crtu/healthofthenation/whatishonos.aspx

3 Intersecting Social Statuses and Psychiatric Disorder: New Conceptual Directions in the Social Epidemiology of Mental Disorder

JOHN CAIRNEY, SCOTT VELDHUIZEN, AND TERRANCE J. WADE

Introduction

Chapters 1 and 2 of this volume together provide an overview of the development of psychiatric epidemiology and establish the context for modern community surveys of mental health in Canada. Chapter 1 also offers an in-depth review of the social theory underpinning Alec Leighton's work in Stirling County. As noted in that chapter, social theory, while an important part of psychiatric epidemiology during the era of Stirling County, occupies a much less prominent position in the field today. It has, however, continued to be a central focus on scholarly activity in areas outside of psychiatry, especially psychology and sociology.

An interesting theoretical innovation, however, is underway in the field of social epidemiology of mental disorder. There is increasing interest in intersecting social status positions, and in the distribution of mental disorder in the population. Some of this work has been conducted in Canada and represents an important contribution by Canadian scholars. In this chapter, we provide a general overview of the social epidemiology of mental disorder, with a particular focus on the processes of social causation and social selection. We then introduce the intersectional approach to social determinants and provide an example using data from two Canadian national surveys.

Social Epidemiology and the Epidemiology of Mental Disorders

Social epidemiology is the study of the distribution of illness and disease across social positions determined by, for example, education, wealth, occupation, gender, and ethnicity. It is the intersection of social science, epidemiology, demography, and biology, and it provides an analytic and methodological framework for the study of social determinants of health and illness. The social epidemiology of mental disorder narrows the focus to outcomes of interest to psychiatry, such as depression, anxiety, and schizophrenia, as well as psychological distress and well-being among people unaffected by major psychiatric disorders.

The long-standing interest in the social determinants of mental health can be traced to a general belief that important etiological messages are to be found by closely attending to the social patterning of morbidity and mortality in the population.[1] Indeed, the persistent associations between social factors and morbidity suggests that social factors may be fundamental causes of illness,$^{\psi}$ as they determine individual behaviour, exposure to noxious environmental risk factors, and access to resources, which in turn influence development of, and recovery from, disorder.[2,3]

In this chapter, we briefly review the literature on social determinants of psychological disorder and distress. We consider the relevance of sociological approaches in the era of biological psychiatry and the genome, and discuss the twin processes of social selection and social causation, the two phenomena capable of explaining the observed links between social position and disorder. We then describe the stress process model and the influence this paradigm has had on our understanding of the social determinants of mental health and well-being. Finally, we show the importance of an intersectional approach by presenting data on gender and family structure, two social location markers known separately to be correlated with distress and disorder.

The Social Epidemiology of Psychological Disorder and Distress

Introduction

The starting point in social epidemiological studies is the oft-reported association between markers of social location (e.g., gender, socioeconomic status (SES), ethnicity, education, wealth, occupation) and morbidity or mortality. Social position is a very powerful predictor of health and well-being in the developed world: a social gradient is not observed in remarkably few chronic diseases. Studies have shown that wherever status hierarchies exist, a health gradient is also evident.[2,4,5] There is, in fact, a 'fine gradient' of SES and illness, as demonstrated in studies such as Whitehall, which reported differences in mortality and morbidity in the occupational hierarchies within the civil service in Britain.[6] Hierarchical systems of social organization, even in relatively homogeneous populations, are thus strongly associated with health and well-being.

The relationship between SES and mental health remains one of the most consistently documented findings in psychiatric epidemiology.[7-15] More recent work has focused not just on socioeconomic status, but on other characteristics that define an individual's place in the social structure. Markers of social location such as gender,[13,14,16] marital status,[17-19] and ethnicity[20] are also risk markers for psychiatric disorder and psychological distress. These studies consistently show that individuals in disadvantaged socioeconomic positions have higher rates of distress and disorder than those occupying more socially and economically advantaged social positions.

Social Causation and Social Selection

This body of work demonstrates that social location is associated with mental health. It does not, however, explain why this relationship exists. Two possibilities have been widely discussed: psychiatric disorder may lead to differences in social position (social selection); or negative factors related to social position may lead, directly or indirectly, to psychiatric disorder (social causation). The most important suspected factor in the social causation model is stress. Exposure to trauma or other adversity have been shown to be important in the development of psychiatric problems, and *DSM-IV* explicitly recognizes the role of stress or trauma in the development or recrudescence of numerous disorders.[21-23] This association is supported by substantial empirical work. The Adverse Childhood Experiences Study by Felitti and colleagues, for example, found cumulative childhood exposure to trauma and maltreatment to be associated with multiple adverse outcomes in adulthood, including mental illness and even mortality.[24,25] This work parallels a wealth of clinical experience demonstrating that life events play an important role in the origin and course of numerous psychiatric disorders. At the same time, however, evidence has also emerged establishing that most disorders are also strongly influenced by genetics and, often, by other biological factors.

The debate over causation versus selection, while an important focus of debate in the 1950s, 1960s, and 1970s, has therefore largely given way to attempts to uncover the nature of interactions between genetics and social environment and to measure their relative importance in the context of specific disorders. It is long been held, for example, that social selection is likely the best explanation for social class differences in the prevalence of schizophrenia,[14,26] which is likely to result in disrupted social achievement. Social causation, however, is more widely accepted as an explanation for observed relationships between class and other conditions such as depression or substance-related disorders.[27] These processes, however, need not be mutually exclusive, and it has been suggested that the two form an interconnected process whereby disorder both produces and is produced by social disadvantage.[28] Even in cases where one process or the other appears at first to predominate, there generally proves to be substantial roles for both. The cases of schizophrenia and post-traumatic stress disorder (PTSD) illustrate this phenomenon.

POST-TRAUMATIC STRESS DISORDER (PTSD)

Perhaps the clearest case of the importance of stress (as has been pointed out, for example, by Dohrenwend[29]) is that of post-traumatic stress disorder (PTSD). PTSD and related conditions, including acute stress reactions, are precipitated by stressful events. These experiences lead, apparently in a straightforward manner, to psychiatric disorder. Exposure to traumatic events, moreover, is not random, but varies by ethnicity, sex, age, and education, as well as with pre-existing psychiatric disorder.[30] PTSD thus seems to clearly demonstrate the importance of stress and of social conditions as necessary, but not sufficient, causal mechanisms.

There are difficulties, however, with the view that PTSD is a pure example of either the stress process or of social causation. Not everyone exposed to a given event will go on to develop PTSD; instead, there seem to be substantial differences in individual vulnerability. Research suggests that this vulnerability is at least partially genetic,[31] and that risk may be mediated by physiological differences, such as hippocampal volume.[32] Even in the case of a disorder with a name that explicitly recognizes the role of stress, therefore, there is a substantial role for other processes. Although poverty, for example, may increase the probability of exposure to stressful events, the association between it and PTSD may still be due to biological factors.

SCHIZOPHRENIA

Although a number of etiological theories have come into and fallen out of fashion over the past century, schizophrenia is now seen as a disorder of brain development. Imaging and post-mortem studies have shown substantial physical changes over time in the brains of affected people,[33] and it is known to be familial, with at least half the risk thought to be genetic[34] – indeed, some have argued that genetic and epigenetic factors may determine risk for the disorder entirely.[35,36] Other biological causes have also been implicated, however, including maternal nutrition,[37] viral infection,[38] perinatal complications,[39] and exposure to toxins.[40] The disorder causes serious functional problems and may be preceded by prodromal symptoms or by various developmental deficits. It is also sometimes accompanied by a decline in cognitive functioning and by other psychiatric symptoms. All of these features of the illness may limit social achievement or cause the loss of positions formerly held. Schizophrenia is therefore widely viewed as a disease whose causes include genetic factors and neuro-developmental insults and whose overrepresentation among people holding lower-status social positions is due to social drift.

There remains, however, a role for social causation in schizophrenia. It is often forgotten that social factors play a role in determining exposure, for example, to developmental insults. Incidence of schizophrenia has been shown to be elevated among people born during or following famines,[41,42] which are typically events with social and political causes. Poor maternal nutrition in the general population is not randomly distributed, but is strongly influenced by economic and social status.[43] Exposure to pathogens or chemical insults may also vary with social status, and even genetic risk may vary with class as the result of multi-generational social drift, assortative mating, and other phenomena.

There is, moreover, some evidence supporting a more direct role for psychosocial stress. Children whose mothers experienced the death of a close relative or family member during the first trimester of pregnancy have been reported to have a greater risk of developing schizophrenia.[44] Other studies have suggested a role for family environment in early life.[45–47] Link, Dohrenwend, and Skodol[12] found that exposure to noisome (e.g., loud, dirty) conditions in a first full-time job increased the risk of onset of schizophrenia, but not major depression, suggesting a unique role for these stressors in the development of psychosis. Muntaner and his colleagues[48] also found support for other kinds of workplace stressors, including job demands and relative control over work, in risk of onset. Finally, a sharp rise in the incidence of schizophrenia, to a level well above the background rates in either the United Kingdom or the Caribbean, has been noted among first- and second-generation Caribbean immigrants to the United Kingdom.[49,50] Exposure to stress arising from social disadvantage (e.g., economic stress, discrimination, stigma) is thought to be one of the mechanisms responsible for the increased risk in this population. Even in the case of schizophrenia, then, there appears to be an etiological role for social environment.

The Stress Process

The exact nature of this association between social stressors and psychiatric disorder has been a major focus of research in the social sciences over the past several decades.[e.g., 51] The result of these endeavours has been the creation of a model that connects stress to psychological outcomes through the mediating influences of several factors: social support, psychosocial resources, and coping skills. This model is commonly referred to as the stress process. While many variations exist,[e.g., 15,52,53] all share a common focus on the effect of stress on psychological distress and disorder and a common goal of clarifying the mediating or moderating effects of social and psychological characteristics in this relationship.[51] Literally hundreds of studies on the effects of stress on health have been published using the stress process paradigm (for reviews see Aneshensel[54] and Thoits[55]).

The work of Pearlin and his colleagues has been particularly influential in developing the stress process model as an explanatory framework for the study of the effect of socially induced stress on psychological distress and disorder. In what is now regarded as a classic article in the field, Pearlin[56] persuasively argued for the importance of the stress process model as a tool for understanding the uniquely sociological features of the stress-distress relationship. He drew attention to the distinction between stress arising from random events (e.g., automobile accidents) and stress arising as a result of normal social relationships, and argued that close examination of the latter provides an important perspective from which to understand how the structure of everyday social life can influence health and well-being. He then identified and reviewed the principal components of the stress process model, including the different varieties of social stressors (life events, chronic strains, childhood adversities), the key psychological con-structs thought to buffer the negative impact of stress (mastery and self-esteem), and the role of social support in resilience to its negative effects. A review of the literature on the development of each of these components in the stress process is beyond the scope of this chapter. A detailed examination of another of Pearlin's influential papers,[15] however, will illustrate one of the more common conceptualizations of the stress process.

In 'The Stress Process,'[15] Pearlin and his colleagues were able to demonstrate the chain of events flowing from a single life event (job loss) to increased rates of depression in a large, prospective study of community dwelling adults. Central to this paper and the stress process was the conceptualization of what would later be termed stress proliferation[57] and the erosion of psychosocial resources, in par-ticular, a sense of personal mastery or control, that flowed from job loss and subsequent economic strain. Pearlin et al. were able to show that the secondary stress of economic instability and uncertainty resulting from job loss eroded feelings of personal control, which led in turn to increases in depressive symptoms. They were also able to identify protective factors that seemed to reduce the negative impact of exposure to stress. For example, among individuals who lost their jobs, those who compared themselves positively with others and those who tended to devalue economic or monetary achievements reported lower levels of economic strain, higher levels of self-esteem, and lower levels of depressive symptoms. Similarly, high levels of perceived emotional support seemed to ameliorate the negative impact of job disruption on subsequent economic strain, and were associated with higher self-esteem and mastery over time. Although there have been many elaborations on this model since the time of the original publi-cations,[55,56,58] the three domains of stress, psychosocial resources, and distress/disorder remain core elements in the model to this day.

Pearlin's uniquely 'sociological' approach to the study of stress pro-vided a valuable theoretical model for researchers interested in under-standing the social distribution of distress and disorder in the popula-tion. In Canada, the model was particularly influential on sociologists such as Jay Turner and Blair Wheaton from the University of Toronto, and Bill Avison and his colleagues from the University of Western Ontario. Both these groups of researchers used the framework to account for social status variations in the epidemiology of depression in Toronto, and to explore reasons for elevated depression in single mothers relative to their married counterparts. For example, in the Toronto Comorbidity Study, which was partially modelled, in that it also used the UM-CIDI, after the first National Comorbidity Survey in the United States,[16] Turner and colleagues were able to show that differential exposure to stress, coupled with a lack of adequate coping and social resources, could explain a good deal of the variation in the relationship between social position (socioeconomic status, gender, marital status) and mental disorder.[23,59-61] So, not only are individuals from low socioeconomic status groups more likely to have greater exposure to stress relative to more socially advantaged groups, they have lower levels of perceived mastery and self-esteem and are less likely to have supportive social networks, which, together, account for their overall higher levels of distress and depression. Similarly, Avison and his colleagues also found that differences in depression between single and married mothers could also be accounted for by elevated exposure to stress, lower self-esteem and mastery, and differences in social support between these groups.[62,63] A consistent picture of social disadvantage leading to greater stress exposure and compromised coping, can be found in this body of work. This account resonates not only with Pearlin's model of stress, but also with social epidemiologists' general interest in the social structure determinants of health and well-being. Turner's work in particular has been extremely influential in the sociology of mental health and in social epidemiology.

Intersectionality and Social Epidemiology

A fair criticism of a large part of this body of work, however, relates to the way in which social structure or social location is conceptualized and treated empirically in analyses. Social location is typically defined in terms of a single or 'master' status. Previous research, for example, has examined the association between gender *or* SES *or* divorce on psychological distress, where other positions (such as race or age) are 'controlled' statistically. The implicit assumption in this work is that social factors are additively associated with distress; so gender, regardless of other social locations, increases the risk of depression, *ceteris paribus*. This research is concerned with the role that stress exposure plays in accounting for gender differences in depression, class differences in distress, and so on. The problem, of course, is that people occupy multiple social locations simultaneously. From the perspective of sociology, the *self* is made of up multiple positions and role combinations. More importantly, certain combinations of disadvantaged social statuses (e.g., gender and poverty) may have greater conse- quences than other combinations. Inequality is thus linked not to a single status but to multiple, intersecting positions. While much of social epidemiology has this 'master status' focus, some recent work has started to consider the problem of intersecting social locations. Indeed, the study of single parents and mental health briefly men- tioned earlier is a step toward 'intersectionality,' although, as we will demonstrate, this work does not go far enough in considering the het- erogeneity that exists within the group of single parents, or the conse- quences of this heterogeneity for our understanding of the epidemiol- ogy of mental disorder in this population.

The intersectional approach begins with the notion that individuals' social positions are defined by many different characteristics: age, sex, income, wealth, occupation, education, ethnicity, language (and accent), culture, religion, and others. In this view, the notion of a simple social gradient defined by wealth or other single indicators of status is discarded. Instead, an intersectional approach poses the ques- tion: how does occupancy of multiple social positions simultaneously influence the incidence of illness within populations? From here, we may also ask, what do these new patterns of associations tell us about the etiology of disorder? The notion that we occupy multiple statuses and roles in society is not a novel one. The interplay of strains associ- ated with these social positions is, however, remarkably understudied.

McMullin[64,65] discusses the importance of theorizing social status positions as intersecting systems of social inequality, using gender and social class as examples. Feminist scholars argue that sociology's tra- ditional concern with the study of class disregards the fact that modern, western societies (along with many others) are patriarchal, meaning that access to resources, economic and social, differs for men and women. Lower class women, in particular, suffer the double dis- advantage of living in both a gendered and class-based system that marginalizes both social locations. McMullan argues that sociologists must reconstruct social theory to include gender, class, and age as fun- damental organizing features of society and, therefore, intersecting social systems that produce inequality. She draws particular attention to the ways in which the labour force is not only structured by gender, but by age as well. In the unskilled occupations (e.g. garment indus- try), older women earn significantly less than their older male coun- terparts, but also younger workers (male and female). The trajectory of earning is clearly influenced by age and class in different ways for men and women. McMullan argues that we must consider how class, age, gender, and ethnicity influence individual experiences simultaneously, rather than focusing on one aspect of social stratification.

Intersectionality:
The Double- and Multiple-Jeopardy Hypotheses

Sociologists interested in examining the mental and physical health consequences of occupying two or more disadvantaged social positions have proposed the double- or multiple-jeopardy hypothesis [e.g., 66–69] In mental health research, Schieman and Plickert[70] employ what they term a 'multiple-hierarchy stratification perspective' to examine the effect of functional disability on depression in older adults, by considering the interactive influences of race, gender, and SES. For example, while increases in limitations were generally associated with increases in depressive symptoms over time among older adults with low SES, non-Latino White men and women were most affected. Drapeau and her colleagues[71] used the concept of 'social anchorage' to explore the effect of gender on mental health service use in a large, representative sample of Canadians. Social anchorage, although not well defined in this study, seems to refer to the kinds of social roles that men and women occupy, presumably with some anchoring them more closely to other persons or their communities than others. These researchers are interested in the ways in which, for example, role or location combinations influence help-seeking. Interestingly, they found that while women, on average, were more than twice as likely to have sought help for mental health reasons in the part year, there were no gender differences in help-seeking among single parents or those who were unemployed. From a conceptual point of view, the importance of this work lies in the recognition that the intersection between variables like age, gender, poverty, and others, leads to unique compounded structural disadvantages.

Intersectionality: The Case of Single Parents

Research on single parents and mental health is another important example of the impact of multiple statuses on health and well-being. Family structure, in North America, represents the intersection of gender, marital status, and parenthood.[62] Family structure and mental health represent an important way in which we can seek to better understand the role of intersecting social locations in population health.

Research from Canada, Great Britain, and the United States has consistently shown that lone mothers are at increased risk for psychiatric disorder and psychological distress.[63,72–78] Until very recently however, research on single parents implicitly meant that comparisons would be drawn between married and single mothers with children. This has as much to do with demographics as anything else. It is estimated, for example, that approximately 15% (about 1.4 million families) of all Canadian families are headed by a single parent,[79] and of these, about 80% are single parent mother families. In Canada, at least, 'single parent' is thus almost synonymous with 'single mother.' However, recent data suggest that single parent father families may be becoming more common.[79,80] Research on this family form is sparse, however, being limited to small, non-representative convenience samples, and focusing primarily on the children rather than the parents.[81]

This shifting demographic trend in family structure allows for the possibility of considering the association between distress and disorder and the intersection of gender and family structure in ways that were not previously possible. Indeed, there are several compelling reasons to assume that the prevalence of disorder and psychological distress differs between single mothers, single fathers, and their married counterparts. First, differences in the economic circumstances of single mother and single father families are substantial. In Canada in 2001, average before-tax household income was $34,530 for single mothers, $40,990 for single fathers, and $73,495 for two-parent families.[80] Even more striking is the average household income of single parent, female-headed families where the parent is not in the labour force ($14, 936).[82] Poverty may be one of the mechanisms linking single parenthood to psychiatric disorder in mothers.[76] While economic differences between single mothers and fathers may be associated with differences in rates of disorder, the pathways into single parenthood are also likely to differ for single mothers and fathers. This difference in trajectories into single-parent status may help further account for any differences between genders. Single fatherhood, for example, is more likely to come about as a result of widowhood, whereas many single mothers become parents through childbirth out of marriage. Previous research has documented the importance of considering differing pathways into single parenthood among women in relation to the prevalence of depression and anxiety.[72,75] It may be that the different pathways into single parenthood also lead to differences in the rates of disorder between men and women in these roles. Finally, any differences between single and married fathers and mothers may also be disorder-specific. Most of the work on single mothers in mental health has focused on depression and anxiety.[62,72,74,76] Men are less likely than women to report these problems, but are more likely to experience problems with substance use,[83] while psychotic and bipolar disorders are thought to be approximately equally prevalent in both sexes.

In order to demonstrate the importance of considering the intersectionality of social roles, we examined the prevalence of several major psychiatric disorders among single and married mothers and fathers using data from three national surveys of Canadians: the National Population Health Survey (NPHS), and cycles 1.1 and 1.2 of the Canadian Community Health Survey (CCHS). The results of these preliminary analyses are shown in tables 3.1 and 3.2. In table 3.1, we present the prevalence of major depression, the only disorder measured in all three surveys, stratified by marital status and gender. Single parent fathers and mothers have consistently higher rates of depression than their married counterparts. Single mothers have the highest rates of all, consistently higher than those among single fathers.

In table 3.2, we present prevalence estimates of a range of disorders using CCHS 1.2, Canada's first national survey of major mental disorders. A pattern similar to that in table 3.1 emerges: single parenthood is associated with higher rates of disorder regardless of gender, and all disorders, with the important exception of substance dependence, are more common among women than men. Among men, single fathers have nearly twice the rate of depression of childless men, and nearly three times the rate of depression of married fathers. The rates of substance dependence, on the other hand, are similar among single fathers, married fathers, and the population of men as a whole.

These results reinforce the importance of considering the intersection of gender, marital, and parental status. In particular, the finding of a two- to three-fold difference in the prevalence of depression between single and married fathers is of interest to those interested in social determinants of psychiatric disorder. One of the most robust findings in the psychiatric epidemiological literature is that the rate of depression is about twice as high in women as men.[84,85] Not surprisingly, this

Table 3.1
12-month prevalence estimates of probable major depressive episode (MDE) among parents by family structure and gender of respondent (public use data files)

Family structure	1994 NPHS[a,c]			CCHS cycle 1.1[a,d]			CCHS cycle 1.2[b,c]		
	Single parent	Married parent	Total population	Single parent	Married	Total population	Single parent	Married	Total population
Total	9.6%	4.5%	5.4%	15.6%	5.6%	7.4%	10.8%	3.9%	4.8%
Male	5.5%	2.5%	3.4%	10.2%	3.7%	5.2%	7.3%	3.0%	3.7%
Female	11.2%	6.5%	7.3%	16.8%	7.6%	9.5%	12.3%	5.1%	5.9%

[a] Used UM-CIDI-SF for case identification.
[b] Used WMH-CIDI for case identification.
[c] 'Single parent' defined as a respondent living with children under 25 but no married or common-law partner. The household may also include other adults.
[d] 'Single parent' defined as a respondent living with children; no other relationships are permitted. Ages of children in household are not specified.

Table 3.2
12-month prevalence estimates of any probable mood disorder, anxiety disorder, substance dependence, and any disorder among parents by family structure and gender of respondent in CCHS cycle 1.2 (public use data files)[a]

Family structure	Mood disorder			Anxiety disorder			Substance dependence[b]			Any disorder		
	Single parent	Married parent	Total population	Single parent	Married parent	Total population	Single parent	Married parent	Total population	Single parent	Married parent	Total population
Total	11.7%	4.3%	5.2%	8.2%	4.3%	4.6%	2.7%	2.5%	2.7%	17.6%	9.3%	10.3%
Male	8.3%	3.6%	4.2%	4.8%	3.4%	3.5%	7.5%	3.9%	4.0%	11.0%	5.8%	9.3%
Female	13.6%	5.3%	6.3%	10.6%	5.4%	5.7%	3.6%	1.3%	1.5%	20.3%	9.4%	11.2%

[a] Used WMH-CIDI for prevalence rates
[b] Used Statistics Canada modified version of WMH-CIDI for alcohol and substance abuse/dependence

has generated interest in biological factors, especially hormonal differences, as a potential mechanism in depression[86,87] (but see Cairney and Wade[88]). Bringing an intersectional approach to the problem, however), suggests that other mechanisms, in particular social and psychological factors, may also be at work. Beiser,[89] for example, examined gender differences in depression among South-east Asian refugees to Canada. In the first few years after immigration, the characteristic two-to-one ratio in depression was reversed – the prevalence being twice as high in men as in women. However, over time, the gender difference came to resemble that among native-born Canadians, with women showing much higher rates than men. The explanation for this, Beiser suggests, is that in the first few years after arrival, men were exposed to many negative stressors, including stigma and discrimination, especially in relation to work, from which married women were largely protected because they stayed home to look after children. Over time, however, men adjusted to these conditions, and began to assimilate into the host culture, whereas women became increasingly isolated both from the larger culture and their own family members. Language, Beiser argued, was one of the reasons for increased isolation. Husbands and children were obliged to learn English, as a condition of work and education, respectively, while women were under much less pressure to do so. We may add single parenthood as another intersecting location that reinforces the need to consider social conditions as risk factors for mood disorder.

In addition to enriching our understanding of the descriptive epidemiology of family structure and mental disorder, an intersectional approach can also be useful for understanding pathways into parenthood, and the impact of life transitions on mental health. Cross-sectional data cannot be used to determine causality, so we cannot conclude from these data that single fathers or single mothers are at greater risk for disorder because of their social circumstances. We cannot, in other words, discount the social selection hypothesis with such data. However, as our discussion of these hypotheses indicated, social selection and social causation are not exclusive. Researchers elsewhere have shown, for example, that both explanations contribute to the effect of marital transitions on depression among mothers.[77,90] In an analysis of the British Household Panel Survey (BHPS), Wade and Pevalin[90] compared transitions out of marriage resulting from separation and divorce to transitions resulting from the death of a spouse. Relative to those who remained married, respondents whose marriages ended in separation or divorce had elevated rates of psychological distress two years prior to and two years after the event. This suggests that the high levels of distress observed among formerly-married respondents is due partly to the process of social selection. Those experiencing marital transition due to the death of a spouse, however, had higher rates of psychological distress only surrounding the year of the death, which is consistent with the process of social causation.

Considering the intersection of gender, marital status, and family structure opens up new possibilities for examining the relative effect of social conditions on well-being and the impact of disorder on social functioning. It may be the case, for example, that social selection is relatively stronger among women than men, owing to the fact that the pathway into single parenthood for men is more frequently the death of a spouse, an event that is neither planned nor 'on time' from a life course perspective. The trauma of losing a spouse, and subsequently finding oneself thrust into the single parent role, may be a key social risk factor leading to disorder. At present, the pathways to single parenthood for women are more heterogeneous, so disorder may play a more significant role in the selection of parental status. For example, early onset of depression has been shown to be associated with a greater likelihood of being a teen parent.[91] In this case, selection based on disorder leads to a precocious transition, itself a factor leading to a disrupted trajectory of social attainment, which increases the likelihood of subsequent poor mental health, as well as of intergenerational downward social drift for the child resulting from the potentially disadvantaged social environment.

Conclusion

There is a long, rich tradition of social epidemiology in psychiatry, dating back to pioneering community studies such as those of Srole[92] and Leighton[93] (see also chapter 4). While the debate over whether social class differences were the cause or consequence of psychiatric disorder long-dominated the research agenda, it is now widely accepted that both processes play a role in the etiology of disorder and impairment. Recent work on genetic-environmental interactions in conditions such as depression[94,95] provide empirical evidence to validate such a claim. In this chapter, we have made a case, however, for stepping back and reconsidering the association between social location and the prevalence of disorder. For too long, we have failed to embrace the fact that an individual's relative position in the social structure is determined by multiple social locations. These intersecting social statuses may compound one's social disadvantage, either additively or multiplicatively, which in turn increases the likelihood of disorder. To illustrate this, we considered the intersection of gender and family structure, the latter itself being the intersection of marital status and parenthood. This is only one example of the broad array of potential combinations of social statuses that may influence disorder. Other combinations, such as age, gender, and ethnicity, or poverty and race, may also be important to examine in the context of psychiatric disorder. In order to truly understand the association between social position and disorder, we must first be assured that we have captured the complexity in the social structure of our society. This is especially true in a country such as Canada, where pluralism based on ethnic identity is not only prevalent, as evidenced by the diverse composition of the population, but an integral part of our identity as Canadians.

NOTES AND REFERENCES

ψ   While some may take exception to the term 'cause,' the use of the term 'fundamental cause' by Link and Phelan[3] is to highlight the fact that the association between social conditions and health outcomes has persisted over time while other risk factors have changed; their permanency, therefore, reflects their status as fundamental causes because, while other risk factors have come and gone, the association between social class and health, for example, has remained unchanged for centuries. Fundamental causes is also used to emphasize the fact that social conditions are risk factors for other risks, many of which are more proximal to disease processes (e.g., smoking or stress exposure). The word 'cause' in this sense is used in the way we might think of exogenous and endogenous variables in a path model. Social conditions are distal causes of disease, operating through other proximal risk factors.

1   Turner RJ. The pursuit of socially modifiable contingencies in mental health. *J Health Soc Behav* 2003;44(1):1–17.
2   Link BG, Phelan JC Social conditions as fundamental causes. *J Health Soc Behav* 1995;35:80-94.
3   Link BG, Phelan JC. 'Fundamental Sources of Inequality.' In: Mechanic D, Rogut LB, Colby DC, Knickman JR, eds. *Policy Challenges in Modern*

Health Care. New Brunswick, New Jersey, and London: Rutgers University Press, 2005.

4. Mackenbach AE, Kunst AE, Cavelaars F, et al. Socioeconomic inequalities in morbidity and mortality in Western Europe. The EU working group on socioeconomic status inequalities in health. *Lancet* 1997;349:1655–9.

5 Wilkinson RG. *Unhealthy Societies: The Afflictions of Inequality.* London: Routledge, 1996.

6 Van Rossum CT, Shipley MJ, van de Mheen H, et al. Employment grade differences in cause specific mortality. A 25-year follow-up of civil servants from the first Whitehall study. *J Epidemiol Community Health* 2000;54(3):178–84.

7 Dohrewend BP, Dohrenwend BS. *Social Status and Psychological Disorder: A Causal Inquiry.* New York: Wiley, 1969.

8 Glenn ND, Weaver CN. Education's effects on psychological well-being. *Public Opin Quart* 1981;45:22–39.

9 Hollingshead AB, Redlich FC. *Social Class and Mental Illness: A Community Study.* New York: Wiley, 1958.

10 Kessler RC. A disaggregation of the relationship between socioeconomic status and psychological distress. *Am Sociol Rev* 1982;47:752–64.

11 Lennon MC, Rosenfield S. Women and mental health: The interaction of job and family conditions. *J Health Soc Behav* 1992;33:316–27.

12 Link BG, Dohrenwend BP, Skodol AC. Socioeconomic status and depression: The role of occupations involving direction, control and planning. *Am J Sociol* 1993;9:1351–87.

13 Mirowsky J, Ross CE. *Social Causes of Psychological Distress.* New York: Aldine de Gruyter; 1989.

14 Mirowsky J, Ross CE. Sex differences in distress: Real or artifact? *Am Sociol Rev* 1995;60:449–68.

15 Pearlin LI, Lieberman MA, Menaghan EG, Mullan JT. The stress process. *J Health Soc Behav* 1981;22:337–56.

16 Kessler RC, McGonagle KA, Zhao S, et al. Lifetime and 12-month prevalence of DSM-III-R psychiatric disorders in the United States: Results from the National Comorbidity Survey. *Arch Gen Psychiatry* 1994;51:8–19.

17 Gove WR. Relationship between sex roles, marital status, and mental-illness. *Soc Forces* 1972;51:34–44.

18 Ross CE, Mirowsky J, Goldstein K. The impact of the family on health: The decade in review. *J Marriage Fam* 1990;52:1059–74.

19 Williams DR, Takeuchi DT, Adair RK. Marital status and psychiatric disorders among Blacks and Whites. *J Health Soc Behav* 1992;33:140–57.

20 Williams DR, Harris-Reid M. Race and mental health: Emerging patterns and promising approaches. In: A Horwitz, and TL Scheid, eds. *A Hand-*

book for the Study of Mental Health. New York: Cambridge University Press, 1999:295–314.

21 Arboleda-Flórez J, Wade TJ. Victimization as a risk factor of major depression. *Int J Law Psychiatry* 2001;24:357–70.

22 Kessler RC, Magee WJ. Childhood adversities and adult depression: Basic patterns of association in a US national survey. *Psychol Med* 1993;23:679–90.

23 Turner RJ, Lloyd DA. Lifetime traumas and mental health: The Significance of cumulative adversity. *J Health Soc Behav* 1995;36:360–76.

24 Felitti VJ, Anda RF, Nordenberg D, et al. Relationship of childhood abuse and household dysfunction to many of the leading causes of death in adults: The Adverse Childhood Experiences (ACE) Study. *Am J Prev Med* 1998;14:245–58.

25 Chapman D, Whitfield C, Felitti VJ, et al. Adverse childhood experiences and the risk of depressive disorders in adulthood. *J Affec Dis* 2004;82:217–25.

26 Ortega ST, Corzine J. Socioeconomic status and mental disorders. *Res Community Ment Health* 1990;6:149–82.

27 Dohrenwend BP, Levay I, Shrout PE, et al. The causation-selection issue. *Science* 1992;255:946–52.

28 Mirowsky J, Ross CE. *Education, Social Status and Health.* Hawthorne, NY: Aldine de Gruyter, 2003.

29 Dohrenwend BP. The role of adversity and stress in psychopathology: Some evidence and its implications for Theory and Research. *J Health Soc Behav* 2000;41:1–19.

30 Breslau N, Davis GC, Andreski P. Risk factors for PTSD-related traumatic events: A prospective analysis. *Am J Psychiatry* 1995;52:529–35.

31 Koenen KC, Nugent NR, Amstadter AB. Gene-environment interaction in posttraumatic stress disorder: Review, strategy and new directions for future research. *Eur Arch Psychiatr Clin Neurosci* 2008;258(2):82–96.

32 Gilbertson MW, Shenton ME, Ciszewski A, et al. Smaller hippocampal volume predicts pathologic vulnerability to psychological trauma. *Nature Neurosci* 2002;5:1242–7.

33 Pearlson G. Structural brain imaging in schizophrenia: A selective review. *Biol Psychiatry* 2003;46:627–49.

34 Riley B, Kendler KS. Molecular genetic studies of schizophrenia. *Eur J Hum Genet* 2006;14:669–80.

35 McGuffin P, Asherson P, Owen M, Farmer A. The strength of the genetic effect. Is there room for an environmental influence in the aetiology of schizophrenia? *Br J Psychiatry* 1994;164:593–9.

36 Petronis A. The origin of schizophrenia: Genetic thesis, epigenetic antithesis, and resolving synthesis. *Biol Psychiatry* 2004;55:965–70.

37 Brown AS, Susser ES, Butler PD, et al. Neurobiological plausibility of prenatal nutritional deprivation as a risk factor for schizophrenia. *J Nerv Ment Dis* 1996;184:71–85.

38 Pearce BD. Schizophrenia and viral infection during neurodevelopment: A focus on mechanisms. *Mol Psychiatry* 2001;6:634–46.

39 Jones PB, Rantakallio P, Hartikainen AL, et al. Schizophrenia as a long-term outcome of pregnancy, delivery, and perinatal complications: A 28-year follow-up of the 1966 North Finland general population birth cohort. *Am J Psychiatry* 1998;155:355–64.

40 Williams JG, Ross L. Consequences of prenatal toxin exposure for mental health in children and adolescents. *Eur Child Adolesc Psychiatry* 2007;16:243–53.

41 Susser E, Lin S. Schizophrenia after prenatal exposure to the Dutch hunger winter of 1944–1945. *Arch Gen Psychiatry* 1992;49:983–8.

42 St Clair D, Mingqing X, Wang P, et al. Rates of adult schizophrenia following prenatal exposure to the Chinese famine of 1959–1961. *JAMA* 2005;294:557–62.

43 Jensen RT, Richter K. Understanding the relationship between poverty and children's health. *Eur Econ Rev* 2001;45:1031–9.

44 Khashan AS, Abel KM, McNamee R, et al. Higher risk of offspring schizophrenia following antenatal maternal exposure to severe adverse life events. *Arch Gen Psychiatry* 2008;65:146–52.

45 Tienari P, Wynne LC, Sorri A, et al. Genotype–environment interaction in schizophrenia-spectrum disorder. Long-term follow-up study of Finnish adoptees. *Br J Psychiatry* 2004;184:216–22.

46 Wahlberg KE, Wynne LC, Oja H, et al. Gene–environment interaction in vulnerability to schizophrenia: Findings from the Finnish Adoptive Family Study of Schizophrenia. *Am J Psychiatry* 1997;154:355–62.

47 Krabbendam L, van Os J. Schizophrenia and urbanicity: A major environmental influence – conditional on genetic risk. *Schiz Bull* 2005;31:795–9.

48 Muntaner C, Tien A, Eaton WW, Garrison R. Occupational characteristics and the occurrence of psychotic disorders. *Social Psych Psychiatric Epidemiol* 1991;26:273–80.

49 Jarvis GE. The social causes of psychosis in North American Psychiatry: A review of a disappearing literature. *Can J Psychiatry* 2007;52:287–94.

50 Cantor-Graae E. The contribution of social factors to the development of schizophrenia: A review of recent findings. *Can J Psychiatry* 2007;52:277–86.

51 Avison WR, Gotlib IH. *Stress and Mental Health: Contemporary Issues and Prospects for the Future.* New York: Plenum Press, 1995.

52 Billings AG, Moos RH. Stressful life events and symptoms: A longitudinal model. *Health Psychol* 1982;1:99–117.

53 Lazarus RS. The stress and coping paradigm. In: Eisdorfer C, Cohen D, Lieinman A, Maxim P., eds. *Models for Clinical Psychopathology.* New York: McGraw Hill, 1981:177–214.

54 Aneshensel CS. Social stress: Theory and research. *Ann Rev Sociol* 1992;18,15–38.

55 Thoits PA. Stress, coping and social support processes: Where are we? What next? *J Health Soc Behav* 1995;39:169–86.

56 Pearlin LI. The sociological study of stress. *J Health Soc Behav* 1989;30:241–56.

57 Pearlin LI, Aneshensel CS, LeBlanc AJ. The forms and mechanisms of stress proliferation: The case of AIDS caregivers. *J Health Soc Behav* 1997;38:223–36.

58 Pearlin LI. Stress and mental health: A conceptual overview. In: Horwitz AV, Scheid TL, eds. *A Handbook for the Study of Mental Health: Social Contexts, Theories and Systems.* Cambridge, UK: Cambridge University Press, 1999:161–75.

59 Turner RJ, Lloyd DA, Roszell P. Personal resources and the social distribution of depression. *Am J Comm Psychol* 1999;27:643–76.

60 Turner RJ, Marino F. Social support and social structure: A descriptive epidemiology. *J Health Soc Behav* 1994;35:193–212.

61 Turner RJ, Wheaton B, Lloyd DA. The epidemiology of social stress. *Am Sociol Rev* 1995;60:104–25.

62 Avison WR. Roles and resources: The effects of family structure and employment on women's psychological resources and psychological distress. *Res Comm Mental Health* 1995;8:233–56.

63 Cairney J, Boyle MH, Offord DA, Racine Y. Stress, social support and depression in single and married mothers. *Soc Psychiatr Psychiatr Epidemiol* 2003;38:442–9.

64 McMullin JA. Theorizing age and gender relations. In: Arber S, Ginn J, eds. *Connecting Gender and Aging: A Sociological Approach.* Philadelphia: Open University Press, 1995:30–41.

65 McMullin JA. Diversity and the state of sociological aging theory. *Gerontologist* 2000;40:517–30.

66 Clark DO, Maddox GL. Racial and social correlates of age-related changes in functioning. *J Gerontol* 1992;47:S222–32.

67 Dowd JJ, Bengston VL. Aging in minority populations: An examination of the double-jeopardy hypothesis. *J Gerontol* 1978;33:427–36.

68   Ferraro FF, Farmer MM. Double jeopardy to health hypothesis for African Americans: Analysis and critique. *J Health Soc Behav* 1996;37:5–33.

69   Markides KS, Timbers DM, Osberg S. Aging and health: A longitudinal study. *Arch Gerontol Geriatr* 1984;3:33–49.

70   Schieman S, Plickert G. Functional limitations and changes in levels of depression among older adults: A multiple-hierarchy stratification perspective. *J Gerontol B Psychol Sci Soc Sci* 2007;62:S36–42.

71   Drapeau A, Lesage A, Boyer R. Is the statistical association between sex and the use of services for mental health reasons confounded or modified by social anchorage? *Can J Psychiatry* 2005;50:599–604.

72   Afifi TO, Cox BJ, Enns MW. Mental health profiles among married, never-married, and separated/divorced mothers in a nationally representative sample. *Soc Psychiatr Psychiatr Epidemiol* 2006;41:122–9.

73   Byrne C, Browne G, Roberts J, et al. Surviving social assistance: 12-month prevalence of depression in sole-support parents receiving social assistance. *CMAJ* 1998;158:881–8.

74   Cairney J, Thorpe C, Rietschlin J, Avison WR. 12-month prevalence of depression among single and married mothers in the 1994 National Population Health Survey. *Can J Public Health* 1999;90:320–5.

75   Cairney J, Pevalin DJ, Wade TJ, et al. A comparison of 12-month prevalence of DSM-III-R psychiatric disorders between single parent and two parent mothers. *Can J Psychiatry* 2006;51:671–6.

76   Lipman EL, Offord DR, Boyle MH. Single mothers in Ontario: Sociodemographic, physical and mental health characteristics. *CMAJ* 1997;156:639–45.

77   Wade TJ, Cairney J. Major depressive disorder and marital transition among mothers: Results from a national panel study. *J Nerv Ment Dis* 2000;188:741–50.

78   Weissman MM, Leaf PJ, Bruce ML. Single parent women. *Soc Psychiatr Psychiatr Epidemiol* 1987;22:29–36.

79   Statistics Canada. *Family Portrait: Continuity and Change in Canadian Families and Households in 2006: National Portrait: Census Families*. 97-553-XWE2006001. 2006. Ottawa, Statistics Canada.

80   Statistics Canada. *Profile of Income of Individuals, Families and Households, Social and Economic Characteristics of Individuals, Families and Households, Housing Costs, and Religion, for Canada, Provinces, Territories, Census Divisions and Census Subdivisions, 2001 Census*. 95F0492XCB2001001. 2001. Ottawa, Statistics Canada.

81   Eggebeen DJ, Snyder AR. Children in single-parent father families in demographic perspective. *J Fam Issues* 1996;17:441–65.

82   Statistics Canada. CANSM II Table 202-0403. [Catalogue #75-202-XIE]. 2002.

83 Aneshensel CS, Rutter CM, Lanchenbruch PA. Social structure, stress, and mental health: Competing conceptual and analytic models. *Am Sociol Rev* 1991;56:166–78.

84 Kessler RC, McGonagle KA, Swartz M., et al. Sex and depression in the National Comorbidity Survey I: Lifetime prevalence, chronicity and recurrence. *J Affec Dis* 1993;29:85–96.

85 Piccinelli M, Wilkinson G. Gender difference in depression. *Br J Psychiatry* 2000;177:486–92.

86 Bebbington PE. The origins of sex differences in depressive disorder: Bridging the gap. *Int Rev Psychiatry* 1996;8:295–332.

87 Bebbington PE. Sex and depression. *Psychol Med* 1998;28:1–8.

88 Cairney J, Wade TJ. The influence of age on gender differences in depression: Further population-based evidence on the relationship between menopause and the sex difference in depression. *Soc Psychiatr Psychiatr Epidemiol* 2002;37:401–8.

89 Beiser M. *Strangers at the Gate: The Boat People's First Ten Years in Canada.* Toronto: University of Toronto Press, 1999.

90 Wade TJ, Pevalin DJ. Marital transitions and mental health. *J Health Soc Behav* 2004;42:155–70.

91 Kovacs M, Krol RS, Voti L. Early onset psychopathology and the risk for teenage pregnancy among clinically referred girls. *J Am Acad Child Adolesc Psychiatry* 1994;33:106–13.

92 Srole L, Langner ST, Michael ST, et al. *Mental Health in the Metropolis: The Midtown Manhattan Study.* New York: McGraw-Hill, 1962.

93 Leighton AH. *The Stirling County Study of Psychiatric Disorder and Sociocultural Environment. Vol. I: My Name Is Legion.* New York: Basic Books, 1959.

94 Thapar A, Harold G, Rice F, et al. The contribution of gene–environment interaction to psychopathology. *Dev Psychopathol* 2007;19:989–1004.

95 Caspi A, Sugden K, Moffitt TE, et al. Influence of life stress on depression: Moderation by a polymorphism in the 5-HTT gene. *Science* 2003;301:386–9.

PART TWO

Methodological Issues

4 Estimating Population Trends through Secondary Data: Attractions and Limitations of National Surveys

TERRANCE J. WADE AND AUGUSTINE BRANNIGAN

Analysis of existing data continues to play an important role in the study of the population determinants of a host of outcomes. In Canada, these include childhood development (National Longitudinal Survey of Children and Youth – NLSCY), labour force dynamics (Survey of Labour and Income Dynamics – SLID), educational attainment (Program for International Student Assessment – PISA), and adolescent labour force entry (Youth in Transition Survey – YITS), to name a few. Among the more recent Statistics Canada surveys are those that analyse mental disorder and addictions. These have made it possible for psychiatric epidemiologists and social scientists to map out the population parameters of mental illness in Canada in ways previously not possible. For example, one of the first national surveys to include mental disorders by Statistics Canada, the National Population Health Survey (NPHS), initiated in 1994, has been used to examine the relationship between age and depression,[1-3] gender differences in the age of onset and cessation of depression,[4,5] the association between physical activity and depression,[6,7] and the association between single-parent and two-parent families and depression, including differences in prevalence,[8] mental health consequences of transitioning into and out of single motherhood,[9] and mental health service utilization.[10] More recently, the Canadian Community Health Survey 1.2 (CCHS 1.2) has been used to examine the epidemiology of a range of mental disorders among older Canadians,[11,12] as well as the determinants of access to care among persons who meet criteria for one or more of the disorders measured in the survey.[13] Outside of psychiatry and epidemiology, secondary data have also been widely used by social scientists in Canada to examine a wide range of issues related to crime and delinquency,[14] welfare, and the economy. Yet, despite its ubiquity as a research tool in these disciplines, relatively little has been written about the methods or the unique challenges associated with using existing data as an analytical tool.

In this chapter, we review the three types of data sources including primary, secondary, and tertiary data. We examine the role of information in the governance of modern societies and the utility of such sources as the census and the general social surveys for the development of state policies. We argue that such information provides academic opportunities in the form of secondary data analysis for testing empirically informed theories of society as well as the examination of the effectiveness of new and innovative social policies. Finally, we caution that any existing data source requires a critical assessment prior to its use. We provide a key set of evaluative questions (who, where, what, when, why, and how) to guide the researcher in the assessment of secondary data sources in order to utilize such information effectively, meaningfully, and judiciously. Although many of the examples are drawn from studies on mental health and addictions, many are not. This is in keeping with the potential wide-range of uses for such data, and the varied interests of the contributing authors.

Primary, Secondary, and Tertiary Data

It is useful to differentiate *secondary* data analysis from both *primary* and *tertiary* data analysis. Primary data analysis refers to research that is designed and implemented by a researcher with his/her resources (often with university, government, or third party support) and on his/her professional initiative. It can be either qualitative or quantitative. Examples of qualitative primary research would include long-term ethnographic studies like *Street Corner Society* in which William F. Whyte lived in the Italian ghetto in Boston to learn about the nature of immigrant social structure and organized crime during the 1930s and 40s.[15] But it could be qualitative observational studies where the researcher undertakes more modest observations of *in situ* behaviour to determine the structures of action in naturalistic settings. These studies are often exploratory in design although there is nothing in principle that would preclude them from being confirmatory (i.e., designed to test specific hypothesis).

Primary data collection also includes quantitative approaches to data collection. Various research methods such as experimental designs or social surveys based on questionnaires and/or interviews can be used to facilitate quantitative data collection. Primary data collection based on a quantitative approach usually involves a specific test of a hypothesis, or set of hypotheses, or the testing of a theoretical model. For example, Hagan and McCarthy (1999) interviewed 750 street people in Toronto and Vancouver to test hypotheses of the causes of homelessness.[16] But these methods of primary data collection can also be exploratory in design such as in much epidemiological work. For example, the Stirling County Study in Atlantic Canada by Alexander Leighton and colleagues was conducted to provide some of the first population estimates of the prevalence of mental disorder in a given population in Canada.[17]

Secondary data analysis is the further analysis or reanalysis of information that was previously collected by a researcher or agency, either public or private, to assist in meeting their specific mandate. Data collected previously by an agency for whatever reason may nonetheless be of utility to the academic researcher, and may provide information that is otherwise difficult and/or costly to assemble. Data sources can be government-based or from private organizations.

A final example using historical data from insurance and company liability is noteworthy. Vivianna Zelizer studied changes in the theory of compensation for wrongful death of children in U.S. cities over the period 1885–1920.[18] When the electric railways were introduced into U.S. urban centres like New York and Chicago, dozens of children who were accustomed to playing in the city streets were killed or injured annually because of the new technology. Zelizer traced how the level of compensation changed qualitatively over time as the basis for settlement shifted. Initially, when child mortality was high, literacy low, and industrial employment was common, replacement of lost wages resulting from the child's death was the basis for compensation. By the end of this period, when childhood survival became the norm, following the abolition of child labour and after a universal educational obligation was adopted, compensation rose dramatically as the sentimental value of the child became the leading issue in compensating accidental child death. Zelizer's work provides an insightful use of secondary data to identify a fundamental shift in the status and value of children in industrial society not possible relying on other means (e.g., narrative records from parents such as diaries, official mortality statistics).

Tertiary data analysis is sometimes referred to as meta-analysis. It is an examination of a series of previous studies on the same question, primary and secondary, to pull together the conclusions of different researchers or, as Gene Glass calls it, an 'analysis of analyses.'[19] It requires the analyst to identify and pool (or average) the various correlations or 'effect' sizes by combining them all together. One of the most famous meta-analyses focused on the classic work of Rosenthal and Jacobsen (*Pygmalion in the Classroom*).[20] They had reported that teachers who had high expectations of student performances in schools actually raised the IQs of those students on objective measures of intelligence. Stephen Raudenbusch conducted a meta-analysis of the 12 main studies and replications and found that the average increase in IQ was 0.11 (z-score).[21] But as any serious student of statistics knows, the mean can easily be biased by outliers. The median increase was a more modest .035 (virtually nothing), and half the findings were in the wrong direction! That is, Raudenbusch found a negative effect where high teacher expectations proved debilitating to the student.

From this example, it is clear that tertiary analysis in the form of meta-analysis permits a rigorous analysis of an aggregation of existing studies and their conclusions without the expense of an entirely new study. In fact, sometimes a new study just adds to the confusion. A synthesis and analysis of the analyses is what is required. But rather than simply relying on a narrative accounting and appraisal of previous work, meta-analysis provides an analytic approach to synthesize sometimes hundreds of research articles on a single topic to gauge the overall correlation or effect size of a phenomenon to either discount it or support it.

Sources, Strengths, and Limits of Secondary Data Analysis

While some of the advantages of using existing data may be obvious, one should not get sentimental or soft-headed about its value. It is a fact of life for many contemporary researchers, even if it is rarely completely satisfactory to meet one's needs. For example, anyone interested in changes in the levels of crime in society has little recourse other than using annual crime statistics collected by governments. Likewise, anyone interested in the changing role of women in society has little recourse other to use the labour force surveys that record the percentage of males and females at every age beyond childhood who are lawfully employed outside the home. Neither crime rates nor labour force measures are perfect. Their utility depend on whether the data set contains the necessary classification of required groups of interest (i.e., inclusion of variables and categories within variables) and whether the degree of error (i.e., over-estimations or under-estimations) is modest enough to render the inferences valid and reliable.

With respect to the identification and classification of groups of interest, limitations occur when state and private bureaucracies are selectively blind (intentionally or unintentionally) to certain kinds of social events. The same caution attaches to the use of official suicide statistics. Since the act of suicide is stigmatized, friends and families of the victims are sometimes reluctant to report such deaths as suicides.[22,23]

This illustrates at least two lessons for the researcher using secondary data. First, as with other information sources, our confidence in the information used is strengthened when the same trends are identified independently across different agencies or data sources, a process referred to as triangulation. Second, where the authors of the original surveys or data source omit categories of interest to the researcher, we have to make allowances for the inherent limitations of secondary sources. The primary collectors of the data may not have collected information for a variable or specific category of a variable for a variety of reasons, such as not having a need for the information for their specific purposes, not having the resources to collect the information, or at that time, the information was not defined as an issue or deemed important to collect. With the value of hindsight, those who *later* wish to analyse the data as a secondary source to address a research question of interest may question how such an important variable or category could be missing. This is a point to which we will return.

Another point to stress is that secondary data, like primary data, may also be qualitative in nature. Historians typically use government documents, historical news accounts, annual reports of various agencies, changes in legislation, treaties, personal letters and diaries, all of which are secondary. In fact, it is hard to think of how historians could engage in primary data collection which was not open to a charge of plagiarism! (see, for example, *The Hitler Diaries*,[24] and the Piltdown forgery).[25] Anthropologists also often use the results of primary ethnographies to identify *comparative* trends in social behaviour that would be unavailable to anyone conducting a primary ethnography.[e.g.,26]

Why Is Secondary Data Analysis of Interest to Researchers? The Population Leverage

There is obviously some critically important information contained in secondary sources (e.g., health service utilization rates, crime trends, labour force participation, basic demographic trends). But beyond that, there are several other reasons to use these surveys. The national secondary data sets, such as the NPHS, CCHS, and NLSCY, permit the researcher to make reliable *population* estimates of social facts that are typically beyond the scope of researcher-initiated primary data collection. For example, it is problematic to try to generalize from a local survey, say, of religiosity and attitudes to abortion, or why three hundred Bay Street lawyers do not like their jobs, or why students in twelve local high schools use marijuana. It is similarly impossible to draw international comparisons from such primary data. However, well-designed surveys such as the CCHS, NPHS and NLSCY permit us to draw out patterns that are valid for the population as a whole and to describe the regional distribution of such traits over the population. Moreover, the large numbers of respondents contained in these surveys permit us to examine unique or exotic subpopulations that are generally absent from most research because of their small numbers. Third, longitudinal components of both the NPHS and NLSCY surveys permit the researcher to track changes over time across the same individuals. Finally, use of such data sets, particularly data acquired with public funds, can be accessed at very moderate costs to the researcher. Primary data collection on a similar scale is simply inconceivable from both a cost and a logistical perspective. However, the use of such surveys must be done with caution – 'buyer beware.'

Politics and Statistics

We have already noted that secondary data analysis based on information collected by a third party is at risk of yielding misleading conclusions because of the explicit or implicit agendas of those who have designed the surveys and gathered the information to meet their own information needs. We should point out that academic research is no less prone to bias because of the agendas of those conducting research, both explicit and implicit. This potential bias exists whether the analysis be based on primary, secondary, or tertiary data. But there is a larger issue that one cannot escape with the use of secondary data sources and something with which we must grapple with explicitly. Information collected by state agencies and bureaucracies is inherently implicated in social control, politics, and government. The term 'statistics' is from the Latin, *statisticus* – 'about politics' from the Latin for state – *status*.[27(p1137)] When the rulers of Normandy conquered the Anglo-Saxons in 1066, they initiated the first national census (since Roman times) that was recorded in *The Domesday Book*. The *Domesday Book* was a statistical inventory of all the property, both private and ecclesiastical, and all the estates and their populations that comprised Anglo-Saxon England. Censuses have historically been used to help raise armies and taxes. Censor and census have the same Latin root – *censere*. The censor was 'one of two magistrates of early Rome acting as census takers, assessors, and inspectors of morals and conduct.'[ψ,27(p180)]

It was not just the state that conducted censuses. The Christian churches throughout European history, kept meticulous records of births, baptisms, marriages, and burials – for they also had a need to raise tithes as well as to administer sacraments. In the nineteenth century, government bureaucracies in the leading European nations – France under Napoleon, Germany under Bismarck, and England under Disraeli – began to develop systematic annual records of the characteristics of civil society to help manage the economic development of their countries. Who were the users of some of this secondary data? Karl Marx pored over the annual reports to the British parliament to trace the development of international capitalism and imperialism in writing his treatises *Das Kapital* and the *Communist Manifesto*.[28,29] Emile Durkheim similarly pored over French records examining, among other things, changes in the prevalence and locations of suicide.[30]

Durkheim's study of suicide was the first and the most important 'empirical' population-based study undertaken by any of the founders of sociology. Durkheim studied the reports of suicide in various areas of France and concluded that the aggregates varied by the religious composition of the regions. He identified differences in the prevalence of suicides by religion, gender, and marital status and drew conclusions about the differential risks of suicide depending on these factors. Suicide, for Durkheim, was a result of pathological social structures, not pathological individuals. All this was based on secondary data analysis. Durkheim's work anticipated the rise of the population health perspective in epidemiology that valorized the macrosociological determinants of individual health.

We should also not forget that the Third Reich, from the very first months of coming to power in Germany in 1933, and throughout its period of European conquest, undertook census surveys to identify the non-Aryans who would subsequently be marked for murder in the Holocaust.[31] Statisticians and the first generation of computer scientists (using IBM card sorting machines) played key roles in the infrastructure of mass murder. Regardless of the purpose or intent, the recognition for the need for data has become increasingly necessary to nation states. Both reprehensible and noble uses are fed by the state's recognition of its need for record keeping to maintain order and control to pursue its own political agenda.

Statistics and National Development in Canada

In Canada, systematic census statistics were compiled from the time of Champlain (1608) and were highly refined by the 1660s – when Louis XIV used the annual census to measure the growth and trade of his colonial properties. In the nineteenth century, there were numerous censuses taken by the various provinces long before Confederation in 1867.[32] In 1867, the *Canada Year Book* was first launched to give a public account of the prosperity in the Dominion in order to attract investment and settlers. It presented a thorough record of the national income and expenditures, the demographic characteristics of the people and provinces, the level of industrial growth and manufacture, the number of acres under tillage and the heads of livestock, the extent of the rail and canal development, the records of criminal convictions, as well as the devotional orientation of the population. All this was done independently in different government departments. Various statistical acts were passed in the late nineteenth century in respect of the collection of agricultural, labour, criminal, and demographic statistics. For example, the 10 year census was initiated in 1871. These efforts were centralized by the creation of a single agency, the *Dominion Bureau of Statistics*, in 1918. This effort to systematically collect national and provincial statistical profiles of Canadian society predated the appearance of the first Canadian chair in Sociology (McGill, 1938) by two decades. If we think back to Durkheim, a case could be made that empirical sociology only became possible *after* the rise of government statistics.

The Second World War created an unprecedented demand for accurate statistics in the areas of industrial production, the behaviour of the domestic economy, and labour force participation.[33] After the war, the demands continued to increase. As an official history of the Dominion Bureau of Statistics aptly noted:

> the increased complexity of the world's social and economic problems in the postwar period, the trend toward social security, the acceptance by governments of responsibilities concerning high employment, all led to increased needs for statistics at the national level. For instance, such policies as government tariffs, taxation, unemployment insurance, old age pensions, etc., must be planned, their incidence studied, and the extent of the burdens they impose in relation to the national economy known before they are put into effect. (Dominion Bureau of Statistics 1952)[cited in 33(p10)]

Increasingly in this process, the expertise of academics had become important in research design and sampling strategies, making academics partners with the state in the creation of secondary data, even though the information collected is in the context of specific national policies which further specific political interests (and may be collected in contexts and under interests that ignore other policy alternatives).

We began this section with a caution to remind us that statistics = politics. However, the statistic collection agencies are becoming increasingly autonomous from state authority but still collect data based largely on political needs. Statistics Canada superseded the Dominion Bureau of Statistics in the 1950s, and now employs thousands of sociologists, economists, demographers, and policy analysts. The need for accurate social statistics has increased with the increasing expansion and complexity of national policies in the areas of education, medicine and health care, international trade, immigration, habitat protection, native treaties, and urbanization. In the next section we outline by way of illustration how national surveys can elevate a particular social problem and illuminate how society might ameliorate it.

The Development of Measurement in Psychiatric Illness and Diagnoses

The area of medicine and health care, specifically as it pertains to psychiatric disorders and mental health care utilization in the Canadian Community Health Survey 1.2 (CCHS 1.2), is of specific interest for this volume (see chapters 1, 2, and 5).

Prior to the CCHS, most epidemiological surveys in Canada were regional (e.g., Ontario, Edmonton). The move from these regional assessments toward a more national approach to the study of mental health and health more generally in Canada was a result of the National Task Force on Health Information (see chapter 5). The Task Force identified a series of problems with currently available information on which to base policy, including its incomplete and fragmented nature, the lack of information sharing across groups and regions, and the lack of analysis of the data for the good of Canada and Canadians.[34] To respond to these needs, Health Canada, the Canadian Institute for Health Information (CIHI), and Statistics Canada joined forces to create the National Health Information Roadmap. With public consultation to guide them, they developed a national health information system and the infrastructure to evaluate and improve the health care system and the health of the Canadian population (see chapter 5). These developments of 'survey' tools to measure mental disorders in a reliable way have made it possible to make precise estimates of the prevalence of mental illnesses and addictions in the population as a whole. Without such innovations in survey methods, such inferences were not possible. This points to one of the major attractions of secondary data analysis to researchers.

The Who, What, Where, When, Why, and How of Secondary Data Analysis

The data available to researchers for secondary analysis are extensive, far surpassing what most would expect. But with this extensive selection also comes an extensive variability in data quality. When searching out secondary data for use to answer research questions, one must be cognizant of the quality of the data as well as its content. In order to assess this, it is useful to ask a series of questions with which to evaluate the various dimensions of the data. We propose framing an inquiry of the data into a series of questions to identify advantages and disadvantages of specific sources of data and to assess the trustworthiness of the results derived from these data. First and foremost, it must be remembered that all data are collected for a *purpose*. This may influence or bias the data in various ways: collection procedures (e.g., interviews versus questionnaires, face-to-face interviews versus telephone interviews), how the respondents are identified, how the terms are defined, how the data are collated and categorized, and/or how the data are weighted—all these decisions can influence the conclusions drawn. Among other advantages, a healthy skepticism about the information provided by others will ensure our confidence in the data that we choose to use to test our hypotheses, and, eventually, to make policy decisions.

What are the problems with surveys? First of all, is it possible to obtain reliable information about sensitive subjects via a telephone survey? Even if we acknowledge that this method is convenient and permits the development of a reliable sampling frame, can we make inferences about differences from such surveys over time? Are households the same size over time or is the population becoming more thinly spread into more units?

A confusion of households and individuals raises another significant problem. Earlier, we distinguished between primary, secondary, and tertiary data. However, we can further distinguish between different types of secondary data: *ecological* data and *individual* data. Ecological data are data collected about population characteristics such as demographic trends, economic trends, and crime trends. The second form focuses primarily on data derived from individuals, which could include politics and voting practices, attitudes and behaviours, health experiences, educational outcomes, and employment experiences. Census information is a form of this type because information is collected from all persons in the population. These data generally focus upon individuals and when collapsed can give an overall impression as to the views, beliefs, and so forth, of a group or population. However, although they are related to one another, at times it can be reckless to infer individual processes from ecological correlations, and ecological processes from individual data (as Durkheim did in his study of suicide). Much of the following discussion pertains more to survey-based secondary data as opposed to administrative or other types.

Returning to the questions we identified, we now discuss how such an approach could be used to assess the adequacy of secondary data to specific research questions/projects.

WHO Collected the Data?

This may be less of a concern when dealing with trustworthy firms, such as Statistics Canada or other similar national agencies whose mandate it is to collect data. For example, in the 1990s, the *Economist* twice identified Statistics Canada as the most reliable data collection agency among the G7 nations. Even here, however, we need to be alert to biases in survey estimates of things like gun ownership, unemployment, and health and educational spending, since they have some political gravity. The 1993 Violence Against Women Survey (VAWS) attracted a lot of criticism because it tended to conflate minor and major offences, and was gender-biased in its specific focus on violence against females as opposed to violence more generally.† Other sources such as polling firms and market researchers may have explicit political orientations, such as surveys commissioned by the Fraser Institute, or the Parkland Institute. It is always advisable to question why a specific topic has been chosen by a specific agency. Surveys conducted by the Canadian Cancer Foundation and Imperial Tobacco about the 'freedom to smoke' in drinking establishments have obvious interest-group agendas. While the potential for bias in this example is obvious, to assess whether there may be more subtle forms of bias present in other cases, it is important to know whether the agency had a vested interest in conducting a survey in the first place.

WHY Were the Data Collected?

This will have a large impact on the trustworthiness of the results and has implications for one's reliance upon the reporting of these data. Did the techniques used assist the researchers to arrive at the conclusions they wanted? For example, were only results supporting a pre-established position reported, while others were suppressed or down-played? This may be evident in certain political party polling where they might only publicly report results that show their candidate in the best light.

WHAT Data Were Collected?

This question can be further expanded to examine the content areas of questions, as well as the structure and ordering of the questions asked. Stewart and Kamins argue the Consumer Price Index (CPI) provides one such case.[35] The CPI is based on prices of about 400 items purchased by an average family (father, aged 38; nonworking mother; boy, aged 13; girl, aged 8) living in an urban area. This index is hardly representative of the expenditures of most of the population, but it continues to be used as a rough guide for tracking increases and decreases in the cost of living. The focus of the survey is also important. For example, the Centre for Addiction and Mental Health – Ontario

Student Drug Use Survey (OSDUS) (formerly the Addiction Research Foundation – Ontario Student Drug Use Survey) asks students to self-report on issues surrounding drugs and alcohol.[36] The majority of questions deal with consumption habits and attitudes towards substance use such as smoking, alcohol, cannabis, and a wide range of hard drugs. Since this survey asks questions that are by their nature very sensitive, students may be inclined to under-report fearing a lack of anonymity. Or, more likely, they may be inclined to over-report use as a lark or to show off to their peers. The architects of this survey included a novel method to detect bias due to over-reporting by including a question about consumption of a fictitious drug. Structured in the same fashion of all the other drugs, they provide both a technical name ('adrenochromes') and a street name ('wagon wheels') for the fictitious drug. Anyone providing a positive response of consumption of 'wagon wheels' on this question is deleted from the survey on the basis that their responses are untrustworthy and unreliable. On average, they found that about 0.5% of students were deleted due to positive responses on this fictitious drug.[36,37]

The structure of the questions and question ordering are issues related to *how the data were collected,* a topic beyond the scope of this chapter (for one example, see Streiner and Norman).[38] However, we provide a few ideas that could influence a response. For example, was the structure of the questions quantitative in nature or qualitative? Was the list of questions all-encompassing to give one a firm understanding of the issues that one was investigating? Did people have the opportunity to provide additional comments if they thought that the questions did not really tap their experiences? Were the scales used to measure specific theoretical constructs using well-validated instruments or were they constructed specifically for this survey? Was the inclusion of specific questions earlier on in the survey likely to influence one's response to subsequent questions? These types of questions and others are helpful in understanding whether the data will be able to provide the level of information required by the secondary researcher to answer his/her questions.

WHERE Were the Data Collected?

This question has implications for the generalizability and applicability of the results. For example, if the survey was conducted in a community in Southern Alberta, can the results be generalized to that community? This will depend upon the sampling procedures and the population target, again an issue of how the data were collected (see Kish for an excellent source on survey sampling[39]). If everyone in the community (or target population) had a *non-zero* chance of being selected for the sample (that is, were included in the sampling frame), then the results (using probability theory) would be generalizable to that community (sampling frame) using some specified weighting scheme. However, a more pressing issue regarding 'where' the data were collected would entail an assessment of the generalizability of these results to the region, province, or country. This is highly unlikely in a pure probabilistic sense. Since others in Alberta and Canada were not part of the sampling frame, there is no way in which they could have participated in the survey. According to probability theory, generalizations to these populations would not be possible. But a researcher might make a theoretical argument suggesting that communities with similar characteristics across the province or country (supported by other secondary data such as census and economic industry) might have attitudes, beliefs, or other characteristics that are similar to those studied in the target population. This argument would be more difficult to make the farther away one gets from the specific population and one would need to discount alternative explanations such as distinctive local or regional effects (e.g., unemployment, industry, history). While this may seem straightforward, this type of over-generalization to other populations is done quite frequently. For example, the Epidemiologic Catchment Area (ECA), a large scale epidemiologic survey of major mental disorders (see chapter 2), was conducted in only five cities across the United States. Yet, these data established accepted prevalence rates for the entire United States providing the benchmark against which all subsequent studies were judged and critiqued (e.g., National Comorbidity Study which was a national probability survey). In Canada, both the Edmonton survey and the Ontario Child Health Survey were used in a similar fashion to provide estimates of the prevalence of mental health problems in the whole country; and these surveys had been the benchmarks in Canada until the advent of the National Task Force on Health Information and the (national) NPHS, NLSCY, and CCHS survey initiatives.

WHEN Were the Data Collected?

The final question is rooted in the contemporary relevance of the available data. Are the data still relevant? If the data were collected five, ten, twenty, or fifty years ago, are they still applicable to the situation today? Also, a longitudinal survey that represents the population fairly accurately in the first panel may become increasingly unrepresentative over time. The original samples for both the NPHS and the NLSCY were established in 1994 based on a national probability sampling strategy. But how representative are these samples of the population more than ten years later? The NLSYC addresses this issue by adding a new cohort of 0–2 year olds to the survey every wave. The NPHS does not add new respondents to its sample; instead its cross-sectional component was replaced by the CCHS cycles.

In addition, were the data collected in a period where there was a great deal of attention on the topic? For example, a survey on neighbourhood safety may obtain very different results if it were conducted during a large public criminal trial or during a rash of neighbourhood break-ins, as opposed to when the level of crime was seemingly quiet. A survey on the sustainability of universal health care in Canada may yield very different results in a period of economic contraction and tax increases versus a period of economic expansion and tax breaks. Similarly, a survey on gun ownership and registration may yield different results following an event such as the Montreal massacre.

Notwithstanding these concerns, there can also be benefits of using historical data. For example, these data may be used to establish a baseline against which to compare current trends or attitudes, in an effort to examine secular changes. This can be more useful when the *same* people are used to establish the baseline that are used to measure trends and changes, as in a panel design like the NLSCY or NPHS. Such designs would make it possible to examine which factors are responsible for any changes observed. Comparison of historical samples with contemporary samples can also provide opportunities to assess the effect of policy and program changes that may occur. The gun ownership surveys provide a potential opportunity to assess the effect of the gun registry legislation assuming one is satisfied with their answers to other issues raised through asking who, why, what, where, and when.

Concluding Comments

From this discussion, it appears as though there are a great many potential pitfalls in using secondary data. One might begin to question whether it is worth the time and effort to conduct research using existing data. We would respond with a resounding *yes*. The availability of high quality secondary data as well as the low cost involved and the quick turn-around time in researching questions makes secondary data analysis an indispensible research tool for inquiry. Instead of taking three to five or more years in which to fund, design, collect, code, enter, clean, and analyse primary data, one can jump right into the analysis without the high cost and effort entailed in conducting the previous stages (keeping the discussed issues in mind, of course). To help make this point, we can get some insight into the users and uses of secondary data from an analysis of the USA General Social Survey (GSS) between 1972 and 1993. For example, Smith and Heaney found that 79.3% of published articles came from people with academic associations.[40] As well, sociology accounted for 62.6% of the articles, covering a very broad range of areas including gerontology, health, demography, religion, urban, stratification, deviance, and research methodology. Many other disciplines also used the GSS. The content of the various surveys has been very diverse collecting information across successive waves on topics too numerous to list.

Finally, throughout this last section, we pose a series of questions and level a series of critiques to evaluate a secondary source of data, but we provide very few answers. This is done intentionally for a number of reasons. First, every data source is unique and has to be evaluated on its own merit based on a series of criteria including but not limited to collection agency, content focus, and methodology. Second, every researcher is unique in the questions she/he poses and this must guide the evaluation of any data source. Third, the availability of secondary data sources is continually growing and it is such a large, moving target that it would take volumes and a number of careers to catalogue and describe all that are available. But there are several organizations that are doing this in specific areas providing archiving services and (varying levels of) access for researchers to utilize these data in Canada, the United States, Europe, and around the world.‡ One is limited only by one's inquisitiveness, time, and persistence.

NOTES AND REFERENCES

ψ   *Note from the Editors*: In fact, the first census was carried out by David (1 Chronicles 27), and he was punished by G-d for it; a lesson all epidemiologists should take to heart.

† A subsequent survey polled both male and female respondents as both potential victims and potential perpetrators.

‡ For example, see <odesi> (Ontario Data Documentation, Extraction Service and Infrastructure Initiative), the latest data archiving initiative by the Ontario Council of University Libraries and OntarioBuys to provide university researchers with access to existing data, full topic search capabilities, and a web-based data extraction system.

1 Wade TJ, Cairney J. Age and depression in a nationally representative sample of Canadians: A preliminary look at the National Population Health Survey. *Can J Public Health* 1997;88:297–304.

2 Wade TJ, Cairney J. The effect of sociodemographics, social stressors, health status and psychosocial resources on the age depression relationship. *Can J Public Health* 2000;91:307–12.

3 Beaudet MP. Depression. *Health Rep* 1996;7:11–22.

4 Wade TJ, Cairney J, Pevalin DJ. The emergence of gender differences in depression among adolescents: National panel results from the USA, Canada and Great Britain. *J Am Acad Child Adolesc Psychiatry* 2002;41:190–8.

5 Cairney J, Wade TJ. The influence of age on gender differences in depression – Further population-based evidence on the relationship between menopause and the sex difference in depression. *Soc Psychiatry Psychiatr Epidemiol* 2002;37:401–8.

6 Wade TJ, Martin JC. The relationship between physical exercise and distress in a national sample of Canadians. *Can J Pub Health* 2000;91:302–6.

7 Cairney J, Hawes R, Corna L, Wade T, McCabe L, Faught B. Physical activity and psychological distress in older adults: A longitudinal analysis. *Gerontologist* 2005;45:360.

8 Cairney J, Thorpe C, Rietschlin J, Avison WR. 12-month prevalence of depression among single and married mothers in the 1994 National Population Health Survey. *Can J Public Health* 1999;90:320–4.

9 Wade TJ, Cairney J. Marital transitions and major depressive episodes: Results from a national panel study. *J Nerv Ment Dis* 2000;188:741–50.

10 Cairney J, Wade T. Are single mothers more likely to use health care services than married mothers? *Soc Psychiatry Psychiatr Epidemiol* 2002;37:190–8.

11 Cairney J, McCabe L, Veldhuizen S, Streiner DL, Hermann N. Epidemiology of social phobia in later life. *Am J Geriatr Psychiatry* 2007;15:224–33.

12 Streiner DL, Cairney J, Veldhuizen S. The epidemiology of psychological problems in the elderly. *Can J Psychiatry* 2006;54:185–91.

13 Urbanoski KA, Cairney J, Bassani DE, Rush B. Perceived unmet need for mental health care among Canadians with co-occurring addiction and mental illness. *Psychiatr Serv* 2008;59:283–9.

14 Wade TJ, Brannigan A. The genesis of adolescent risk-taking: Pathways through family, school, and peers. *Can J Sociol* 1998;23:1–19.

15 Whyte WF. *Street Corner Society*. Chicago: University of Chicago Press, 1943.

16 Hagan J, McCarthy B. *Mean Streets: Youth Crime and Homelessness*. New York: Cambridge University Press, 1999.

17 Leighton DC, Harding JS, Macklin DB, Macmillan AM, Leighton AH. *The Character of Danger: Psychiatric Symptoms in Selected Communities*. New York: Basic Books, 1963.

18 Zelizer V. *Pricing the Priceless Child*. New York: Basic Books, 1985.

19 Glass GV. Primary, secondary, and meta-analysis of research. *Educational Researcher* 1976;5:3–8.

20 Rosenthal R, Jacobson L. *Pygmalion in the Classroom: Teacher Expectations and Pupils' Intellectual Development*. New York: Holt, Reinhart and Winston, 1969.

21 Raudenbusch SW. Magnitude of teacher expectancy effects on pupil IQ as a function of the credibility of expectancy induction: A synthesis of findings from 18 experiments. *J Educ Psychol* 1984;76:85–97.

22 Wilkins J. Producing suicides. *Am Behav Sci* 1970;14:185–201.

23 Wilkins J. Suicidal behavior. *Am Sociol Rev* 1967;32:286–98.

24 Hamilton C. *The Hitler Diaries: Fakes That Fooled the World*. Lexington: University Press of Kentucky, 1991.

25 Walsh JE. *Unraveling Piltdown*. New York: Random House, 1996.

26 MacAndrew C, Edgerton RB. *Drunken Comportment*. Chicago: Aldine, 1969.

27 *Webster's New Collegiate Dictionary*, 1977.

28 Marx K, Engels F. *The Communist Manifesto*. New York: International Publishers, 1948.

29 Marx K. *Capital: A Critique of Political Economy*. New York: International Publishers, 1948.

30 Durkheim E. *Suicide; A Study in Sociology*. New York: Free Press, 1951.

31 Black E. *IBM and the Holocaust*. New York: Crown Books, 2001.

32 Curtis B. *The Politics of Population*. Toronto, Ontario: University of Toronto Press, 2001.

33 Warton DA. *The Dominion Bureau of Statistics*. Kingston, Ontario: Queen's University Press, 1998.

34 Health Canada. *Health Information Roadmap Responding to Needs*. Ottawa: Statistics Canada, 1991.

35 Stewart DW, Kamins MA. *Secondary Research: Information, Sources and Methods.* (2nd ed). Newbury Park: Sage, 1993.
36 Adlaf EM., Smart RG, Walsh GW. *Ontario Student Drug Use Survey, 1977–1993.* Toronto, Addiction Research Foundation of Ontario, 1993.
37 Vingilis E, Wade TJ, Adlaf E. What factors predict student self-rated physical health? *J Adolesc* 1998;21:83–97.
38 Streiner DL, Norman GR. *Health Measurement Scales: A Practical Guide to Their Development and Use.* 4th ed. Oxford: Oxford University Press, 2008.
39 Kish L. *Survey Sampling.* New York: Wiley & Sons, 1965.
40 Smith TW, Heaney K. *Who, What, When, Where, and Why: An Analysis of Usage of the General Social Survey, 1972–93.* University of Chicago, National Opinion Research Center, 1996.

5 The Canadian Community Health Survey: Mental Health and Well-Being

RONALD GRAVEL AND YVES BÉLAND

The Canadian Community Health Survey: Mental Health and Well-Being (CCHS)[1] is funded as part of the Health Information Roadmap Initiative,[2] a plan to modernize and standardize health information across the country. Statistics Canada, the CIHI, and Health Canada jointly support the series of projects that make up the Roadmap Initiative. The CCHS has a two-year collection cycle comprising two surveys: a regional survey in the first year (cycle 1.1) and a province-level survey in the second (cycle 1.2). Each second year of the survey cycle is designed to focus in depth on a particular topic. During consultations for the development of the CCHS,[3] mental health was frequently identified as a high-priority topic to be measured. Consequently, mental health and well-being was the focus of the provincial component of the first CCHS cycle (cycle 1.2), which took place in 2002.

Because information on mental disorders in Canada was incomplete and fragmented, the major objectives of the CCHS 1.2 were as follows: (1) to determine prevalence rates of selected mental disorders to assess the burden of illness; (2) to examine links between mental health and social, demographic, geographic, and economic variables or characteristics; (3) to juxtapose use of mental health services and perceived needs, and (4) to assess the disability associated with mental health problems in regard to individuals and society.

Content

Consultation Process

Topics for the CCHS 1.2 were selected through extensive consultations with regional, provincial, and federal representatives and the research community. Expert consultation was seen as integral to content development. The selection of priority areas in terms of mental disorders and mental well-being was informed by discussions with the Statistics Canada Population Health Surveys Advisory Committee and with a Mental Health Expert Group assembled to advise on the survey. Consultations also included contacts with representatives of the WHO, academia, international, federal, and provincial governments, consumers, and professional associations.

Mental Health Disorders

Mental health disorders were selected according to the criteria that their 12-month anticipated prevalence rate would be at least 1%, that they could be measured with a widely recognized and validated instrument, and that they were amenable to intervention. The impact of the selected disorder on response burden (that is, interview length and clarity of concepts and questions) was also considered. The selected disorders were major depression, mania, panic disorder, social phobia, and agoraphobia.

Interview questions for these disorders were based on the WMH 2000 Project. The WMH 2000 Project is an international initiative responsible for the development of a new version of the CIDI (the WMH-CIDI). The WMH-CIDI is a lay-administered instrument oriented to mental diagnosis that generates a lifetime and past-12-month profile of persons with a disorder defined partly according to both the ICD-10 and the *DSM-IV*. For the purposes of the CCHS 1.2, mental disorders were partially coded to the *DSM-IV* only.

The CCHS 1.2 team, with the support of the Mental Health Expert Group and the WMH 2000 Project, made some modifications to the content of the disorder modules to reduce response burden and clarify concepts. Since the end of the CCHS 1.2 data collection, the WMH 2000 Project has adopted some of these changes and has also introduced additional ones. As a result, comparing the CCHS 1.2 and the WMH-CIDI modules is a challenging task.

Mental Health Problems and Correlates

Other CCHS content areas include eating troubles and behaviours, gambling problems, suicidal ideation and behaviours, and alcohol or illicit drug use and dependence. Instruments used to measure these mental health problems were based on instruments used in Statistics Canada surveys such as the NPHS, the CCHS 1.1, and the HPS. Table 4.2 of the CCHS 1.2 User Guide[4] gives a detailed breakdown of sources and changes from earlier use in the CCHS and NPHS.

Regardless of their answers to the modules on mental disorders and mental health problems, all survey respondents were asked questions on mental health service use, medication, and mental health correlates or determinants. To address mental health issues, many questions on mental health correlates, such as two-week disability or restricted activity, were adapted from material used in the former CCHS and NPHS. For example, in the CCHS 1.2, data collected on two-week disability identified whether the disability was attributed to a mental or to a physical cause. Questions pertaining to the impact or cost of mental health problems were not addressed in relation to the specific surveyed mental disorders or problems. Rather, the survey used the generic terminology of 'mental health, problems with emotions, drugs, and alcohol' to refer to any mental disorders or problems experienced by the respondent. Table 5.1 presents in alphabetical order the list of all modules included in the CCHS 1.2.

Qualitative Testing

The CCHS 1.2 questionnaire was developed in consultation with Statistics Canada's Questionnaire Design Resource Centre. It was reviewed and tested in the field in pre-tests and focus groups, in both English and French. The qualitative testing aimed to evaluate respondent reactions with regard to the sensitivity of the subject matter and their ability to understand and willingness to respond to the questions. Cognitive testing and focus-group testing took place during the summer of 2001. The focus groups were convened in Ottawa, Ontario; Montreal, Quebec; and Edmonton and Red Deer, Alberta.

In the qualitative testing, both individuals with known mental disorders and participants from the general population responded to the survey and provided feedback on their experience. As part of the qualitative testing, 50 face-to-face interviews were conducted. Mental health experts at St Joseph's Hospital in Hamilton, Ontario, and L'Hôpital L-H Lafontaine in Montreal, Quebec, conducted cognitive tests with target groups of participants diagnosed with a mental disorder. The ethical review bodies within each host organization reviewed and approved these tests.

Table 5.1
CCHS 1.2 Questionnaire Modules (alphabetical order)

Administration	Medication use
Agoraphobia	Mental health services
Alcohol dependence	Panic disorder
Alcohol use	Pathological gambling
Chronic conditions	Physical activities
Distress	Psychological well-being manifestation
Eating troubles assessment	scale
General health	Restriction of activities
Height and weight	Screening section
Household contact and demographics	Sociodemographic characteristics
Illicit drug use and dependence	Social phobia
Income	Spiritual values
Labour force	Stress
Major depression	Two-week disability
Mania	Work stress

Qualitative testing identified general acceptance and support of the study. 'It's about time' was a phrase commonly stated. We found the interview to be too long, specific questions too verbose, and some screening criteria too broad. All these findings were addressed, and as a result, a much more respondent-friendly questionnaire emerged.

Sample Design

Target Population

This CCHS component covered only persons aged 15 years or over and living in private dwellings in the 10 Canadian provinces. Excluded from the target population were those living in the three territories, on Indian reserves and Crown lands, clientele of institutions, the full-time members of the Canadian Forces, and residents of some remote areas. Members of the Canadian Forces were part of a separate survey component conducted parallel to the CCHS 1.2.

Sample Size and Allocation

To satisfy reliability criteria for the key mental disorders for specified subpopulations, a total sample size of 30,000 responding sample units was targeted. To balance the reliability for provincial estimates with the national estimates, the sample of 30,000 units was allocated to the provinces using the root-N approach,[5] with the exception that 1,000 sample units were allocated to the province of Prince Edward Island.

Prior to data collection, the provinces of Ontario and Nova Scotia provided extra funds so that a larger sample of dwellings could be selected. The purpose of these 'buy-ins' was to obtain a sample size that would provide reliable estimates for sub-provincial geographic areas. Ontario added 7702 sample units, and Nova Scotia added 790 units, bringing the total target sample to 38,492.

Table 5.2 gives the details of the targeted and observed sample sizes, as well as observed response rates by province, for the CCHS 1.2.

Sample Frame and Household Sampling

The CCHS 1.2 sample was randomly selected from an area probability frame. As designed for the Labour Force Survey (LFS), this area frame covered almost the entire country, from which a sample of dwellings was selected under a multistage stratified cluster design.[6] For areas selected in the first stage of the design, a list of dwellings was prepared and maintained in the field. At the second stage, a sample of dwellings was then selected from each list. The households in the selected dwellings then formed the sample of households. To get a base sample of 38,492 responding households, approximately 48,000 dwellings were selected from the area frame to account for anticipated vacant dwellings and non-response (15% and 20%, respectively).

Sampling of Persons

To accommodate user needs, cost, efficiency of the design, response burden, and operational constraints, it was decided to select one person per household, but with unequal probability. The selection of the individual was designed to ensure overrepresentation of those aged 15 to 24 years. To improve the representativeness of this age group, the rule for selection was determined as follows: Those aged 15 to 24 years had a probability of $2.6/(2.6 * n + m)$ of being selected, and the others had a probability of $1/(2.6 * n + m)$, where n is the number of those aged 15 to 24 years and m represents the number of persons aged 25 years or over.

Table 5.2
CCHS 1.2 Provincial sample sizes and response rates

Province	Targeted sample n	Response rate %	Observed sample n
NL	1,525	82.3	1,562
PE	1,000	81.7	1,002
NS	2,765	70.1	2,785
NB	1,750	78.1	1,706
QC	5,500	78.1	5,332
ON	14,427	73.4	13,184
MB	2,150	82.4	2,230
SK	2,050	80.1	2,045
AB	3,375	77.1	3,236
BC	3,950	77.7	3,902
Canada	38,492	77.0	36,984

Note: Prior to data collection, the targeted sample sizes were inflated to account for non-response and vacant dwellings. Response rate includes both household and person level response rates.

Interviewer Training and Data Collection

Interviewer Training

CCHS 1.2 respondents were asked to share their thoughts, feelings, and experiences about issues that might be perceived as sensitive and personal. Therefore, special attention was given to collection strategies that would minimize negative public reaction, address privacy concerns, and ensure greater security of information.

The two key elements of the CCHS 1.2 interviewer training and support program were related to sensitivity training and ongoing support for the interviewers. Statistics Canada interviewer training addressed specific requirements that focused on three elements: computer assisted personal interviewing (CAPI) application; survey content; and sensitivity to, and awareness of, mental health issues.

Training on the awareness and sensitivity aspect of the survey was developed by the Centre for Addiction and Mental Health (CAMH) and was integrated into Statistics Canada's training. Through the collaboration of five regional experts in mental health, the CAMH also provided ongoing support for interviewers during the collection period. Sensitivity training was intended to raise interviewer awareness about mental illness and to ensure that interviews were conducted in a sensitive, yet professional, manner. The Canadian Mental Health Association (CMHA) supported Statistics Canada by offering helpful information that included general material on mental health and resources and the identification of local help numbers for anyone asking for immediate help. Statistics Canada also sought the support and advice of the following associations in regard to adequately addressing respondents' needs for information and help: the Canadian Medical Association (CMA), the Canadian Psychiatric Association, the Canadian Psychological Association, the CMHA, and Canadian Alliance on Mental Illness and Mental Health (CAMIMH).

Pilot Test

Because this survey was complex and sensitive, a pilot test was conducted prior to the decision to launch the study. The pilot test objectives were, once again, to measure public reaction, to determine the effectiveness of the training and communication strategies, to test the pacing and timing of the training, to provide a preliminary indication of the response rates, and to test the computer application. To meet these criteria, a sample of 600 households was planned. To avoid any bias, the pilot (carried out in February 2002) was conducted in both English and French throughout the provinces of Quebec and Saskatchewan.

Data Collection

To balance interviewer workload, the initial sample of dwellings was equally and randomly allocated within each region over three collection periods. The first collection period covered three months (Q1 covered May to July 2002), and the other two collection periods covered two months each (Q2 covered August and September 2002; and Q3 covered October and November 2002). More time was allowed for the first collection period, compared with the other two periods, to allow interviewers to become more familiar with the survey. Owing to operational constraints, all the dwellings in a primary sampling unit were assigned to the same collection period. It is also important to mention that data collection continued until the end of December to improve response rates. Final combined provincial response rates (that is, household and person-level rates) ranged from 73.4% in Ontario to 82.4% in Manitoba. The overall combined response rate for Canada was 77.0%.

A computer assisted interviewing (CAI) application was used to administer the CCHS 1.2 questionnaire. This method offers several data quality advantages over other collection methods. With CAI, the interview can be controlled according to the respondent's answers. On-screen prompts are shown when an invalid entry is recorded, and thus, immediate feedback is available. Another enhancement is the automatic insertion of reference periods based on current dates. Pre-filling of text- or data-based information gathered during the interview allows one to proceed without having to search for previous answers. This type of prefill includes such data as correct name or sex within the questions themselves. Allowable ranges or answers based on data collected during interviews can also be programmed. In other words, questionnaires can be customized to respondents according to data collected at that time or during a previous interview. Finally, questions that are not applicable to the respondent are automatically skipped.

Interviewing

The CAPI was used to interview respondents in English and French. In all selected dwellings, a knowledgeable household member was asked to supply basic demographic information for all residents. Depending on the household's composition, one member aged 15 years or over was then selected for a more in-depth interview. CAPI interviewers were trained to make an initial personal contact with each sampled dwelling. When this initial visit resulted in non-response, telephone follow-ups were permitted. Every effort was made to conduct face-to-face interviews. Data collection by telephone was authorized only when travel was prohibitive or the respondent refused to conduct the interview in person. Household contact and respondent selection by telephone were also allowed after an initial in-person contact was attempted unsuccessfully. Ultimately, 14% of the interviews nationally were completed by telephone (with a slightly higher rate in Ontario). No proxy interviews were permitted for this survey. The average length for all interviews was a little less than 70 minutes.

Special Circumstances during CCHS 1.2 Collection

For the CCHS 1.2, the total workload imposed by the lengthy interview, complex content, and difficult respondent burden in some cases was expected to pose a potential challenge for the data collection infrastructure. To ensure successful collection, several strategies were put in place. In addition to customized interviewer training and special support vis-à-vis mental health issues, a monitoring system was created to ensure that data quality was maintained during collection. Various aspects related to the interview process, such as average interview time and item non-response, were monitored at the interviewer level. Regular weekly feedback from the head office to the regional offices helped to maintain good quality data and to correct problems as they occurred. A validation process was also put in place in the field to monitor the quality of the interviewers' work.

The various strategies adopted by Statistics Canada were proven successful. Item non-response was not found to be higher for this study. Share and link rates were also comparable to other health surveys: observed rates were 94.2% and 87.3%, respectively.

Data Computation and Coding

Creation of Derived and Grouped Variables

To facilitate data analysis, several variables on the data files were derived from items found on the CCHS 1.2 questionnaire. In some cases, the derived variables are straightforward, involving collapsing of response categories. In other cases, several variables have been combined to create a new variable.

For the mental disorders and problems, well over 200 derived variables were created. The process of creating, reviewing, and testing the algorithms for these derived variables was complex. In addition to the questionnaire differences between the CCHS 1.2 and the World Mental Health-Composite International Diagnostic Interview (WMH-CIDI), there were also variations in the way the derived variables for each of the WMH disorders were computed, which represents an additional challenge for data comparison.

The differences between the CCHS and the WMH-CIDI were inevitable. Interpreting and employing mental health concepts is challenging in any environment. For this reason, complete survey data as well as interim and final derived variables are available on the data files. The available documentation also provides the specifications for each derived variable created.

While the derived variables for the five selected disorders have been employed to partly meet the *DSM-IV* classification criteria, alcohol and illicit drug dependencies are both coded to partly meet *DSM-III-R* criteria. The algorithms for the selected five disorders were reviewed and tested by the CCHS analysts; by several mental health experts familiar with this subject matter, including the Ontario Mental Health Survey team; and by the WMH 2000 Project team. The CCHS analysts also reviewed the algorithms for the other mental health problems and correlates. Feedback from the authors of specific instruments was also obtained.

Imputation

Owing to some technical problems in certain skip patterns associated with the suicide questions, some respondents were not asked the questions required for the calculation of the derived variables '12-month suicidal thought' and '12-month suicidal attempt.' Consequently, important information is missing for these individuals (about 5% of all respondents for the 12-month suicidal thought and about 1% of all respondents for the 12-month suicidal attempt). Because of their profiles, these individuals are more likely to have had a 12-month suicidal thought or a 12-month suicidal attempt; therefore, the lack of this information will have resulted in an underestimation of the prevalence. To fill in these missing responses, the following approaches were used to impute values. Two methods of imputation were used: a deterministic method and one based on a logistic regression model. For some respondents, it was possible to derive the missing value directly from other responses, and therefore, a deterministic imputation method was first used. This was the case for all missing values for the variable 12-month suicidal attempt and for about one-fourth of the missing values for the variable 12-month suicidal thought. To derive the missing values of the variable 12-month suicidal thought, a logistic regression imputation method was used. To impute the variable 12-month suicidal thought, a logistic regression model was fitted with correlated characteristics drawn from respondents without missing values who were similar to those requiring imputation. From the fitted model, a probability of response (yes or no) was calculated for each respondent who needed imputation; a response based on that probability was then imputed.

Technical Support

As part of its commitment to support data analysis, Statistics Canada provides a complete set of documentation, including a data dictionary and derived variable document, to all Public Use Microdata File users to help explain the survey content and sampling strategy.

Further information about this survey, in addition to summary results, can be found on Statistics Canada's Web site at www.statcan.ca. Survey information is also available from cchs-escc@statcan.ca.

NOTES AND REFERENCES

This chapter was originally published in the *Canadian Journal of Psychiatry*, as part of a special edition (edited by the editors of this collection) showcasing recent research conducted using the Canadian Community Health Survey 1.2, Canada's first national prevalence study of several major psychiatric disorders. Given the centrality of this survey to current research in psychiatric epidemiology in this country; the important role that secondary data sources, especially those collected by Statistics Canada, has played in the development of the discipline; and the fact that several of the chapters in this collection use data derived from this survey, we felt it important to have a chapter devoted to describing this history and methods used in the CCHS 1.2. Readers of the original article may note that the last section, dealing with an earlier survey, has been omitted, as it is not relevant to the results presented in this book. With the kind permission of the journal, we have re-printed the article here.

We thank Jennifer Ali and Marc Hamel from the Health Statistics Division at Statistics Canada for their useful comments.

1 Gravel R, Connolly D, Bédard M. *Canadian Community Health Survey: Mental Health and Well-Being.* Catalogue 82-617-XIE. www.statcan.ca/english/freepub/82-617-XIE/. Accessed Jul 7, 2005.
2 Canadian Institute for Health Information. *Health Information Roadmap:*

Beginning the Journey. Canadian Institute for Health Information, 1999. http://secure.cihi.ca/cihiweb/en/downloads/profile_roadmap_e_eng-beg.pdf. Accessed Jul 26, 2005.

3 Béland Y, Bailie L, Catlin G, et al. CCHS and NPHS. An improved health survey program at Statistics Canada. *Proceedings of the Survey Methods Section*. American Statistical Association, 2000. www.amstat.org/sections/srms/Proceedings/y2000f.html. Accessed Jul 26, 2005.

4 *CCHS 1.2 User Guide in English*. http://data.library.ubc.ca/datalib/survey/statscan/cchs/cycle1.2/guide _e.pdf. Accessed Jul 7, 2005.

5 Bankier M. Power allocations: Determining sample sizes for subnational areas. *Am Stat* 1988;42:174–7.

6 Statistics Canada. *Methodology of the Canadian Labour Force Survey*. Ottawa: Statistics Canada, 1998. Catalogue nr. 71-526-XPB.

7 Starkes JM, Poulin C, Kisely SR. Unmet need for the treatment of depression in Atlantic Canada. *Can J Psychiatry* 2005;50:580–90.

PART THREE

Epidemiology of Disorders

6 Affective Disorders in Canada

SCOTT B. PATTEN

From the perspective of public health, affective disorders are among the most important health conditions. Their importance derives from a combination of two factors: high prevalence and their considerable impact on psychosocial functioning and mortality. For many years, the full significance of these disorders was under-appreciated. This changed with publication of the first (1990) Global Burden of Disease report, which ranked Unipolar Major Depressive Disorder as the fourth leading cause of disease burden and as the world's leading single cause of disability.[1] The Global Burden of Disease report projected that the relative burden of major depression would increase in subsequent decades. These findings were reinforced by the 2000 iteration of the Global Burden of Disease project.[2]

The terms 'affective disorder' and 'mood disorder' describe a group of mental disorders in which disturbances in mood and affect are predominant features. In the fourth edition of the American Psychiatric Association's *Diagnostic and Statistical Manual of Mental Disorders* (*DSM-IV*),[3] these disorders are assembled in a 'Mood Disorders' chapter. In the tenth edition of the *International Classification of Disease* (ICD-10), the term 'affective disorder' continues to be used synonymously with the term 'mood disorder.'[4]

Depression is the most common form of affective disturbance, but not all instances of depression represent a depressive disorder. In order to be considered a mental disorder, certain general characteristics should be present. In *DSM-IV*, mood disorder definitions align with a set of general requirements for the diagnosis of a mental disorder: there must be a clinically significant behavioural or psychological syndrome or pattern that must be associated either with present distress or disability or with a significantly increased risk of suffering death, pain, disability, or an important loss of freedom. The diagnostic criteria in *DSM-IV* and ICD-10 are designed to assist with the distinction between normal and abnormal affective changes. This is accomplished by the application of some criteria that are symptom based, and other criteria that refer either to the duration, presumed etiology, or clinical significance of the symptoms.

Bereavement is an example of an attempt in *DSM-IV* to differentiate affective disorders from normal emotional reactions. Bereavement is not considered a disorder (although a *DSM-IV* diagnostic code is available for bereavement as a condition not attributable to a mental disorder). Similarly, mild and self-limited reactions to stressful events are excluded by the diagnostic criteria. Such reactions may be diagnosed as adjustment disorders if they are associated with marked distress or significant dysfunction. The main categories of mood disorder in *DSM-IV* are: major depressive disorder, bipolar I disorder, bipolar II disorder, cyclothymia, and dysthymia. Depressive disorders with an identifiable organic etiology and substance-induced disorders or mood disorders due to a general medical condition are also contained in the mood disorder chapter in *DSM-IV*. In order to diagnose a disorder as being due to a general medical condition, it is necessary for there to be evidence from the history, physical examination, or laboratory findings that the disturbance is the direct physiological consequence of the general medical condition.[3]

By far the most studied category of mood disorder in Canada is major depression. Some prevalence data for bipolar disorder are also available, but the distinction between bipolar I and bipolar II has been difficult to address in epidemiological studies. Very limited information about dysthymia is available, and cyclothymia has not been studied at all. The two 'organic' categories may be conceptually flawed, and reliable epidemiological data about these two conditions are not available.

The ICD-10 classification is similar in many respects to that of *DSM-IV*, but does not exactly coincide. ICD-10 contains codes for depressive, manic, hypomanic, and mixed episodes, which contribute to definitions for recurrent depressive disorder and bipolar affective disorder. Cyclothymia and dysthymia are also present in the classification. ICD-10 includes one category, recurrent brief depressive disorder, which does not appear in *DSM-IV*. This condition is characterized by depressive episodes lasting less than two weeks, and which occur about once per month. There are no epidemiological data about recurrent brief depressive disorder in Canada.

Depressive disorders are associated with elevated risk of suicide. Suicide accounts for 1.7% of deaths in Canada, and a cause-specific mortality rate of 12 per 100,000.[†] Furthermore, major depression is a predictor of mortality after myocardial infarction[5] and in type 2 diabetes.[6]

The Stirling County Study under the leadership of Alexander Leighton and Jane Murphy was a pioneering investigation that in some ways set the stage for subsequent psychiatric epidemiological studies around the world. This project has been associated with Dohrenwend's 'second generation' of epidemiological studies,[7] but can also be regarded as a precursor of the 'third generation' – those based on *DSM-III* or later diagnostic criteria[8] because it pioneered case ascertainment methods based on largely non-theoretical diagnostic criteria. Several developments led to an acceleration of epidemiological research in the 1980s and 1990s. These included the emergence of *DSM-III* in 1980 as an empirical diagnostic system, and the associated development of structured diagnostic interviews that could be administered by trained non-clinician interviewers, making epidemiological research much more feasible. Studies published in this period confirmed the high prevalence of mood disorders in community populations and pointed towards considerable under-utilization of treatment.[e.g. see 9,10] This era coincided with an expansion of therapeutic options for treatment, most prominently the emergence of specific serotonin re-uptake inhibiting antidepressants, alternatives to lithium for bipolar disorder, and the publication of randomized controlled trials confirming the effectiveness of cognitive and interpersonal therapies for major depression.

Beyond prevalence, unmet need, and clinical effectiveness, some additional questions have begun to emerge during the past decade. There has been a rapid expansion of treatment for mood disorders. Antidepressant medications are now among the most frequently prescribed of all medications. According to the 2002 Canadian Community Health Survey 1.2 (Mental Health and Well-Being), 4.7% of the

---

[†]   Source: Statistics Canada, Health Statistics Division. Selected leading causes of death, by sex. Age-standardized mortality rate per 100,000 population. http://www40.statcan.ca/l01/cst01/health36.htm.

population 15 years of age or older took an antidepressant in the two days preceding their interview.[11] One Alberta-based telephone survey reported a 7.2% frequency.[12] A Canadian longitudinal study, the National Population Health Survey (NPHS), provides an opportunity to evaluate changes in the frequency of use over time. The NPHS interview included a short form version of the Composite International Diagnostic Interview for major depression (CIDI-SFMD).[13] In 1994, fewer than 15% of subjects with a major depressive episode in the preceding year were taking an antidepressant at the time of the interview, but this had doubled by 2000.[14] The increased use of antidepressant medications has also been observed in prescription monitoring systems, making the trend unlikely to be just an artifact of self-reporting or recall bias, inherent to community-based surveys.[15]

As antidepressants shorten the duration of major depressive episodes, and protect against recurrence, one might expect that increased treatment would lead to a diminished burden of mood disorder morbidity in the population.[16] There is, unfortunately, no solid evidence that this has occurred. It is possible that positive effects of treatment have been offset by increased incidence, or changing prognosis. It is also possible that antidepressant treatments are less effective in 'real world' clinical practice than in clinical trials. It has been suggested that services need to be realigned away from an emphasis on acute treatment and towards a chronic disease orientation if the benefits of treatment are to be more fully realized.[17,19]

Psychiatric epidemiology is a discipline in evolution, and a simple recounting of published prevalence estimates can no longer provide an adequate summary of the available data. In 1983, Spitzer wondered whether the development of structured diagnostic interviews might some day make clinicians unnecessary.[19] Two decades later, the basic validity of such instruments is being challenged [20] and debated.[21,22] The diagnostic boundaries of the mood disorders themselves are topics of debate.[23,24] It has been shown using data from American surveys that sizable differences in prevalence estimates can arise due to relatively minor differences in the treatment of items assessing clinical significance in structured interviews.[25] Clinical significance items include help-seeking behaviours and interference with life activities. The importance and subtlety of such considerations serves as a reminder that assessment of mood disorders in epidemiological research remains a challenging task.

In the following sections, a brief review of Canadian epidemiological data about affective disorder epidemiology is presented. An effort will be made to understand the results of earlier studies in light of more recent findings, keeping in mind results from the international literature, and also various unresolved methodological and nosological concerns.

Major Depression

The Stirling County Study (see also chapters 1 and 2) is sometimes omitted from discussions of major depression epidemiology because the diagnostic interview employed (called DPAX-1 and DPAX-2) in the project predated and was not designed to accommodate *DSM-III* or *DSM-IV* classification. The 1992 sample was administered the Diagnostic Interview Schedule (DIS), a structured diagnostic interview that was used in the American Epidemiological Catchment Area (ECA) studies, and also by Bland et al. in a landmark survey conducted in Edmonton (discussed later). The Stirling County Study is unique in providing a long-term view of depressive disorder epidemiology. This study did not identify any change in the point prevalence of depression over time, but did identify a change in the use of terminology for describing dysphoria, with the phrase 'low spirits' being less frequently endorsed in more recent years.[26]

Major depression data from a study by Bland et al., which has come to be known as the 'Edmonton Study,' was reported in detail by Spaner, Bland, and Newman in 1994.[27] The lifetime prevalence of major depression was 8.6%, which was higher than that reported by the methodologically similar ECA studies in the United States, raising the possibility of a prevalence difference between the two countries. An opportunity to confirm the apparently higher prevalence of major depression in Canada arose with conduct of a subsequent study: the Mental Health Supplement of the Ontario Health Survey.[28] This study used a different diagnostic instrument, the Composite International Diagnostic Interview (CIDI). The CIDI is related to the DIS, and was intended to provide a more portable international alternative to it.[29] While it maintained the fully structured format of the DIS, the CIDI was capable of supporting ICD as well as *DSM* (now *DSM-IIIR* rather than *DSM-III*) diagnoses. The Ontario study used one of several versions of the CIDI; one that was developed at the University of Michigan (called the UM-CIDI). This is the same version that was used in the first National Comorbidity Survey (NCS) in the United States.[30] It produced *DSM-IIIR* rather than *DSM-III* diagnoses. The UM-CIDI included a modification that involved the movement of screening questions for entry into detailed assessment modules to a screening section at the start of the interview. The intention was that respondents could not learn to avoid questions by providing negative answers to screening items. This, combined with a different treatment of clinical significance items,[25] apparently contributed to a dramatically higher set of prevalence estimates in the NCS than had been reported by the ECA studies. However, the Ontario annual major depression prevalence estimate (4.1%) resembled that of the Edmonton study (4.6%), but was considerably lower than that of the NCS (10.3%).

The considerable variation between these early major depression prevalence estimates confirmed that psychiatric epidemiological results were not as replicable as had been previously assumed, or hoped. Changes to the ordering of interview items, or the algorithms used to score the interviews, could apparently lead to significant changes in prevalence estimates. While these observations subsequently encouraged efforts to refine diagnostic instruments such as the CIDI (using for example, cognitive interviewing techniques),[22] they also illustrated certain practical realities. All in all, it seems best to consider structured diagnostic interviews as being a somewhat crude type of diagnostic measure. Some confirmatory evidence of this was reported in a follow-up to the Edmonton study. In this follow-up, the DIS was used to evaluate (among other things) incidence, but subjects who were eligible for the denominator of the incidence calculation (i.e., no episode preceding an initial interview) sometimes reported an episode at their second interview in which the onset date preceded the first interview.[31]

In the United Kingdom, psychiatric epidemiologists have tended to view clinical judgment as being the missing ingredient accounting for the apparent limitations of fully structured interviews such as the DIS and CIDI. In the United Kingdom, the use of semi-structured interviews such as the SCAN[32] has often been favoured over the fully-structured approach to assessment. Aside from the expense of this approach (semi-structured interviews must generally be administered by a trained clinician), there are some other difficulties with this solution. One of the most basic tenets of epidemiological research is that the determinants of disease can be elucidated by studying their distributions in populations. Ideally, epidemiological estimates can bring empirical support to clinical and public health decisions and judgments. There is an obvious danger, then, in allowing the epidemiological estimates themselves to be determined by judgments made by clinicians.[33]

The first national estimates of major depression prevalence for Canada derive from the CCHS 1.2, which was conducted in 2002 by Statistics Canada. This study used the latest version of the CIDI (the World Mental Health 2000 CIDI, or WMH-CIDI).[34] The pattern of prevalence was the expected one, with a 4.8% annual prevalence and 1.8% 30-day prevalence.[35] These estimates, interestingly, are quite consistent with earlier ones from Edmonton and Ontario. Prevalence was higher in women and declined with age in most demographic groups. Of respondents with past-year major depression, 40.4% reported taking an antidepressant at the time of the survey.[36]

While prevalence, typically period prevalence, has been the focus of most Canadian studies, incidence is another parameter of interest. Prevalence can be regarded as a steady state outcome of incidence and prognosis, being approximately equivalent to the product of incidence and duration. Duration, in turn, is influenced by recovery and mortality. Experience with the use of structured interviews organized around the concept of lifetime prevalence does not appear to be a promising strategy for studying incidence, although this was attempted as a part of the ECA.[37] The European NEMESIS study has used more detailed life history methods to identify longitudinal patterns over a three-interview survey cycle.[38] In Canada, the only ongoing source of longitudinal data is the NPHS, which included only a brief measure of major depression – the CIDI Short Form.[13]

The NPHS has carried out interviews every two years on a cohort initially consisting of a representative sample of 17,262 household residents. The NPHS also collects episode duration data using an item that asks about weeks spent in the depressed state during the past year. The frequency with which subjects who are disease-free at one cycle and then have a major depressive episode at the next cycle were combined with the episode duration data to produce a Markov model predicting incidence and recovery probability estimates.[39] The estimated episode incidence from the NPHS was 3.1%, coinciding with a pooled analysis by Waraich et al.[40] The most interesting result of these modelling studies was confirmation of a finding originally described by Keller et al.[41] that the recovery rate declines with increasing episode duration. The same result was presented in another way by a modelling project using NEMESIS and Australian data, which depicted the recovery pattern using a lognormal distribution.[18,42] The pattern suggests that many depressive episodes in the community are short lived, resolving within a few weeks, whereas those that persist longer have a diminishing probability of recovery over time. The NPHS model placed the mean duration of episodes at 17 weeks, consistent with the four-month figure presented in the text of *DSM-IV*,[3] yet it also shows that the mean duration is misleading if it is interpreted as a typical or characteristic duration. Most episodes are much shorter than this, and a smaller proportion of episodes are much longer. Here, the median may be a better indicator of central tendency. According to the NPHS data, the median duration of episodes is between six and seven weeks.[43]

Major depression has a seasonal subtype wherein seasonal episodes substantially outnumber non-seasonal episodes.[3] The prevalence of seasonal major depressive episode was assessed in a Toronto telephone survey that used a non-standard structured diagnostic interview, the Depression and Seasonality Interview – Toronto version,[44] to identify seasonal disorders. The criteria used were not exactly consistent with the *DSM-IV* criteria; the study required that non-seasonal episodes be 'rare' rather than that they be substantially outnumbered by seasonal episodes. By this standard, 11% of major depression was found to be of the seasonal type,[44] the overall lifetime prevalence of this subtype being 2.9%.

It has been hypothesized that major depression may have a higher prevalence in urban as opposed to rural areas. This question was addressed by Kovess et al. in Quebec, using a diagnostic algorithm for major depression that was derived from a symptom rating scale. Higher prevalence in an urban area was observed, and the difference persisted after adjustment for a variety of covariates.[45] The differences were related predominantly to unemployment, which was more strongly associated with depression in urban men, and to marital status (lack of a current partner), which was more strongly associated with depression in urban women. A county administrative centre in the predominantly rural area had a prevalence that more closely resembled that of rural subjects.

Parikh et al. used population density to differentiate between urban and rural residence using data from the Mental Health Supplement of the Ontario Health Survey. A non-significant difference in major depression prevalence – 4.2% urban versus 3.2% rural – was reported.[46] A non-significant difference was also reported by Wang, using data from the National Population Health Survey. However, after adjustment for potential confounders, a significant difference emerged in this analysis.[47] Wang reported that there were two factors associated with a higher prevalence of major depression that were more common in an urban setting: unemployment and divorced, widowed, or separated marital status. However, two factors associated with a lower prevalence – being an immigrant and being in a 'non-white' racial category – were also more frequent in the urban residents. In a logistic regression model, the latter effects predominated and the adjusted odds ratio for rural residence was 0.80. Small differences were also observed in a comparison of an urban health region in Alberta to a neighbouring predominantly rural health region[48] and by D'Arcy et al. in the Saskatchewan Health and Dynamics Survey.[49] As this literature accumulates, it appears increasingly likely that the negative results are due to type II error and that the prevalence of major depression is slightly higher in urban than in rural Canada.

Another question of interest to Canada is the possibility that prevalence may differ depending on language. An analysis of CCHS 1.2 data for subjects 55+ years old by Streiner et al. found a higher major depression prevalence in francophone subjects than anglophone subjects.[50] A higher francophone prevalence was also reported by Cairney and Krause in an analysis of 55+ year old respondents in the 1994 NPHS data.[51]

According to the CCHS 1.2, annual prevalence of major depression declines with age in Canada.[35,50] This corroborates a report based on CCHS 1.1 by Afifi et al.,[52] and with data reported by Wade and Cairney[53] from the first wave of the NPHS, where age differences were also investigated. Notably, a higher prevalence in women was evident in the Afifi et al. study, which examined the 12-to-19-year-old age group. This indicates that the sex difference in major depression prevalence becomes established early in life. Longitudinal analyses by Wade, Cairney, and Pevalin used data collected in three different countries and found that the sex difference becomes established by age fourteen.[54] The result was consistent across a variety of different measures of depression, including both dimensional and categorical ones.

Risk factors for major depression are difficult to study since many factors that may contribute to the etiology of depression may also be a result of depression. This reality was illustrated by Wade and Cairney's analysis of marital status transitions using longitudinal data from the NPHS. Whereas most prior literature had focused on the possibility that marital status transitions (e.g., from married to separated or divorced status) may cause depression, this analysis found that women (with children) who were depressed in the initial NPHS cycle were more likely to subsequently have a marital status transition.[55] Beaudet used longitudinal data from the National Population Health Survey to identify predictors of major depression, finding significant associations, after adjustment in a multiple regression model, for age, being in school (men only), being a smoker, having a chronic medical condition (women only in this analysis), low social support (women only), and having low levels of psychological resources (women only).[56] The effect of chronic medical conditions may be related both to an effect on incidence and recurrence,[57] and seems strongest for conditions associated with pain.[58] An association of childhood traumas with adult major depression prevalence has been reported both by De Marco[59] using Ontario data, and by Arboleda-Flórez and Wade[60] using the NPHS. MacMillan et al. found that this association may be stronger in women than in men.[61] Stressful life events have been found to be strongly associated with major depression prevalence in cross-sectional Canadian studies.[48,59,62–64]

Dysthymia

Dysthymic disorder is a chronic form of depression. By definition, the symptoms must last at least two years, and there must be no major depressive episodes during the first two years of the disturbance. The disturbance tends to be a persistent one, and *DSM-IV* specifies that during the two year period required for the diagnosis, there should be no period lasting longer than two months when the person is free of depressive symptoms. In Canada, dysthymia has been far less extensively studied than major depression, but several prevalence estimates are available. As noted, the third sample of the Stirling County Study was administered the DIS. This resulted in a 1992 estimate of dysthymia (without major depression) prevalence of 2.9%.[26] The estimate is not far from the lifetime prevalence reported by the Edmonton study, at 3.7%,[65] but both estimates differ from the 0.8% reported by the Ontario survey.[28] The Alberta Mental Health Survey was a province-wide telephone survey that included an abbreviated diagnostic interview with a dysthymia module, the Mini

Neuropsychiatric Interview (MINI). The MINI was administered to a sample of 5383 subjects in 2003, and a prevalence of 1.2% was found for dysthymia.[66]

Bipolar Disorder

The assessment of bipolar disorder in population surveys has been problematic. In the Edmonton survey, the lifetime prevalence of manic episodes was 0.6%[67] and the one-year prevalence in the Ontario study[28] and Edmonton study[67] was 0.6%. The WMH-CIDI used in the CCHS 1.2 included a module for manic episode, but this was not entirely consistent with the *DSM-IV* definition. One important difference was the duration requirement: whereas *DSM-IV* requires a symptom duration of one week (in the absence of need for hospitalization),[3] the WMH-CIDI requires only 'several days' of symptoms. As such, the interview probably detects a mixture of manic and hypomanic episodes, possibly also with the detection of some mixed episodes. The net effect on the estimates of prevalence is unknown, but the lifetime prevalence of bipolar disorder in the CCHS 1.2 was 2.6% of subjects aged 25 to 64.[68] A revised prevalence estimate is offered by Schaffer et al.[69] Like the earlier analysis, these investigators used data from the CCHS 1.2. However, in this study, exclusion criteria for organic etiology were incorporated into the diagnostic algorithms, resulting in an estimated lifetime prevalence of 2.2%. Both of these estimates are higher than the traditionally accepted rate of approximately 1%.[40] However, they are in line with recent international trends toward expansion of the bipolar disorder category. For example, the National Comorbidity Survey Replication in the United States found a 0.6% prevalence for bipolar I disorder, but reported an overall prevalence of 'any bipolar disorder' of 4.4% by adding bipolar II and subthreshold cases.[70] No data concerning the incidence of bipolar disorder have been collected in Canada.

The frequency of seasonal bipolar disorders was assessed in one Ontario telephone survey.[71] The sample consisted of 1605 respondents, 63 (3.9%) of whom were identified as having bipolar disorder by a structured diagnostic interview. Fourteen of these 62 subjects had a seasonal pattern, which was too small a number to support detailed analyses. However, it was reported that the subjects with a seasonal pattern were more likely to have bipolar I than bipolar II disorder.

'Organic' Mood Disorders

Generally, the philosophy of *DSM-IV* is empirical, and the manual attempts to avoid the inclusion of etiological or theory-driven judgments in its sets of diagnostic criteria, at least to the extent that this is practically possible. The categories concerned with organic mood disorders represent a departure from this philosophy, since they depend almost entirely on clinical judgments about etiology. *DSM-IV* has two relevant categories: substance induced mood disorder and mood disorder due to a general medical condition. To make a diagnosis of substance induced mood disorder, *DSM-IV* requires evidence from the history, physical examination, or laboratory findings that a severe disturbance of mood (which can follow either a depressed, manic, or mixed pattern) developed during or within a month of substance intoxication or withdrawal, or that medication use was etiologically related to the disturbance.[3] These categories are problematic because the pathophysiology of mood disturbance is not well understood, so it is not clear that such judgments can be reliably made, let alone how they could be based on evidence from the history, physical examination, or laboratory findings. The intention is apparently to support the formulation of a differential diagnosis that includes organic etiologies.

As already noted, disease definitions that make explicit reference to etiology subvert some of the basic tenants of epidemiology as an empirical science.[33] Some practical issues also emerge in the application of such definitions in epidemiological research. If clinical judgment is relied upon, by incorporating an instrument such as the SCAN, then the data collected will represent clinical opinion and will not necessarily be able to challenge or add to the existing state of knowledge. On the other hand, the problems are no less acute when fully structured interviews are used. The WMH-CIDI that was used in the CCHS 1.2, for example, asks subjects whether they thought that their symptoms were always due to an organic cause, essentially sampling their opinions about etiology. Previous versions of the CIDI asked whether a health professional had made such an attribution.[72] The ways in which the responses to such items are incorporated into diagnostic algorithms are often not clarified in epidemiological reports. In the CCHS, approximately 12% of subjects with major depression attributed the etiology of their symptoms 'always' to physical causes. However, many of these could not be regarded as etiologically meaningful attributions; e.g., 'chemical imbalance' or 'exhaustion.' It has generally remained unclear how such responses have been dealt with in studies that report taking them 'into account.'[e.g.73]

The various categories of organic depression appear to be conceptually flawed. There is only one Canadian study that examined associations between medications and the major depressive syndrome (without etiologic exclusions) in a population sample.[74] This study found an association between major depression and corticosteroid use, but did not find convincing evidence of other associations. The association of corticosteroids with major depression is consistent with an existing literature of clinical studies.[75]

Conclusions

Canada has a long tradition of psychiatric epidemiological research. With the release of the CCHS 1.2, there are now solid national estimates for the prevalence of a set of specific mental disorders, including major depression. For this condition, the prevalence figures have been quite consistent across different studies – almost all annual prevalence estimates falling within the 4%–5% range. For dysthymia and bipolar disorder there is considerably less consistency and very little is known about the remaining affective disorder categories.

Typically, the maturation of an epidemiological literature involves a progression from basic descriptive work towards analytically oriented studies that can guide clinical and public health action. This progression can be seen in the literature about affective disorders, most notably major depression, in Canada. Gradually, there has been a shift in emphasis from the description of the frequency of disorders in the population to efforts to use epidemiological data to identify unmet needs in the population. This transition has stimulated efforts to increase access to services and diminish stigma associated with mental disorders. Several paradoxes have emerged in the course of this transition. One of these is the apparently high frequency of antidepressant use (approximately 5%–7% of the general population) combined with low proportions of those with disorders receiving treatment (less than 50%). Another paradox is that an apparently large increase in treatment has not been accompanied by evidence of reduced prevalence.

The low proportion of people with past-year episodes who are receiving treatment is at least partially a methodological artifact resulting from simplistic methods of estimating this parameter.[76] It is probably also partially due to the rapid resolution of some major depressive episodes. A related factor has been a growing awareness that *DSM*-based diagnoses are not as effective as proxies for clinical need as may have previously been assumed.[77]

The failure of prevalence to decline with increasing treatment coverage, however, remains unexplained. This would appear to be a critical issue since the ultimate goal of epidemiologic research is to improve population health. Much work concerning the epidemiology of affective disorders remains to be done.

REFERENCES

1 Murray CJL, Lopez AC. *Global Burden of Disease and Injury*. Boston: Harvard School of Public Health, 1996.
2 Ayuso-Mateos JL. *Global Burden of Unipolar Depressive Disorders in the Year 2000*. Report No.: Global Burden of Disease Draft 28-05-03. World Health Organization Global Program on Evidence for Health Policy (GPE), 2003.
3 American Psychiatric Association. *Diagnostic and Statistical Manual of Mental Disorders (DSM-IV-TR)*. Washington: American Psychiatric Association, 2000.
4 World Health Organization. *ICD-10 Classification of Mental and Behavioural Disorders, with Glossary and Diagnostic Criteria for Research*. Edinburgh: Churchill Livingstone, 1994.
5 Lesperance F, Frasure-Smith N, Talajic M. Major depression before and after myocardial infarction: Its nature and consequences. *Psychosom Med* 1996;58:99–110.
6 Katon WJ, Rutter C, Simon G, et al. The association of comorbid depression with mortality in patients with type 2 diabetes. *Diabetes Care* 2005;28:2668–72.
7 Dohrenwend BP, Dohrenwend BS. Perspectives on the past and future of psychiatric epidemiology. The 1981 Rema Lapouse Lecture. *Am J Publ Hlth* 1982;72:1271–9.
8 Dohrenwend BP. A psychosocial perspective on the past and future of psychiatric epidemiology. *Am J Epidemiol* 1998;147:222–31.
9 Bland RC, Newman SC, Orn H. Help-seeking for psychiatric disorders. *Can J Psychiatry* 1997;42:935–42.
10 Galbaud du Fort G, Newman SC, Boothroyd LJ, et al. Treatment seeking for depression: Role of depressive symptoms and comorbid psychiatric diagnoses. *J Affect Disord* 1999;52:31–40.

11 Beck CA, Williams JVA, Wang JL, et al. Psychotropic medication use in Canada. *Can J Psychiatry* 2005;50:605–13.

12 Patten SB, Williams JVA, Wang JL, et al. Antidepressant pharmacoepidemiology in a general population sample. *J Clin Psychopharmacol* 2005;25:285–6.

13 Kessler RC, Andrews G, Mroczek D, et al. The World Health Organization Composite International Diagnostic Interview Short-Form (CIDI-SF). *Int J Methods Psychiatr Res* 1998;7:171–85.

14 Patten SB, Beck CA. Major depression and mental health care utilization in Canada: 1994–2000. *Can J Psychiatry* 2004;49:303–9.

15 Hemels MEH, Koren G, Einarson TR. Increased use of antidepressants in Canada: 1981–2000. *Ann Pharmacother* 2002;36:1375–9.

16 Katon W, Von Korff M, Lin E, et al. Population-based care of depression: Effective disease management strategies to decrease prevalence. *Gen Hosp Psychiatry* 1997;19:169–78.

17 Andrews G. Should depression be managed as a chronic disease? *Br Med J* 2001;332:419–21.

18 Vos T, Haby MM, Berendregt JJ, et al. The burden of major depression avoidable by longer-term treatment strategies. *Arch Gen Psychiatry* 2004;61:1097–103.

19 Spitzer RL. Psychiatric diagnosis: Are clinicians still necessary? *Comp Psychiatry* 1983;24:399–411.

20 Brugha TS, Jenkins R, Taub N, et al. A general population comparison of the Composite International Diagnostic Interview (CIDI) and the Schedules for Clinical Assessment in Neuropsychiatry (SCAN). *Psychol Med* 2001;31:1001–13.

21 Brugha TS, Bebbington PE, Jenkins R. A difference that matters: Comparisons of structured and semi-structured psychiatric diagnostic interviews in the general populations. *Psychol Med* 1999;29:1013–20.

22 Wittchen H-U, Ustun TB, Kessler RC. Diagnosing mental disorders in the community. A difference that matters? *Psychol Med* 1999;29:1021–7.

23 Akiskal HS, Bourgeois ML, Angst J, et al. Re-evaluating the prevalence of and diagnostic composition within the broad clinical spectrum of bipolar disorders. *J Affect Disord* 2000;59(suppl): S5–S30.

24 Baldessarini RJ. A plea for integrity of the bipolar disorder concept. *Bipolar Disord* 2000;2:3–7.

25 Narrow WE, Rae DS, Robins LN, et al. Revised prevalence estimates of mental disorders in the United States: Using a clinical significance criterion to reconcile 2 surveys' estimates. *Arch Gen Psychiatry* 2002;59:115–23.

26 Murphy JM, Laird NM, Monson RR, et al. A 40-year perspective on the prevalence of depression. *Arch Gen Psychiatry* 2000;57:209–15.

27 Spaner D, Bland RC, Newman SC. Major depressive disorder. *Acta Psychiatr Scand* 1994;376(suppl):7–15.

28 Offord DR, Boyle MH, Campbell D, et al. One year prevalence of psychiatric disorder in Ontarians 15 to 64 years of age. *Can J Psychiatry* 1996;41:559–63.

29 Robins LN, Wing J, Wittchen H-U, et al. The Composite International Diagnostic Interview. An epidemiological instrument suitable for use in conjunction with different diagnostic systems and in different cultures. *Arch Gen Psychiatry* 1988;45:1069–77.

30 Blazer DG, Kessler RC, McGonagle KA, et al. The prevalence and distribution of major depression in a national community sample: The National Comorbidity Survey. *Am J Psychiatry* 1994;151:979–86.

31 Newman SC, Bland RC. Incidence of mental disorders in Edmonton: Estimates of rates and methodological issues. *J Psychiatr Res* 1998;32:273–82.

32 Wing JK, Babor T, Brugha T, et al. SCAN. Schedules for Clinical Assessment in Neuropsychiatry. *Arch Gen Psychiatry* 1990;47:589–93.

33 Rothman KJ. Epidemiology in clinical settings. In *Epidemiology. An Introduction*. Oxford: Oxford University Press, 2002: 198–217.

34 Kessler RC, Ustun TB. The World Mental Health (WMH) Survey Initiative Version of the World Health Organization (WHO) Composite International Diagnostic Interview (CIDI). *Int J Methods Psychiatr Res* 2004;13:83–121.

35 Patten SB, Wang JL, Williams JVA, et al. Descriptive epidemiology of major depression in Canada. *Can J Psychiatry* 2006;51:84–90.

36 Beck CA, Patten SB, Williams JVA, et al. Antidepressant utilization in Canada. *Soc Psychiatry Psychiatr Epidemiol* 2005;40:799–807.

37 Bruce ML, Takeuchi DT, Leaf PJ. Poverty and psychiatric status. Longitudinal evidence from the New Haven Epidemiological Catchment Area Study. *Arch Gen Psychiatry* 1991;48:470–4.

38 Bijl RV, van Zessen G, Ravelli A, et al. The Netherlands Mental Health Survey and Incidence Study (NEMESIS): Objectives and design. *Soc Psychiatry Psychiatr Epidemiol* 1998;33:581–6.

39 Patten SB, Lee RC. Refining estimates of major depression incidence and episode duration in Canada using a Monte Carlo Markov model. *Med Decis Making* 2004;24:351–8.

40 Waraich PS, Goldner EM, Somers JM, et al. Prevalence and incidence studies of mood disorders: A systematic review of the literature. *Can J Psychiatry* 2004;49:124–38.

41 Keller MB, Lavori PW, Mueller TI, et al. Time to recovery, chronicity, and
    levels of psychopathology in major depression. A 5-year prospective
    follow-up of 431 subjects. *Arch Gen Psychiatry* 1992;49:809–16.
42 Kruijshaar ME, Barendregt J, Vos T, et al. Lifetime prevalence estimates of
    major depression: An indirect estimation method and a quantification of
    recall bias. *Eur J Epidemiol* 2005;20:103–11.
43 Patten SB. A major depression prognosis calculator based on episode
    duration. *Clin Pract Epidemiol Mental Hlth* 2006;2:13.
44 Levitt AJ, Boyle MH, Joffe RT, et al. Estimated prevalence of the seasonal
    subtype of major depression in a Canadian community sample. *Can J
    Psychiatry* 2000;45:650–4.
45 Kovess V, Murphy HBM, Tousignant M. Urban-rural comparisons of
    depressive disorders in French Canada. *J Nerv Ment Dis* 1987;175:457–65.
46 Parikh SV, Wasylenki D, Goering P, et al. Mood disorders: Rural/urban
    differences in prevalence, health care utilization, and disability in
    Ontario. *J Affect Disord* 1996;38:57–65.
47 Wang JL. Rural-urban differences in the prevalence of major depression
    and associated impairment. *Soc Psychiatry Psychiatr Epidemiol*
    2004;39:19–25.
48 Patten SB, Stuart HL, Russell ML, et al. Epidemiology of depression in a
    predominantly rural health region. *Soc Psychiatry Psychiatr Epidemiol*
    2003;38:360–5.
49 D'Arcy C, Kosteniuk J, Smith P, et al. Depression in Saskatchewan: An
    analysis of the Saskatchewan Population Health and Dynamics Survey
    1999–2000. *Applied Research/Psychiatry,* 2004.
50 Streiner DL, Cairney J, Veldhuizen S. The epidemiology of psychological
    problems in the elderly. *Can J Psychiatry* 2006;52:185–91.
51 Cairney J, Krause N. The social distribution of psychological distress and
    depression in older adults. *J Aging Health* 2005;17:807–35.
52 Afifi T, Enns MW, Cox BJ, et al. Investigating health correlates of adoles-
    cent depression in Canada. *Can J Pub Health* 2005;96:427–31.
53 Wade TJ, Cairney J. Age and depression in a nationally representative
    sample of Canadians: A preliminary look at the National Population
    Health Survey. *Can J Pub Health* 1997;88:297–302.
54 Wade DT, Cairney J, Pevalin DJ. Emergence of gender differences in
    depression during adolescence: National panel results from three coun-
    tries. *J Am Acad Child Adolesc Psychiatry* 2002;41:190–8.
55 Wade TJ, Cairney J. Major depressive disorder and marital transition
    among mothers: Results from a national panel study. *J Nerv Ment Dis*
    2000;188:741–50.

56 Beaudet MP. Psychological health – depression. *Health Rep* 1999;11: 63–75.
57 Patten SB. An analysis of data from two general health surveys found that increased incidence and duration contributed to elevated prevalence of major depression in persons with chronic medical conditions. *J Clin Epidemiol* 2005;58:184–9.
58 Patten SB, Beck CA, Kassam A, et al. Long-term medical conditions and major depression: Strength of association in the general population. *Can J Psychiatry* 2005;50:195–202.
59 De Marco RR. The epidemiology of major depression: Implications of occurrence, recurrence, and stress in a Canadian community sample. *Can J Psychiatry* 2000;45:67–74.
60 Arboleda-Flórez J, Wade TJ. Childhood and adult victimization as risk factor for major depression. *Law & Psychiatry* 2001;24:357–70.
61 MacMillan HL, Fleming JE, Streiner DL, et al. Childhood abuse and lifetime psychopathology in a community sample. *Am J Psychiatry* 2001;158:1878–83.
62 Newman SC, Bland RC. Life events and the 1-year prevalence of major depressive episode, generalized anxiety disorder, and panic disorder in a community sample. *Compr Psychiatry* 1994;35:76–82.
63 Patten SB. Descriptive epidemiology of a depressive syndrome in a western Canadian community population. *Can J Pub Health* 2001;92:392–5.
64 Turner RJ, Wheaton B, Lloyd DA. The epidemiology of social stress. *Am Sociol Rev* 1995;60:104–25.
65 Bland RC, Newman SC, Orn H. Period prevalence of psychiatric disorders in Edmonton. *Acta Psychiatr Scand* 1988;338(suppl):33–42.
66 Patten SB, Adair CE, Williams JVA, et al. Assessment of mental health and illness by telephone survey: Experience with an Alberta Mental Health Survey. *Chron Dis Canada* 2006;27:99–109.
67 Bland RC, Orn H, Newman SC. Lifetime prevalence of psychiatric disorders in Edmonton. *Acta Psychiatr Scand* 1988;338(suppl):24–32.
68 Wilkins K. Bipolar I disorder, social support and work. *Health Rep* 2004;15(suppl):21–30.
69 Schaffer A, Cairney J, Cheung A, et al. Community survey of bipolar disorder in Canada: Lifetime prevalence and illness characteristics. *Can J Psychiatry* 2006;51:9–16.
70 Merikangas KR, Akiskal HS, Angst J, et al. Lifetime and 12-month prevalence of bipolar spectrum disorder in the National Comorbidity Survey Replication. *Arch Gen Psychiatry* 2007;64:543–52.

71 Schaffer A, Levitt AJ, Boyle M. Influence of season and latitude in a community sample of subjects with bipolar disorder. *Can J Psychiatry* 2003;48:277–80.

72 World Health Organization. *The Composite International Diagnostic Interview, Version 1.1, Researcher's Manual.* Geneva: World Health Organization, 1994.

73 ESEMeD/MHEDEA 2000 Investigators. Prevalence of mental disorders in Europe: Results from the European Study of the Epidemiology of Mental Disorders (ESEMeD) project. *Acta Psychiatr Scand* 2004;109(suppl 420):21–7.

74 Patten SB, Lavorato DH. Medication use and major depressive syndrome in a community population. *Compr Psychiatry* 2001;42:124–31.

75 Patten SB, Barbui C. Drug-induced depression: A systematic review to inform clinical practice. *Psychother Psychosom* 2004;73:207–15.

76 Beck CA, Patten SB. Adjustment of antidepressant utilization rates to account for major depression in remission. *Comp Psychiatry* 2004;45:268–74.

77 Mechanic D. Is the prevalence of mental disorders a good measure of the need for services? *Health Aff* 2003;22:8–20.

7 Anxiety Disorders in Canada

TRACIE O. AFIFI, BRIAN J. COX, AND JITENDER SAREEN

Anxiety disorders are a category of psychiatric disorders identified in the *Diagnostic and Statistical Manual of Mental Disorders*, fourth edition (*DSM-IV*), which includes panic disorder (panic attacks), agoraphobia, specific phobia, social phobia, obsessive compulsive disorder (OCD), posttraumatic stress disorder (PTSD), acute stress disorder, generalized anxiety disorder (GAD), anxiety disorder due to a general medical condition, substance-induced anxiety disorder, and anxiety disorder not otherwise specified.[1,2] The identification of *DSM* diagnoses in general population samples are commonly obtained using the Composite International Diagnostic Interview (CIDI), a structured interview developed by the World Health Organization based on the Diagnostic Interview Schedule (DIS) and the Present State Examination, which is often administered by trained interviewers.[3] Anxiety disorders have been found to be highly prevalent in general population samples[4] and have a negative impact on quality of life and psychosocial functioning.[5] A systematic review of prevalence studies published worldwide between 1980 and 2004 estimated the pooled past-year and lifetime prevalence of any anxiety disorder to be 10.6% (95% confidence interval [CI] = 7.5%–14.3% and 16.6%, 95% CI = 12.7%–21.1%), respectively.[6] In addition, the results from this review indicated that women are more likely to experience anxiety disorders than men, anxiety disorders remain prevalent throughout adulthood (18 to 64 years), and limited information is available with regard to incidence.[6]

Information on the incidence of anxiety disorders requires prospective longitudinal survey designs, which to date, have not been conducted in Canada. Epidemiologic cross-sectional surveys are often used to understand the prevalence and correlates of anxiety disorders.

To date, several cross-sectional surveys using Canadian community samples have been conducted to further our understanding of psychopathology, including anxiety disorders. The purpose of the present chapter is to not only report the prevalence of anxiety disorders in Canada, but also to review the characteristics and correlates of anxiety disorders in Canadian community settings. Such a discussion will provide a more representative profile than would be available by only examining clinical samples and will have especially important public health implications.

Surveys and Samples Used to Assess Anxiety Disorders in Canada

A description of all the surveys assessing anxiety disorders in Canada is presented in table 7.1. The earliest data on anxiety disorders in Canada came from several epidemiologic cross-sectional surveys using community samples from Alberta, Ontario, Winnipeg, and the Montreal area. The first large scale epidemiologic survey was conducted in Edmonton between 1983 and 1986 using a two-stage sampling design and included assessments of several anxiety disorders.[7] Several years later, in 1990, data on several anxiety disorders were collected for the Ontario Health Survey – Mental Health Supplement (OHS-MHS) using a community sample of Ontario residents.[8] In 1992 to 1993, a two-stage sampling design was used to collect data to assess panic attacks and GAD among east-end Montreal residents.[9] A year later in 1994, data were collected by way of a two-stage sampling design for two cross-sectional epidemiologic survey samples, one from Winnipeg (Winnipeg Area Study) and one from Calgary, Edmonton, and rural Alberta (Alberta Survey) to assess OCD and PTSD.[10,11] The same methods were used, 1996 to 1997, to collect two new samples for the Winnipeg Area Survey and Alberta Survey to assess social phobia.[12] More recently, in 2002, estimates of agoraphobia, social phobia, and panic disorder at the national level in Canada were made possible for the first time by way of the Canadian Community Health Survey cycle 1.2 – Mental Health and Well-Being (CCHS 1.2; see chapter 5).[13]

Comparing prevalence rates from different samples is limited because city- and province-wide are not representative of Canada. Second, data from the epidemiologic cross-sectional surveys in Canada were collected at different times spanning a 19-year period

Table 7.1
A comparison of the surveys assessing anxiety disorders in Canada

Survey	Year of data collection	Sample size	Age range	Response rate %	Diagnostic criteria	Interview schedule	Anxiety diagnoses included
Edmonton (Orn et al.)[7]	1983–6	3,258	18 +	71.6	DSM-III	DIS	Agoraphobia, social phobia, simple phobia, panic disorder, OCD
(OHS-MHS) Ontario (Offord et al.)[8]	1990	8,116	15–64	76.5	DSM-III-R	CIDI	Agoraphobia, social phobia, simple phobia, panic disorder, GAD
Montreal Area (Fournier et al.)[9]	1992–3	893	18 +	63.6	DSM-III-R	CIDIS	Panic attacks and GAD
Winnipeg Area Study and Alberta Survey (Stein et al.)[10,11]	1994	1,002 (Wpg) 1,259 (AB)	18 +	72 (Wpg) 73 (AB)	DSM-IV	CIDI	OCD, PTSD (Wpg only)
Winnipeg Area Study and Alberta Survey (Stein et al.)[12]	1996–7	750 (Wpg) 1,206 (AB)	18 +	62 (AB) 74 (Wpg)	DSM-IV	CIDI	Social phobia
(CCHS 1.2) Canada (Gravel et al.)[13]	2002	36,984	15 +	77	DSM-IV	WMH-CIDI	Agoraphobia, social phobia, panic disorder

from 1983 to 2002. The year the data were collected determines which diagnostic tools and criteria were used to assess anxiety disorders.

Panic Attacks and Panic Disorder

A panic attack is defined as a short period of intense feelings of apprehension, fear, terror, and doom while experiencing symptoms of shortness of breath, palpitations, chest pain, choking sensations, and fear of losing control.[1] Panic disorder is characterized by recurrent unexpected panic attacks.[1] Panic disorder can occur with or without agoraphobia. The prevalence of panic disorder and panic attacks are presented in table 7.2. Results from the earlier Edmonton survey of psychiatric disorders found that lifetime prevalence of panic disorder increases after age 25 and declines after the age of 65 years.[14] Women were at least two times more likely than men to experience panic disorder.[15] The study also determined that the mean age of onset of panic disorder for males and females was 19.3 years and 21.5 years, respectively. Data from the Edmonton sample also indicated that 13.9% of individuals with a lifetime diagnosis of panic disorder attempted suicide one or more times and that the lifetime rate of panic disorder was significantly higher in attempters compared to non-attempters (risk ratio 17.4).[16] Similar to findings from the Edmonton study, the sample from the Montreal area indicated that panic attacks were more common among women than men.[9] In addition, data from the OHS-MHS indicated that individuals with a lifetime diagnosis of panic disorder had increased odds of lifetime use of hallucinogens (odds ratio [OR] = 3.62, 95% CI = 1.80–7.29) after adjusting for age, sex, and education.[17]

Results from the CCHS 1.2 indicated that 21% of the population aged 15 years or older had suffered from a panic attack at some point during their lifetime. Women relative to men, and younger compared to older age cohorts, were more likely to experience attacks.[18] Females were also more likely to experience lifetime (4.6% versus 2.8%) and past-12-month (2.0% versus 1.0%) panic disorder relative to males. The average age of onset for individuals with panic disorder was 25 years, with 75% of individuals experiencing panic disorder by age 33. Panic disorder was more common among individuals who were separated or divorced compared to those who were married or common-law, and more likely among those who had low to lower-middle income compared to upper-middle to high levels of income.

Table 7.2
Lifetime and 12-month Prevalence of Anxiety Disorders in Canada

Dataset and/or place of collection (authors)	Type of sample	12-month prevalence % (SE)	Lifetime prevalence % (SE)
Panic disorder			
Edmonton (Bland et al.)[14,27]	Community	0.7 (N/A)	1.2 (0.2)
(OHS-MHS) Ontario (Offord et al.)[8]	Community	1.1 (0.2)	N/A
Montreal Area (Fournier et al.)[9]	Community	N/A	3.3 (2.1–4.5)[a]
(CCHS 1.2) Canada (Ramage-Morin)[18]	National	1.5 (N/A)	3.7 (N/A)
Agoraphobia			
Edmonton (Bland et al.)[14]	Community	(N/A)	2.9 (0.3)
(OHS) Ontario (Offord et al.)[8]	Community	1.6 (0.2)	N/A
(CCHS 1.2) Canada Original analysis[b]	National	0.74 (0.07)	1.53 (0.1)
Social phobia			
Edmonton (Bland et al.)[14]	Community	N/A	1.7 (0.3)
(OHS-MHS) Ontario (Offord et al.)[8]	Community	6.7 (0.5)	N/A
(OHS-MHS) Ontario (Stein et al.)[22]	Community	6.7 (0.5)	13.0 (0.6)
Winnipeg and Alberta (Stein et al.)[12]	Community	7.2 (0.6)	N/A
(CCHS 1.2) Canada (Shields)[25]	National	3.0 (N/A)	8.1 (N/A)
Specific phobia			
Edmonton (Bland et al.)[14]	Community	N/A	7.2 (0.5)
(OHS-MHS) Ontario (Offord et al.)[8]	Community	6.4 (0.5)	N/A
Obsessive compulsive disorder (OCD)			
Edmonton (Bland et al.)[14,27]	Community	1.8 (N/A)	3.0 (0.3)
Winnipeg and Alberta (Stein et al.)[10]	Community	Past month 0.6 (0.3–0.8)	N/A
Posttraumatic stress disorder (PTSD)			
Winnipeg (Stein et al.)[11]	Community	Past month 2.7 (♀) 1.2 (♂)	N/A
Generalized anxiety disorder (GAD)			
(OHS-MHS) Ontario (Offord et al.)[8]	Community	N/A	1.1 (0.2)
(OHS-MHS) Ontario (Stein et al.)[30]	Community	0.7 (0.1)	1.2 (0.2)
Montreal Area (Fournier et al.)[9]	Community	N/A	11.5 (9.4–13.6)
Any anxiety disorder[c]			
Edmonton (Bland et al.)[14,27]	Community	7.6 (N/A)	11.2 (0.6)
(OHS-MHS) Ontario (Offord et al.)[8]	Community	12.2 (0.6)	N/A
(CCHS 1.2) Canada Original analysis[b]	National	4.8 (0.2)	11.5 (0.3)

[a] Panic attacks not panic disorder
[b] Original analysis conducted by the authors of this chapter
[c] Prevalence figures for any anxiety disorder are not comparable across studies because they are based on anxiety disorders included in the specific study (Bland study = agoraphobia, social phobia, specific phobia, panic disorder, OCD, and somatization; Offord study = agoraphobia, social phobia, specific phobia, panic disorder, and GAD; Original analysis = agoraphobia, social phobia, and panic disorder)

Negative correlates among individuals with panic disorder included social withdrawal, increased smoking, drinking, and illicit drug use.

The past-12-month and lifetime prevalence of panic disorder reported in all studies are somewhat similar. Overall, the past-12-month and lifetime prevalence of panic disorders from all studies ranges from 0.7% to 1.5% and 1.2% to 3.7%, respectively.[8,9,14,18] However, since the surveys use different samples and diagnostic criteria, it is difficult to directly compare the findings. Very little is known about the incidence of panic disorder in Canada. A study using a community sample from Edmonton indicated that the incidence of panic disorder in males and females to be 1.2 per 1,000 (standard error [SE] = 0.6) and 10.2 per 1,000 (SE = 1.9), respectively.[19]

Agoraphobia

Agoraphobia is described as avoiding and having anxiety about places or situations that may be difficult to escape, that may create embarrassment, or that may lack access to help if panic ensues.[1,2] Agoraphobia occurs either with or without panic disorder. The prevalence of agoraphobia is reported in table 7.2. Little attention has been paid specifically to agoraphobia using Canadian samples. For example, data from the Edmonton Survey found the lifetime prevalence of agoraphobia to be 1.5% (SE 0.4%) among males and 4.3% (SE 0.5%) among females.[14] Further analysis of these data determined that the mean age of onset of first phobic symptom among those with agoraphobia was 13.7 years (standard deviation [SD] = 11.3 years) with women (12.5 years, SD = 11.5 years) experiencing onset earlier than men (17.9 years, SD = 9.9 years) and 50% of the combined male and female sample experiencing their first symptom by age 10.[20] Data from the OHS-MHS indicated the past-year prevalence of agoraphobia to be 0.7% (SE = 0.2%) and 2.5% (SE = 0.4%) among males and females, respectively.[8] The lifetime prevalence of agoraphobia seems to remain relatively stable throughout adulthood.[14] Furthermore, data from the OHS-MHS indicated that individuals with a lifetime diagnosis of agoraphobia had increased odds of lifetime use of hallucinogens (OR = 3.09, 95% CI = 1.82–5.25) after adjusting for age, sex, and education.[17]

To understand agoraphobia from a national level in Canada using CCHS 1.2 data, an analysis was done specifically for this chapter. It showed that the lifetime prevalence of agoraphobia was higher among women (2.2%, SE = 0.2) than men (0.8%, SE = 0.1). With regard to age of onset, 60% of individuals with agoraphobia had experienced their first agoraphobic fear before the age of 25, 77% before the age of 35, and 95% before the age of 50. In addition, 14.9% (SE = 2.5%) of individuals with a past-12-month diagnosis of agoraphobia thought about suicide in the previous year compared to 3.6% (SE = 0.2%) without this diagnosis. Similarly, 5.0% (SE = 1.9%) of individuals with a diagnosis of agoraphobia (12 month) attempted suicide in the preceding 12-month period compared to 0.5% (SE = 0.05%) of those without this diagnosis. Finally, individuals with a past-12-month diagnosis of agoraphobia compared to those without this diagnosis were more likely to report past-two week disability [32.1% (SE = 4.2%) versus 13.1% (SE = 0.2%)], long-term reduction in activities [49.5% (SE = 4.7% versus 21.6% (SE = 0.31%)], poor psychological well-being [83.1% (SE = 3.1%) versus 49.3% (SE = 0.4)], and greater distress [84.6% (SE = 3.1) versus 43.5% (SE = 0.4%)]. The past-12-month and lifetime prevalence of agoraphobia reported in all studies are somewhat similar. Overall, the past-12-month and lifetime prevalence of agoraphobia from all studies ranges from 0.7% to 1.6% and 1.5% to 2.9%, respectively.[8,14]

Social Phobia

Social phobia is defined as significant anxiety generated by exposure to social and performance situations leading to avoidance of such situations.[1,2] Avoidance characteristic of social phobia makes this disorder difficult to study, especially in the general population. The types of situations that individuals with social phobia tend to avoid are those where they feel they may be scrutinized.[21] Lifetime and 12-month prevalence of social phobia derived from numerous Canadian samples are presented in table 7.2. Early research using data from Edmonton indicated that the lifetime prevalence of social phobia among women and men was 2.0% (SE = 0.4) and 1.4% (SE = 0.4), respectively[14] and that the prevalence of social phobia remains stable between the ages of 18 and 54 years and then declines.[20] In addition, the mean age of onset of first phobic symptoms among those with social phobia was 9.5 years (SD = 7.4 years) with females [8.4 years (SD = 7.0 years)] experiencing first symptoms earlier than males [11.7 years (SD = 7.8 years)] and 50% of the sample experiencing their first symptom by age 6.5 years.[20]

The OHS-MHS found that individuals with a lifetime diagnosis of social phobia relative to those without, had increased odds of dissatisfaction with several domains of life and poor well-being after adjusting for age, sex, social class, and major depression.[22] In addition, it indicated that individuals with a lifetime diagnosis of social phobia had increased odds of lifetime use of stimulants (OR = 2.16, 95% CI = 1.38–3.39), cocaine use (OR = 2.42, 95% CI = 1.67–3.51), and hallucinogens (OR = 2.30, 95% CI = 1.70–3.11) after adjusting for the effects of age, sex, and education.[17] Social phobia was significantly associated with hazardous alcohol use, with age onset of social phobia preceding a diagnosis of alcohol abuse in 85% of the cases.[23] A study using community data from the Winnipeg Area Study and Alberta Survey found that individuals with social phobia experienced greater functional impairment than those with sub-threshold social fear, which had a negative impact on educational and employment pursuits and personal life after adjusting for age and sex.[12] Research has indicated that 50% of individuals with social phobia recover (mean length of illness of 25 years) with late age of onset of social fears being the strongest predictor of recovery.[24]

The most contemporary data available on social phobia in Canada come from a Statistics Canada report using the CCHS 1.2 survey,[25] which indicated that the average age of onset of fear or avoidance of social situations among those with a lifetime diagnosis of social phobia was 13 years, with the average duration of symptoms lasting 20 years.[25] Women relative to men had a higher prevalence of lifetime (8.7% versus 7.5%) and past-year diagnosis (3.4% versus 2.6%) of social phobia. Individuals with lifetime and past-year social phobia were more likely to have never married and to be divorced or separated versus married. In addition, those living in low to lower-middle income households compared to upper-middle to high income households had higher prevalence rates of lifetime and past-year social phobia. Finally, according to data from the CCHS 1.2, individuals with past-12-month and lifetime diagnosis of social phobia compared to those without this diagnosis were more likely to report low social support, long-term disability, reduction in activities, fair or poor self-perceived physical health, fair or poor self-perceived mental health and dissatisfaction with life.[25] The increased odds of the poor outcomes associated with lifetime and past-12-month social phobia remained statistically significant even after adjusting for sex, age, marital status, education, household income, major depressive disorder, panic disorder, substance dependency, and chronic physical conditions.[25]

The past-12-month and lifetime prevalence of social phobia reported in all studies are not very similar. Overall, the past-12-month and lifetime prevalence of agoraphobia from all studies ranges from 3.0% to 7.2% and 1.7% to 13.0%, respectively.[8,12,14,22] The variability in prevalence may be due to differences in samples and diagnostic criteria. Further research at the national level in Canada is required to clarify the prevalence of social phobia.

Specific Phobia

Specific phobia is the experience of clinically significant anxiety due to the exposure to a certain object or situation.[1,2] To date, two community samples have provided information on specific phobia in Canada. The lifetime and past-12-month prevalence rates from these two studies are reported in table 7.2. Data from the Edmonton sample found that lifetime prevalence estimates of specific phobia increase after age 25 and decline after age 55.[14] Results from this study also determined that females (9.8%, SE = 0.8%) were more likely to have a diagnosis of specific phobia than males (4.6%, SE = 0.6). Similarly, findings from the OHS-MHS from Ontario also reported a higher prevalence of specific phobia (past 12 months) among females (8.9%, SE = 0.8%) than males (4.1%, SE = 0.5%).[8] With regard to marital status, data from the Edmonton sample found that lifetime specific phobia was more prevalent among individuals who were widowed, separated, or divorced (9.5%, SE = 1.3%) compared to those who were married (7.6%, SE = 0.7%) or never married (5.5%, SE = 0.9%).[14] The mean age of onset of first phobic symptoms among those with specific phobia was 10.5 years (SD = 9.4 years) with women experiencing their first symptom earlier than men [9.3 years (SD = 8.4 years) versus 14.4 years (SD = 11.3 years)] and 50% of the combined male and female sample experiencing their first symptom by age 7.5 years.[20]

In addition, data from the OHS-MHS indicated that individuals with a lifetime diagnosis of specific phobia had increased odds of lifetime use of stimulants (OR = 2.30, 95% CI = 1.35–3.94) and hallucinogens (OR = 2.27, 95% CI = 1.57–3.29) after adjusting for the effects of age, sex, and education.[17] Another study using OHS-MHS data found a significant association between specific phobia and hazardous alcohol use, with age of onset of specific phobia preceding a diagnosis of alcohol abuse in 90% of the cases.[23] Specific phobia was not assessed in the CCHS 1.2 and, therefore, the prevalence of specific phobia at the national level in Canada is not known.

Obsessive Compulsive Disorder (OCD)

Obsessive compulsive disorder (OCD) is described as obsessive thoughts that create anxiety or distress, which is relieved by engaging in compulsive behaviours.[1,2] Prevalence rates of OCD in Canada are presented in table 7.2. To date, few studies in Canada have included the assessment of OCD. Data from the Edmonton Survey found that the lifetime prevalence rates for OCD did not differ among males (2.8%, SE = 0.5%) and females (3.1%, SE = 0.4%).[14] As well, data from this sample indicated that the prevalence of OCD increases after the age of 25 and remains prevalent in older age brackets. Few differences between males and females were noted with regard to age of onset. More specifically, it was determined that 50% of males with OCD are diagnosed by age 20 and 50% of females are diagnosed by age 19.[26] Other findings indicated that the highest prevalence of OCD is found among those who are widowed, separated, or divorced (6.6%, SE = 1.1%) relative to those who are married (2.2%, SE = 0.4%) or never married (2.6%, SE = 0.6%).[14] Data from the Edmonton sample also indicated that 14.8% of individuals with a lifetime diagnosis of OCD attempted suicide one or more times and that the lifetime rate of OCD was significantly higher in attempters compared to non-attempters (risk ratio 5.9, p < .01).[16]

The only other study to investigate OCD in Canada was conducted using the Winnipeg Area Study and the Alberta Survey.[10] The study by Stein and colleagues initially found the past-month prevalence of OCD to be 3.1% based on *DSM-IV* criteria, but after clinical reappraisal, the past-month prevalence of OCD decreased to 0.6% (95% CI = 0.3%–0.8%) with an additional 0.6% (95% CI = 0.3%–0.8%) of individuals experiencing a sub-clinical diagnosis. They concluded that over-diagnosis of OCD by lay interviewers was due to misidentification of worries and concerns as obsessions and overestimating distress or interference related to symptoms.[10] The authors suggested that the prevalence of OCD found in other surveys may be somewhat overestimated; however, further research is necessary before firm conclusions can be made.[10] Indeed, earlier data from the Edmonton survey reported the past-month prevalence of OCD to be 1.2%,[27] twice the rate of 0.6% found in the study by Stein et al.[10] However, it cannot be interpreted that the prevalence of OCD has decreased over time since the samples are not readily comparable due to different criteria and methods for assessing OCD. National Canadian data on OCD are currently unavailable.

Posttraumatic Stress Disorder (PTSD)

PTSD is characterized by re-experiencing a traumatic event along with increased arousal and avoidance of reminders of the trauma.[1,2] To date, only a small amount of research has been conducted on PTSD in Canada. The first study to estimate the prevalence of PTSD was conducted in 1994 using the Winnipeg Area Study,[11] which found that 2.7% of women and 1.2% of men met *DSM-IV* criteria for a past-month diagnosis of PTSD. It was also found that an additional 3.4% of women and 0.3% of men had a past-month sub-threshold PTSD diagnosis. Sub-threshold or partial PTSD has been defined in different ways, but generally speaking, it is when an individual lacks one to a few specified criteria required to meet the full *DSM* diagnosis.[11] The data also indicated that many individuals from the community sample had been exposed to one (74.2% among women and 81.3% among men) or two or more traumatic events (45.8% among women and 55.4% among men) with the most common events being the violent death of a friend or family member, and being physically attacked.[11] The data also indicated that women were not more likely than men to experience more types of traumatic events; however, women were more likely to experience full or sub-threshold PTSD after experiencing nonsexual assaultive violence than were men.[28] Stein and colleagues also found that the level of impairment at work or school increased as severity increased from those with no PTSD, to sub-threshold PTSD, to full PTSD diagnosis.[11]

Data on PTSD in Canada are limited by the use of small community samples that are not representative of the national population. Therefore, data about the lifetime or past-12-month prevalence of a *DSM* diagnosis of PTSD at the national level in Canada do not exist. To date, only national estimates of PTSD based on survey respondents self-report of a PTSD diagnosis by a health professional are available. Using this method it is estimated that the prevalence is 1%[29] and that after adjusting for socio-demographic factors and mental and physical disorders, the presence of PTSD was associated with an increased likelihood of poor quality of life, high levels of distress, and disability.

Generalized Anxiety Disorder (GAD)

GAD is described as six-months or more of excessive anxiety and worry.[1,2] Prevalence figures for GAD are reported in table 7.2. The OHS-MHS was the first data available on GAD in Canada and determined that the lifetime prevalence of GAD was 0.9% (SE 0.2%) among men and 1.2% (SE 0.3%) among women, indicating no significant gender differences.[8] Further, lifetime GAD was associated with dissatisfaction with job or school activity (OR = 5.15, 95% CI = 2.04–12.97), family life (OR 5.64, 95% CI = 2.35–13.51), and low overall perceived well-being (OR = 4.06, 95% CI = 2.80–5.89) after adjusting for the effects of age, sex, social class, and lifetime dysthymia.[30] In addition, another study using data from the OHS-MHS indicated that individuals with a lifetime diagnosis of GAD had increased odds of lifetime use of hallucinogens (OR = 5.09, 95% CI = 2.81–9.13) after adjusting for the effects of age, sex, and education.[17]

Another study examining GAD in Canada was conducted using residents from the Montreal area.[9] The past-6-month prevalence of GAD in this sample was 3.7% (95% CI = 2.4%–4.9%) with no significant differences in past-6-month GAD prevalence rates between males (4.1%, 95% CI = 2.2%–6.0%) and females (3.3%, 95% CI = 1.7%–4.9%).

Anxiety Disorders among Adolescents and Young Adults

Anxiety disorders do occur in younger cohorts, although to date, only one study at the national level has been conducted specifically on anxiety disorders among young Canadians. The study examined the prevalence and correlates of anxiety disorders using a sample of adolescents and young adults (n = 5,673) aged 15 to 24 years from the CCHS 1.2.[31] Results from this study determined that the lifetime and past-12-month prevalence of anxiety disorders (panic disorder, agoraphobia, and social phobia) were 12.1% and 6.5%, respectively. Females were more likely than males to experience both lifetime and past-year prevalence of anxiety disorders. The odds of experiencing any anxiety disorders were similar among 15 to 19 year olds and 20 to 24 year olds. However, adolescents who endorsed experiencing extreme levels of stress were more likely to have an anxiety disorder than those experiencing average stress levels.[31]

Comorbidity

Current epidemiological research indicates that comorbidity of psychiatric disorders is common among those with anxiety disorders. When using cross-sectional data, information regarding the age of onset of disorders is required to determine which of the comorbid conditions is more likely to occur first. To properly investigate which disorder was the primary diagnosis or if conditions developed concurrently, prospective longitudinal data or reliable documentation of the age of onset of disorders is required.

With regard to panic disorder, data from the Edmonton Survey determined that 90.4% of respondents with a lifetime diagnosis of panic disorder also met criteria for another lifetime psychiatric disorder.[15] More specifically, the lifetime mental disorders found to be highly comorbid with lifetime panic disorder were a major depressive episode (73.4%), alcohol abuse/dependence (54.2%), drug abuse/dependence (43.0%), and phobic disorders (44.2%).[15] Using the CCHS 1.2, it was found that 48% of those with a past-year diagnosis of panic disorder also met criteria for another past-year mental disorder.[18]

Comorbid psychiatric conditions were also found to be highly prevalent among individuals with agoraphobia. An analysis conducted for the current chapter using CCHS 1.2 data indicated that a large proportion of respondents who met criteria for a past-12-month diagnosis of agoraphobia also met criteria for other past-year diagnoses including alcohol dependence (6.8% SE = 1.6%), drug dependence (5.0% SE = 1.4%), major depression (30.4% SE = 4.0%), mania (13.0% SE = 3.2%), panic attacks (51.8% SE = 4.7%), panic disorder (18.4% SE = 3.0%), and social phobia (23.5% SE = 3.5%).

The OHS-MHS data from Ontario determined that 52% of individuals with a diagnosis of lifetime social phobia had at least one other lifetime psychiatric disorder, with the greatest odds of comorbidity found with bipolar disorder (OR = 8.95, 95% CI = 4.31–18.57), dysthymia (OR = 8.24, 95% CI = 5.09–13.35), agoraphobia (OR = 7.20, 95% CI = 4.88–10.64) and GAD (OR = 6.78, 95% CI = 4.14–11.10) after adjusting for age, sex, and level of education.[32] The study also found that the mean age of onset for social fears was 13 years among those with social phobia, which preceded the age of onset of the comorbid disorder in 32% of those with a comorbid anxiety disorder, 71% of those with a comorbid affective disorder, and 80% of those with a comorbid substance abuse/dependence disorder. In addition, data from the CCHS

1.2 indicated that individuals with a lifetime or past-12-month diagnosis of social phobia were more likely to experience comorbid major depressive disorder, panic disorder, and substance dependency.[25]

Using data from the Edmonton sample collected in the mid 1980s, it was determined that comorbidity of other psychiatric disorders was prevalent among those with OCD. More specifically, it was found that 73.9% of those with an OCD diagnosis also had an additional psychiatric diagnosis with the most common comorbid disorders being phobias (44.7%), alcohol abuse/dependence (35.9%), depression (29.6%), drug abuse/dependence (26.5%), depression (29.6%), dysthymia (12.4), schizophrenia (11.4%), and antisocial personality (10.1).[26]

Limited information is available on GAD and comorbid conditions. However, the OHS-MHS data showed that almost half of those with GAD also met criteria for major depressive disorder.[30]

The study from the Montreal area found that 50.7% of individuals with a past-6-month diagnosis of any anxiety disorder (including panic attacks and GAD) also had a past-6-month affective disorder (including major depressive episode and dysthymia).[9] As well, data from the OHS-MHS indicated that any lifetime anxiety disorder was associated with any lifetime antisocial diagnosis (OR = 1.72, 95% CI = 1.07–2.77) after adjusting for the effects of age, sex, education, lifetime major depression, and lifetime alcohol and substance abuse or dependence.[33]

An analysis conducted for the current chapter using CCHS 1.2 data indicated that a large proportion of respondents who met criteria for a past-12-month diagnosis of any anxiety disorder also met criteria for other past-year diagnoses including alcohol dependence (7.1%, SE = 0.7%), drug dependence (3.6%, SE = 0.5%), major depression (29.2%, SE = 1.6%), and mania (9.6%, SE = 0.9%).

Clinical Interventions, Public Policy, and Directions for Further Research

Research studies on anxiety disorders in Canada have important implications for interventions, policy, and future research. First, research has shown that anxiety disorders have an early age of onset with first symptoms sometimes occurring in childhood or adolescence. Evidence of early onset of anxiety disorders points to the need for timely interventions for children, adolescents, and young adults who experience anxiety symptoms. In addition, more research is required on early detection of children who experience anxiety and how to prevent anxious symptoms from developing into diagnosable disorders. Prevention of anxiety disorders among children, adolescents, and young adults would have a beneficial impact on Canadian society. Simply stated, more needs to be done for anxious youth and appropriate resources should be directed towards anxiety among youth. Likewise, it is also important to study anxiety disorders in other populations such as the elderly, as Cairney, Streiner, and colleagues have done (see chapter 11). As well, to have a more complete understanding of anxiety disorders with regard to disease incidence and course, longitudinal data in Canada are required. Many important research questions in psychiatric epidemiology research can only be answered using a prospective longitudinal survey design.

Second, anxiety disorders have a negative impact on quality of life, are associated with reduced functioning and psychiatric comorbidity, and often precede other disorders.[15,22,23,26,32] For example, the onset of anxiety disorders often occurs at an early age and may lead to subsequent depression, alcohol problems, suicide, and other negative events. In such cases, the detection of an anxiety disorder may facilitate the secondary prevention of other psychiatric disorders, suicidal behaviour, and other negative consequences.

Third, although several studies have been conducted on anxiety disorders in Canada, further research at the national level is required to better understand the prevalence, correlates, and comorbidity of all anxiety disorders. More specifically, future research needs to include the assessment of all anxiety disorders to truly understand the prevalence and impact anxiety disorders have in the Canadian community context. PTSD is an important anxiety disorder that is associated with negative outcomes. However, to date, research on PTSD using *DSM* criteria and a nationally representative Canadian sample is unavailable and addressing this limitation represents an important avenue for future research. In addition, comorbidity of mental health disorders is an important concept in psychiatric epidemiology research. Without the inclusion of more anxiety disorders in surveys, the ability to detect and understand psychiatric comorbidity is limited.

From a public health perspective, it may also be important to study sub-threshold diagnosis of anxiety disorders. Research has indicated that independent of a *DSM* diagnosis, self-perceived need for mental health treatment and help-seeking for mental health problems is associated with elevated levels of distress, disability, and suicide ideation.[34,35] Individuals who perceive a need for mental health treatment but do not meet criteria for a *DSM* diagnosis may experience some symptoms or have a sub-threshold *DSM* diagnosis and could potentially benefit from treatment. The study of sub-threshold anxiety disorders may provide insight into the assessment of the need for mental health intervention in the Canadian community context.

NOTES AND REFERENCES

Ms. Tracie Afifi was supported by the Social Sciences and Humanities Research Council of Canada's Canada Graduate Scholarship. Dr. Brian Cox was supported by the Canada Research Chairs Program. Dr. Jitender Sareen was supported by a Canadian Institutes of Health Research New Investigator Award and Manitoba Research Council Establishment Grant. The authors thank Jina Pagura for her thoughtful review of the chapter.

1 American Psychiatric Association. *Diagnostic Criteria from DSM-IV-TR*. Washington, DC: American Psychiatric Association, 2000.
2 American Psychiatric Association. *Diagnostic and Statistical Manual for Mental Disorders (DSM)*, 4th ed. Washington, DC: American Psychiatric Association, 1994.
3 Kessler RC, Wittchen H-U, Abelson JM, et al. Methodological studies of the Composite International Diagnostic Interview (CIDI) in the US National Comorbidity Survey (NCS). *Int J Methods Psychiatr Res* 1998;7:33–55.
4 Kessler RC, Chiu WT, Demler O, et al. Prevalence, severity, and comorbidity of 12-month DSM-IV disorders in the National Comorbidity Survey Replication. *Arch Gen Psychiatry* 2005;62:617–27.
5 Mendlowicz MV, Stein MB. Quality of life in individuals with anxiety disorders. *Am J Psychiatry* 2000;157:669–82.
6 Somers JM, Goldner EM, Waraich P, et al. Prevalence and incidence studies of anxiety disorders: A systematic review of the literature. *Can J Psychiatry* 2006;51:100–13.
7 Orn H, Newman SC, Bland RC. Design and field methods of the Edmonton survey of psychiatric disorders. *Acta Psychiatr Scand* 1988;77 (suppl 338):17–23.
8 Offord DR, Boyle MH, Campbell D, et al. One-year prevalence of psychi-

atric disorder in Ontarians 15 to 64 years of age. *Can J Psychiatry* 1996;41:559–63.

9 Fournier L, Lesage AD, Toupin J, et al. Telephone surveys as an alternative for estimating prevalence of mental disorders and service utilization: A Montreal catchment area study. *Can J Psychiatry* 1997;42:737–43.

10 Stein MB, Forde DR, Anderson G, et al. Obsessive-compulsive disorder in the community: An epidemiologic survey with clinical reappraisal. *Am J Psychiatry* 1997;154:1120–6.

11 Stein MB, Walker JR, Hazen AL, et al. Full and partial posttraumatic stress disorder: Findings from a community survey. *Am J Psychiatry* 1997;154:1114–9.

12 Stein MB, Torgrud LJ, Walker JW. Social phobia symptoms, subtypes, and severity: Findings from a community survey. *Arch Gen Psychiatry* 2000;57:1046–52.

13 Gravel R, Béland Y. The Canadian Community Health Survey: Mental health and well-being. *Can J Psychiatry* 2005;50:573–9.

14 Bland RC, Orn H, Newman SC. Lifetime prevalence of psychiatric disorders in Edmonton. *Acta Psychiatr Scand* 1988;77(suppl 338):24–32.

15 Dick CL, Bland RC, Newman SC. Panic disorder. *Acta Psychiatr Scand* 1994;(suppl 376):45–53.

16 Dyck RJ, Bland RC, Newman SC, et al. Suicide attempts and psychiatric disorders in Edmonton. *Acta Psychiatr Scand* 1988;77(suppl 338):64–71.

17 Sareen J, Chartier MJ, Paulus MP, et al. Illicit drug use and anxiety disorders: Findings from two community surveys. *Psychiatry Res* 2006;142:11–7.

18 Ramage-Morin PL. *Panic Disorder and Coping*. Ottawa, ON: Statistics Canada, 2004. Report No.: Catalogue 82-003.

19 Newman SC, Bland RC. Incidence of mental disorders in Edmonton: Estimates of rates and methodological issues. *J Psychiatr Res* 1998;32:273–82.

20 Dick CL, Sowa B, Bland RC, et al. Phobic disorders. *Acta Psychiatr Scand* 1994;(suppl 376):36–44.

21 Stein MB. Phenomenology and epidemiology of social phobia. *Int Clin Psychopharmacoly* 1997;12(suppl 6):S23–S26.

22 Stein MB, Kean YM. Disability and quality of life in social phobia: Epidemiologic findings. *Am J Psychiatry* 2000;157:1606–13.

23 Sareen J, Chartier M, Kjernisted KD, et al. Comorbidity of phobic disorders with alcoholism in a Canadian community sample. *Can J Psychiatry* 2001;46:679–86.

24 Dewit DJ, Ogborne A, Offord DR, et al. Antecedents of the risk of recovery from DSM-III-R social phobia. *Psychol Med* 1999;29:569–82.

25 Shields M. *Social Anxiety Disorder: Beyond Shyness*. Ottawa, ON: Statistics Canada, 2004. Report No.: Catalogue 82-003.

26 Kolada JL, Bland RC, Newman SC. Obsessive-complusive disorder. *Acta Psychiatr Scand* 1994;(suppl 376):24–35.

27 Bland RC, Newman SC, Orn H. Period prevalence of psychiatric disorders in Edmonton. *Acta Psychiatr Scand* 1988;77(suppl 338):33–42.

28 Stein MB, Walker JR, Forde DR. Gender differences in susceptibility to posttraumatic stress disorder. *Behav Res Ther* 2000;38:619–28.

29 Sareen J, Cox BJ, Stein MB, et al. Comorbidity, disability and suicidal behavior associated with posttraumatic stress disorder in a large Canadian community sample. *Psychosom Med* 2007;69:242–8.

30 Stein MB, Heimberg RG. Well-being and life satisfaction in generalized anxiety disorder: Comparison to major depressive disorder in a community sample. *J Affect Disord* 2004;79:161–6.

31 Nguyen CT, Fournier L, Bergeron L, et al. Correlates of depressive and anxiety disorders among young Canadians. *Can J Psychiatry* 2005;50:620–8.

32 Chartier MJ, Walker JR, Stein MB. Considering comorbidity in social phobia. *Soc Psychiatry Psychiatr Epidemiol* 2003;38:728–34.

33 Sareen J, Stein MB, Cox BJ, et al. Understanding comorbidity of anxiety disorders and antisocial behavior: Findings from two large community surveys. *J Nerv Ment Dis* 2004;192:178–86.

34 Sareen J, Cox BJ, Afifi TO, et al. Perceived need for mental health treatment in a nationally representative Canadian sample. *Can J Psychiatry* 2005;50:643–51.

35 Sareen J, Stein MB, Campbell DW, et al. The relation between perceived need for mental health treatment, DSM diagnosis, and quality of life: A Canadian population-based survey. *Can J Psychiatry* 2005;50:87–94.

8 Contribution of Psychiatric Epidemiology to the Study of the Adult Severely Mentally Ill

ALAIN D. LESAGE

Introduction

When trying to apply a set of seventeen definitions that have been suggested to define adult severe mental illness (SMI) to a sample of patients in contact with a specific psychiatric services clinic in Philadelphia, Schinnar et al.[1] found an estimated prevalence of serious mental illness among this specialists' care clinical population ranging from 4% to 88 %! Since then, efforts have been made to either validate definitions of SMI in populations of patients in contact with specialist services in order to establish their internal and external validity, or to use different sampling frames to evaluate definitions and produce estimates. Both of these reflect different aspects of classical epidemiology.

The NIMH definition,[2] presented in table 8.1, is representative of those used in studies that yielded estimates in the middle range of 45% to 55%. This definition highlights three dimensions that will repeatedly appear in defining SMI: (1) diagnosis, (2) disability, and (3) duration. In addition to the two key dimensions of the presence of a mental disorder and disability, the dimension of duration has been added. This proposed dimension relates not only to the duration per se, but also to having required more intensive care than outpatient treatment, possibly even psychiatric residential care. For the purposes of clarity, it would be wise to further break down this category into two – duration and need.

A first general proposal of the dimensions to help define SMI from a clinical services perspective is illustrated in figure 8.1. The first three key dimensions contrast somewhat with those proposed by researchers who have tried to define need for care and SMI from pop-

Table 8.1
NIMH definition of severe mental illness (SMI)

Diagnosis
A major mental disorder according to DSM-III-R: a schizophrenic, major affective, paranoid, organic, or other psychotic disorder or a disorder that may lead to a chronic disability such as a borderline personality disorder

Disability
Severe recurrent disability resulting from mental illness. The disability results in functional limitations in major life activities. Individuals typically meet at least two of the following criteria on a continuing or intermittent basis:
- Is unemployed, is employed in a sheltered setting or supportive work situation, or has markedly limited skills and a poor work history
- Requires public financial assistance for out-of-hospital maintenance and may be unable to procure such assistance without help
- Has difficulty in establishing or maintaining a personal social support system
- Requires help in basic living skills such as hygiene, food preparation, or money management
- Exhibits inappropriate behaviour which results in intervention by the mental and/or judicial system

Duration
Treatment history meets one or both of the following criteria:
- Has undergone psychiatric treatment more intensive than outpatient care more than once in a lifetime (e.g. crisis response services, alternative home care, partial hospitalization, or inpatient hospitalization)
- Has experienced an episode of continuous, supportive residential care, other than hospitalization, for a period long enough to have significantly disrupted the normal living situation.

---

ulation surveys: they have used the dimension of psychological distress and not duration; presence of disorder and disablement were also key dimensions. In the United States, it has been suggested that these efforts to define SMI stem from the flow of federal funds in the mid-1980s tagged for 'severely mentally ill'[3] but without a sufficiently precise operational definition. Definitions that existed could not be applied to the patients already in contact with specialist services, as shown in the Schinnar et al. exercise[1], or, as we will see, with population-based surveys. Shapiro et al.[4], on the basis of data from a community survey to assess the number of people who may present emotional or mental disorders of significance, and hence in need of care, considered three dimensions – presence of a disorder, disability, and distress; duration was not considered. Their results are based on the beginning of the 1980s Epidemiological Catchment Area (ECA)

Figure 8.1. Dimensions for defining severe mental illness: A clinical services perspective proposal

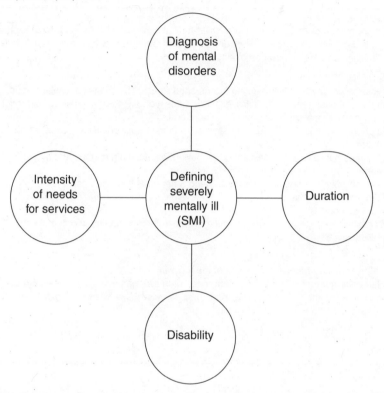

surveys in five U.S. urban centres and are illustrated in figure 8.2. One possible definition of SMI would be the group presenting a disorder in the past 12 months, disability and distress – about 2.7% of the population. Other combinations of disorder with disability or distress or singly could be used to define less seriously ill groups who are potentially in need of care.

These results could be replicated with a survey such as the Canadian Community Health Survey cycle 1.2 that has been presented in chapter 5 of this book, but exact figures would differ because: (1) for disorders, the coverage of mental disorders investigated, the instrument that was used, the diagnostic criteria, the sampling frame, population investigated, and period differ; (2) for social dysfunction and psychological

Figure 8.2 Epidemiological surveys perspective on severity of disorders and needs for care – assessment according to three dimensions (Shapiro et al., 1985)

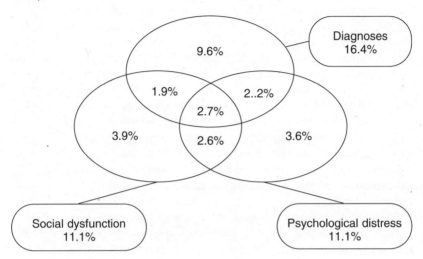

distress, the questions used and threshold employed would be crucial in determining the respective figures; and finally, (3) it is not clear which of the dimensions should be reported as indicating greater need: those with disorder, disablement, and distress; or those with disorder and/or distress and disablement? Further, what interventions, services, duration, and benefits should be considered? As indicated by Regier,[5] one must also take into account information regarding need for mental health care and services. Examination of these often-proposed dimensions to assess both SMI as well as the significance of the presence of a mental disorder indicates that the definition is not related only to the presence or, for that matter, the nature of the mental disorder, but also considers the disability: the definition is not only related to the strictly medical but necessarily entails a social dimension.

If one considers the origin of the term SMI, most authors[6–13] align with Barker and Grégoire,[14] who showed that in the United States, there was a historical evolution since deinstitutionalization in the 1960s and a large development of outpatient care in the 1970s and 1980s through community mental health centres. However, there was some degree of failure to deliver care for the most severely mentally ill, despite a 1987 regulation for federal funding for programs targeted to them. This group of patients would be considered a priority for planning and organization of services because of their greater need of services. This was associated with a series of commissioned works by U.S. psychiatric epidemiologists to try to define SMI. In the United Kingdom, other European countries, and in Canada[15-18] priority of policies during that period and until recently were on people who have been considered SMI, those who would have been admitted to psychiatric hospitals in the past. Hence, the SMI have remained a focus of mental health policies until recently when attention has shifted to people suffering from common mental disorders who could benefit from evidence-based treatments, with a proposal to call this latter group 'moderate mental illness' (MMI).[3] Both SMI and MMI can be associated with a notion of need for care and services and the issue of prioritization where those with greatest needs would be allocated more resources.

Drawing from the work of sociologists and economists, social psychiatrist and epidemiologist John Wing[19] proposed that need for care and services can be defined for planning and service organizational purposes 'in terms of problems for which state of the art solution exist.'[19(p8)] Wing also made a distinction between need for care (interventions) and need for services (agents, programs, service settings).[16,20] Allocation of resources according to need leads to the situation where need cannot be defined only by the presence or nature of the mental disorder or by the disability, but also by the existence of forms of treatment that have evidence for their efficacy. Modern balanced mental health care systems[21] would include an array of services for people with mental disorders who could benefit from interventions and models of care that are evidenced-based. Even though similar levels of evidence do not exist for all interventions and forms of care, most of the services can be justified so that the majority of people with SMI could live in the community with support and not be segregated in psychiatric hospitals; however, hospitalization remains as one required component of a balanced mental health system of care and services.[21]

The discussion on allocation of resources would be incomplete without taking into account the public health perspective of the needs of those patients presenting 'sub-clinical syndromes' who may represent a sizeable proportion of the population who are incapacitated due to mental disorders, and are at risk for moderate mental and physical

Table 8.2
Simulation of the number of places and people in need of specialist care in a balanced mental heath care system

	Costs of a good system of care for severely mentally ill patients (catchment area size – 100,000 inhabitants)		
	People/places	Cost/person/year	Total/year
Long-term hospitalization	15	$ 89,078	$ 1,336,170
Acute care beds	25	$ 109,438	$ 2,735,950
Day hospital places	60	$ 7,229	$ 433,740
Nursing homes	22	$ 65,521	$ 1,441,462
Hostels	14	$ 35,616	$ 498,624
Foster families	26	$ 7,746	$ 201,396
Supervised group homes	28	$ 49,793	$ 1,394,204
Supervised apartments	48	$ 19,348	$ 928,704
PACT	70	$ 7,410	$ 518,700
Intensive home care	120	$ 4,711	$ 565,320
Outpatients	1,072	$ 1,638	$ 1,755,936
Total	1,500		$ 11,810,206
Per capita			$ 118

disorders and excess mortality.[22] We do not know what would be the right balance between allocations for prevention, treatment, and rehabilitation.[23]

The contribution of psychiatric epidemiology in counting and translating needs for services for the SMI was well illustrated in the following simulations inspired by Wing (see table 30 in[24]). This simulation, shown in table 8.2 and figure 8.3, is drawn for the prevalence figures from benchmarks suggested by Wing et al.[19] and Lesage et al.,[25,26] with cost estimations drawn from economic appraisals within the Canadian situation,[27,28] and for adults aged less than 65. They illustrate, first, that a balanced mental health care system of specialist services would include, for a minority of cases, long term hospitalization or tertiary psychiatric residential care alternatives, acute care hospitalization, some supervised residential facilities, community assertive treatment, and intensive homecare (about .5% of the population); and, second, for the majority who would live at home, outpatient-based interventions (about 1% of the population). Yet, the group requiring forms of psychiatric residential care (i.e., hospitalization, supervised residential facilities), about 0.25% of the population, would use almost 2/3 of the

Figure 8.3. Estimated cost distribution for specialist care budget in a balanced mental health care system (total 100%)

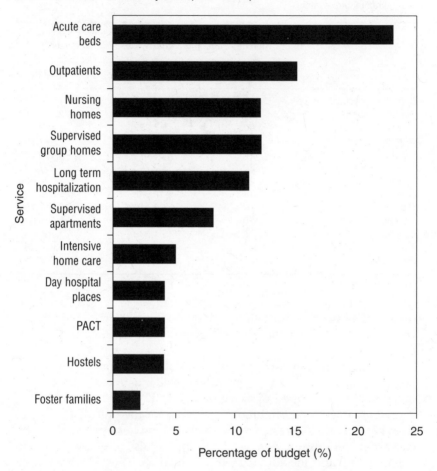

specialists' mental health care budget; the group requiring intensive home care support (0.25%) would use 10% of the budget; and those 1% of the population requiring only outpatient care would take the remaining 15% of a balanced specialist mental health care budget. A confirmation of the simulation comes from Italy where in best practice areas like Verona, that have applied radical community care reform and closure of psychiatric hospitals, over 60% of the cost of the specialist mental health care system is associated with hospitalization (one-third of the 60% or 20% overall) and supervised psychiatric residential care (two-thirds of the 60% or 40% overall).[29]

The prevalence figures of need for specialist services suggested here should recognize that needs may vary between regions or between catchments areas of cosmopolitan cities with 50,000–250,000 inhabitants by a factor of up to 3,[30–32] with greater need associated with more socioeconomically disadvantaged areas. Estimates of the number of persons or places in services settings, as well as costs proposed for each of them, could be subjected to a sensitivity analysis. Costs will vary within and between countries, and may change over time.[33,34] Needs cannot be seen in absolute terms within a given country and vary relatively between regions because of services and societal issues. These societal and cultural issues appear much more clearly in international comparisons among industrialized countries.

The EPSILON project, which compared care for people with schizophrenia in five urban catchment areas of the United Kingdom, Denmark, Netherlands, Italy, and Spain, examined the existing services provided in relation to outcomes.[35] A large inter-country difference in provision of services was found: hospital indefinite stay beds ranged from 14/100,000 population in London to 75/100,000 in Santander, with Copenhagen at 67/100,000; but 24-hour support residential facilities numbered a remarkable high of 147 in Copenhagen to a floor of 4 in Santander, and London at 33; Copenhagen also counted 91 daily support residential facilities and none in Santander; overall bedspaces in hospital and community settings ranged from a low of 92 in Santander, to 106 in London and Verona; 195 in Amsterdam and 529 in Copenhagen.

Thornicroft and Tansella[36] pointed out that values influence planning decisions, determination of need, and priorities. They delineated nine values that can be abbreviated by the acronym 3 ACEs: autonomy, accountability, access, comprehensiveness, continuity, coordination, equity, effectiveness, efficiency. The autonomy value differs among countries and is related to the social role relatives are ready to play in supporting severely mentally ill patients – lower needs were identified in countries like Spain and Italy, higher in the Scandinavian countries. This differentiated role of families where many more Italian patients live with families than their U.S. or Canadian or fellow French-Canadian citizens has been well described between Italian and U.S. or Canadian mental health systems contexts.[37–39]

It is tempting to conclude that the 0.5% of the population described here in high contact with psychiatric services fully meet the NIMH[2] criteria of need proposed for SMI, and to call them the most severely mentally ill, if one were sure that all those are in contact with specialists services; but some may be homeless.[40] It may be found that a proportion of the psychiatric outpatients would meet criteria of duration, disability, and certainly of presenting a mental disorder, and this 1% could be in general associated with SMI. However, more people can be counted as seriously mentally ill during one year and requiring specialist care, but are in contact only with primary care services, or not at all. Only community surveys and analysis of administrative databases of physician billings could illuminate these numbers that may be found among patients who would be considered among the 10% to 15% of the general population as 'moderately mentally ill.'[3] Numbers and concepts may now seem to be too many for the readers to follow, and it may be useful, before moving on to examples of operationalization and testing of definitions of severe mental illness from various sources, to ensure that a fuller perspective in the definition of SMI is achieved.

1. Defining Severely Mentally Ill –
   A Case for What, for Whom, and When?

In his contribution to estimating needs for mental health care, Fryers[41] underlined a key principle in epidemiology, that the definition of a case depends on the question being asked: a case for what purpose? The definition and work on the concept of SMI came mostly from the need of planners and decision makers. Epidemiology, as we have seen elsewhere in this book, can be used for etiological studies and for study of the evolution of disorders. The efforts in defining the dimensions of disability and duration and need for care and services may help etiological research on specific mental disorder, or for the description of such disorders' outcome. Schizophrenia research includes many examples of longitudinal studies that have used a series of simple indicators of social status, disability, and duration and utilization of services. These have been used to create a composite outcome for course of recovery, ranging from mild to severe.[42–45]

A Case for Whom and When

The heuristic matrix model of Thornicroft and Tansella[36] for evaluating and viewing mental health care systems will help draw attention to the issue that the need to establish the number of persons who are severely mentally ill is different for national or regional planners and decision makers than it is for local health and social services clinical teams. Their matrix model is composed of two axes: a temporal one of input, processes, and results; and a geographical one of national/regional. The local and individual/clinical level are also described by Donabedian[46] as system, programmatic, and individual. In order to assess and meet needs for care and services of a population, both top-down and bottom-up approaches are relevant.[19] The two approaches described so far in assessing the number of SMI have drawn from approaches that can best be described as top down.

At the individual and local level, identifying SMI in order to set priorities may require considering other dimensions in addition to those described so far. For example, the Care Program Approach in the United Kingdom[47] could not be based solely on top-down criteria of, say non-affective psychotic disorder (disorder dimension); high level of disability (on the Global Assessment Functioning (GAF) scale [see following for definition] lower than 60 or 50); and duration of contact with services of more than two years to determine the level of intensity of services to be offered to individuals by the local programs. The approach also had to take into account the service providers' perspective, the informal carers, and the patients themselves, and dimensions of risk to self and others.[9,48] The addition of these dimensions clearly point toward the shortcomings and the impossibility of applying national standardized definitions of needs at the local level.[14]

State/provincial and regional planners are in a similar predicament. Socioeconomic and cultural factors are powerful determinants of the prevalence of disorders, from mild to severe, and of needs for care and services. Benchmarks emerging from best practices or national epidemiological surveys are often too imprecise at the state/provincial level and are always too imprecise at the regional and local level to be the basis for the equitable allocation of resources. In the examples of operationalization below, we will see some strategies that are being tried to bridge information available at various levels.

In deciding what a case is, an epidemiologist will need to consider where the request comes from: Is it from the national, provincial, regional, local, or, even, the individual level? He or she will need, also, to consider the context of the request and the timeline. More often than not, sufficient information is available in existing data sources, surveys, or, simply, in the literature already published (such as in this book) to answer the needs for estimates of SMI in a sufficiently precise manner to allow planning and organization of services to go ahead. In other circumstances, commissioning will be inspired by the examples below.

2. Operational Definitions of Severely Mentally Ill to Help Counting Them at a National, Provincial/State, Regional and Local Level

Key elements in operational definitions are: (1) What dimensions will be included: disorder, disability, duration, need, danger to self and others, etc; (2) the measures of each dimension and threshold used; and (3) the sources of information. We began by discussing dimensions; now we will elaborate on sources of information and follow with a discussion of measurement issues.

A key epidemiological principle is to ensure coverage of the universe, which means to ensure that all those in the designated area meeting the general definition of whatever is being surveyed (in our discussion, SMI) are counted. When counting the SMI, not all will be found in contact with specialist services, nor will surveys that cover the majority, but not all the population, complete the picture. Figure 8.4 illustrates this situation by delineating other areas and situations where the severely mentally ill may be found. Figure 8.4 draws from work undertaken to track the most severely mentally ill patients (those in need of intensive treatment and rehabilitation) in the Eastern Townships of Quebec, a region of about 250,000 inhabitants that was functioning without a psychiatric hospital. It illustrates where community surveys of households and the examination of all those in contact with specialist mental health services will miss those who are: (1) homeless; (2) in non-specialist mental health service facilities such as nursing homes; and (3) in prison; and (4) it will not have taken into account those who have died prematurely of suicide or preventable deaths.

3. Four Examples of Operational Definitions of Severe Mental Illness and the Population Count Obtained.

Testing and Comparing a Definition of Severe and Persistent Mental Illness Applicable at the Local and Regional Level

In the study by Ruggeri et al., the source was all people in contact with public specialist services in two European catchments areas. They

Figure 8.4 A more comprehensive sampling frame to count SMI at the local, regional, provincial/state, and nation level

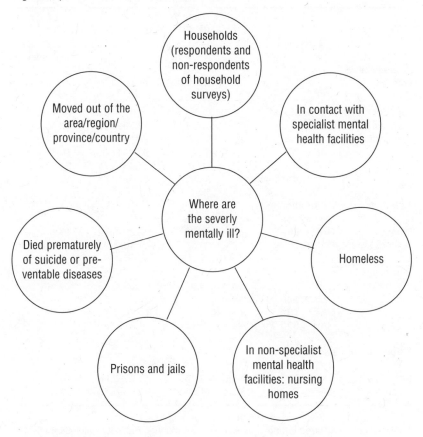

created two definitions based on the NIMH dimensions (table 8.1).[2] For the diagnosis dimension, one definition included the psychoses, and the other added non-psychotic disorders. The duration of service dimension was defined as contact for more than two years; and for disability, a score of less than 50 on the Global Assessment of Functioning (GAF). The instrument includes the severity of symptoms, abnormal and dangerous behaviours, and social functioning to produce a global assessment. The results are shown in table 8.3 for the South-Verona, Italy, catchment area.

Table 8.3
Results of the South-Verona catchment area

Operationalized criteria			South Verona (62,240 inhabitants over 18) (n=933)[a]		
			Rate per 1,000	95 % CI	Estimated percentage of all cases
One-dimensional definitions					
Diagnosis of psychosis			3.41	2.79–4.02	23 %
Dysfunction					
	GAF ≤ 70		10.54	9.22–11.86	70 %
	GAF ≤ 50		3.11	2.43–3.79	21 %
	Duration: ≥ 2 years		10.00	8.96–11.04	67 %
Two-dimensional definitions					
	Dysfunction				
Diagnosis of	GAF ≤ 70		2.85	2.29–3.42	19 %
psychosis	GAF ≤ 50		1.51	1.10–1.93	10 %
Diagnosis of		Duration			
psychosis		≥ 2 years	3.01	2.53–3.49	20 %
	Dysfunction	Duration			
	GAF ≤ 70	≥ 2 years	6.77	5.78–7.77	45 %
	GAF ≤ 50	≥ 2 years	2.33	1.77–2.89	16 %
Three-dimensional definition					
	Dysfunction	Duration			
Diagnosis of	GAF ≤ 70	≥ 2 years	2.45	1.92–2.98	16 %
psychosis	GAF ≤ 50	≥ 2 years	1.34	0.95–1.73	9 %

GAF, score on the Global Assessment of Functioning Scale
[a] 933 patients registered in one year; 578 in three months. Basis for estimation of three-month rates: 353 valid cases for dysfunction, 532 for duration, 341 for both duration and dysfunction. Rates adjusted to one year

In combining in the first definition diagnosis of psychosis, dysfunction, and duration in South Verona, 1.34 cases per 1,000 inhabitants were found; the figures for London were 2.55 per 1,000. A second definition that would include non-psychotic disorders in addition to psychotic disorders would add 0.98 cases per 1,000 for a total of 2.42 in Verona: one third of a per cent of the general population that they would later call 'severe and persistently mentally ill.'[49] Thus, not all people in contact with these public specialist services (including people who have been in contact for more than two years), would be considered SMI using the definition proposed here; only 1/3 of them. The count of people in contact with specialist services may vary in countries between 1% to 3% and was estimated in the mid-1990s in France and Quebec to be about 1.2% to 1.5% of the population based on data emerging from administrative data basis or population surveys.[16,31] There may have been an increase up to 3% in some jurisdictions according to trends seen in the United States,[8] and is related to the increase in resources for specialist services; not to be confounded with inter-regional or intra-regional variations associated for decades with greater prevalence in socioeconomically disadvantaged areas.

Some validation of the approach and findings in Canada was found in a program evaluation survey of the psychiatric outpatients of an east-end catchment area of Montreal.[50] In the representative sample of 1173 of all the 5867 patients in contact with the catchment area's services in one year, 32% had a non-affective psychosis diagnosis, and 31% had a GAF score lower than 50.

Establishing the National Prevalence of Adults with Serious Mental Illness for Securing Block Grant Funding in the United States[51]

Over two decades ago, U.S. legislation established block grants for states to fund community mental health services for adults and children with SMI; the legislation also mandated that states would include SMI in their funding applications, and that the Substance Abuse and Mental Health Services Administration (SAMHSA) would develop an operational definition for use by the states. The law minimally stated a definition of 12-month *Diagnostic and Statistical Manual* (*DSM*) disorder and 'serious impairment.' A taskforce was to estimate the prevalence of SMI in the country as a whole and to examine sociodemographic correlates of SMI for state/regional estimates. The following description shows how national estimates were recently established.

The recent replication of the U.S. National Co-morbidity survey served as the representative U.S. household population of English speakers 18 years and older. *DSM-IV* diagnoses were based on a structured interview administered by lay people, and 12-month disorders were considered (including anxiety, mood, impulse control, and substance use disorders). Severity was classified as 'serious' if any of the following were present:

- A suicide attempt within the last 12 months with serious lethality intent
- Work disability or substantial limitation due to a mental or substance disorder
- Positive screen results for non-affective psychosis
- Bipolar I or II disorder
- Substance dependence with serious role impairment (as defined by disorder-specific impairment questions)
- Impulse control disorder with repeated serious violence
- Any disorder that resulted in 30 or more days out of role in the year

Cases were defined as 'moderate' if they had any of the following:

- Suicidal gesture, plan, or ideation
- Substance dependence without serious role impairment
- At least moderate work limitation due to a mental or substance disorder
- Any disorder with at least moderate role impairment in two or more domains of a scale used when a disorder was identified (the Sheehan Disability Scale assessed disability in work role performance, household maintenance, social life, and intimate relationships on 0-10 visual analog scale, and score of 4 and higher being moderate, severe, or very severe).

All other cases were classified as mild.

The U.S. prevalences of mental disorders, serious, moderate, and mild mental disorders among adults living in households and speaking English obtained, according to these definitions, are shown in table 8.4.

An earlier estimate that uses almost the same definition, estimated that 5.4% of the U.S. non-institutionalized population met criteria for SMI during the past year,[6] but a majority were not in receipt of care. In this U.S. population survey,[52] it was observed that 20% of those with a disorder reported receiving services for their emotional problems, and 40% among those with serious mental disorder.

Table 8.4
Estimates of severe mental disorders in the past year based on a national population survey in the United States (2007)[51]

Severe mental disorder	5.8%
Moderate mental disorder	9.8%
Mild mental disorder	10.5%
Any disorder	26.2%

Establishing the State/Regional Numbers of Adults with Serious Mental Illness for Securing Block Grant Funding in the United States[53]

A key issue with the application of the results of national surveys' definition of SMI is the level of precision at the state, regional, and local levels. In Canada, the Canadian Community Health Survey (CCHS), cycle 1.2 on mental health and well-being (see chapter 5) had a sample of 35,000 that was drawn to ensure reasonable estimates at the provincial level for disorders with prevalences above 1%. Ontario asked for extra cases to be able to run estimates at the regional level. For example, provincial comparisons of CCHS 1.2 showed for depression in Canada estimates of 4.8 (with 95% confidence intervals between 4.5% and 5.1%); Nova Scotia estimates were 4.6 (95% CI 3.6%–5.5%) with a provincial sample of 1119; while for drug dependence, figures were of 0.8% (95% CI 0.6%–0.9%) and 0.6% (95% CI of 0.3%–0.9%).[54] For Nova Scotia planners, the estimate varies three-fold for drug dependence. Imagine the estimates precision for, say, the Halifax region from which fewer than 300 respondents were drawn; there would be too much imprecision to reliably assess the prevalence.

The dilemma for regional planners is two-fold here. Greater numbers are required to ensure more precision of estimates, and extensive mental health surveys are not run regularly. In the United States, the U.S. National Co-morbidity survey was repeated 10 years apart, and Australia has a similar survey schedule (1997 and 2007). There are plans to run a Canadian national mental health survey again in 2012, 10 years after CCHS 1.2. It is likely that, at this time, prevalence of disorders may change. If the sample were to be as large as the full CCHS cycles x.1, and to be repeated every two years with a national sample of over 130,000 respondents, and if these omnibus health surveys were to contain screening questions to estimate some mental disorders, possibly even SMI, then timely and precise estimates would be available at the state/regional level. If this were to happen, then, regional planners could commission less expensive regional surveys that could include brief screening questions to obtain reasonably precise local area estimates and changes over time.

In the United States, SAMHSA funded a methodological study that considered three measures as screens for SMI: the first was a truncated version of the Composite International Diagnostic Interview; the second measure was a modified version of the K10/K6 scales, where 6 or 10 questions measure psychological distress (as in figure 8.2) in the past month; and the third measure was a truncated version of the World Health Organisation Disability Assessment Schedule, covering illness-related impairments in a variety of social domains in the past month. A two-stage design was used, where a sample of 1,000 respondents to telephone interviews were screened for SMI as defined in table 8.1; in a second stage, in-depth standardized face-to-face interviews were conducted by trained clinical interviewers with a sample of 155 respondents. The 6-question psychological distress scale K6 proved the best predictor of SMI, with a sensitivity of .36; specificity of .96, and total classification accuracy of .92.

The authors warned against using such results and automatically applying the cut-off found for use in state level estimates without using calibration measure to take into account that variation in rates influences the precision and estimates. At that stage, too, numbers in the calibration were much too small and are still considered preliminary[55] because the results were based on a relatively small non-probability sample. The authors suggest that with the largest calibration studies being conducted as part of the World Mental Health series of national surveys, with more than 200,000 respondents, more precise calibration of K10/K6 scales could be accomplished. However, other issues will arise in relation to the reliability and validity of estimates with standardized questionnaires being used in many different countries and cultures. As discussed, local planners and clinicians are wary of national definitions of SMI; imagine if the definitions were drawn from international studies!

Estimating Regional and Local Area Needs for Severely Mentally Ill Using Social Indicators

Beyond counting the number of severely mentally ill, regional and local planners are concerned that resources are equitably distributed.

Planners want information that will help them ensure that the array of services required, such as those enumerated in table 8.2 and figure 8.3, are available and sufficient in various areas, recognizing that some areas may have a greater proportion of people with SMI. It is known from population surveys that urban areas and, within those, socioeconomically disadvantaged areas, have higher rates of persons with psychosis.[56] A long tradition of studies as far back as Faris and Dunham in 1939[57] showed a relationship between rates of admissions for psychosis and intensity of social disadvantage in local areas. Socioeconomic indicator modelling has a long tradition and has been applied in the United Kingdom for at least a decade for proportional allocation of resources, in recognition that regions and local areas with greater social disadvantage would have more people with SMI and thus a greater need for resources.[30] The size of the area will determine the magnitude of the differences: for example, Faris and Dunham, in 1939, observed up to a 99-fold difference in rates between small areas of about 5000 inhabitants. In our own socioeconomic indicators modelling in east-end Montreal, we found a similar 100-fold difference among census tracts, but a three- to four-fold difference for larger local health areas (about 75,000 inhabitants).[31] Indeed, in benchmarks for the variety of required number of places for an array of services in areas of 250,000 inhabitants, Wing et al.[19] suggested a range with a three-fold difference, taking into account knowledge of this amount of variation observed and modelled in the United Kingdom for services likely to be required by SMI.

Applying socioeconomic modelling to national, regional, or local areas can be rather inexpensively conducted in Canada, without any new data collection, using population census survey data and administrative hospitalization databases that are available in each province. Provincial or regional health analysts here in Canada would do well to reproduce the regression analysis methods used in the United Kingdom.[31,58]

Montreal regional planners and researchers conducted a modelling exercise to serve in allocating resources across local health and social services areas (approximately 75,000 to 100,000 inhabitants); it was conducted for the whole region (about 1.8 million inhabitants).[59] Two variables (population proportions of married persons over 15% and employment rates) predicted 69% of the variance in admissions rates in the 94 forward sortation areas (FSA) of Montreal. The parameters of the regression equation allowed them to estimate the relative predicted rate of admission vis à vis the average regional one; and when

Figure 8.5 Modelled and observed prevalence of psychiatric hospitalization in Montreal's local health and social services (CLSC) areas (total population 1.8 million inhabitants) for adults (per 1,000 inhabitants.)[60]

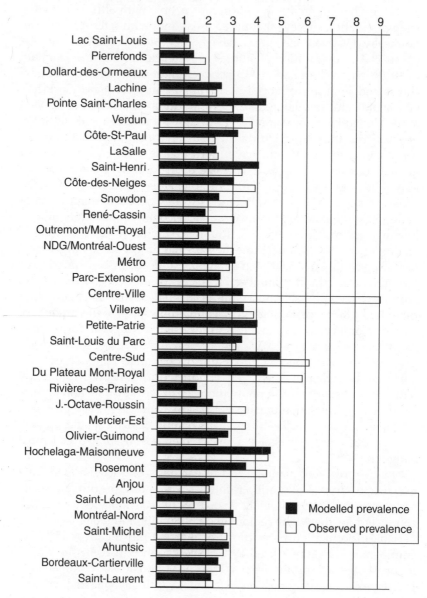

aggregating the FSAs of respective local areas, to produce an expected rate, and a relative predicted rate. The results are shown in figure 8.5.

A 4:1 difference was observed in modelled rates (when grouping into 6 sub-regions, a three-fold difference would remain between affluent West-Island and downtown Montreal). Moreover, the model results were close to the actual situation, except for the very downtown area, the most disadvantaged area of Montreal. Indeed, Croudace[32] warned that such linear regression modelling would underestimate needs for very affluent and very disadvantaged areas.

With these limitations, these modelled rates can serve as an indicator of relative need for specialist services. As we saw in table 8.2 and figure 8.3, hospital services comprise almost 40% of the specialist resources in a balanced mental health care system. It is therefore valid and useful to be able to measure regularly and precisely the relative need for services, at least to ensure equitable allocation of resources that a province or a region would be ready to allocate for specialist mental health services and SMI patients. Using national epidemiologically based surveys of SMI to estimate at the regional and local levels would simply be too imprecise; a two- to three-fold decrease in precision of the estimates would cause havoc in services for the most SMI; and using screening tests as shown in the preceding example from the United States is simply too preliminary. The present method is currently used in the United Kingdom to allocate part of the mental health budget to regions.[60]

A Proposal in Defining and Counting Severely Mentally Ill with Four Dimensions of Need for Services

In the end, is there a contribution from Canadian psychiatric epidemiology to defining and counting SMI? There have been no approaches that have simultaneously been able to take into account the four dimensions; there are no precise definitions that have wide recognition; and no operational definitions have robustly demonstrated their validity, with the exception of the socioeconomic indicators approach. But this approach only provides good estimates of relative needs; it does not estimate which of the array of services and interventions would be useful, nor their numbers and rates. It's not just about counting anymore.[61]

This state of affairs has led UK opinion leaders, such as Sir David Goldberg,[62] to make proposals that describe more the outlines, rather than the precise figures, of needs for mental health services. This is

Table 8.5
A proposal for defining, counting, and outlining the needs of severely mentally ill among an adult mental health population

	Proportion in the community	Dominant services	Diagnoses	Current disability	Duration
I. Severe and persistent	0.5%	Specialist	Psychoses	Severe and persistent	Lifetime
II. Severe	1.0%	Specialist with primary	50-50% non-affective psychotic disorders/bipolar disorders and 50% other mental disorders	Severe	Chronic and acute
III. Serious	3.5%	Primary with specialist	Other mental disorders with comorbidity	Serious	Acute and chronic
IV. Moderate	10%	Primary	Anxiety, depressive, impulse control and substance abuse disorders	Moderate to mild	Episodic
V. Mild	15%	Primary/ public health	Anxiety, depressive, impulse control and substance abuse disorders; adjustment/psychological distress	Mild to none	Transient but at risk

despite some benchmarks for needs for the array of specialist services with provision for a range that recognizes variation in absolute numbers related to socioeconomic disadvantage (e.g., Wing)[19,24] for an audience of clinical decision makers at the national, regional, and local levels.

Our proposal (see table 8.5) is therefore one based on expert opinion. It introduces a distinction between severe and persistent mental illness and just severe, drawing from the work of Italian colleagues.[49] It is based on the findings that most people with very severe mental disorders are likely to be in contact with specialist services during any one year in public managed care systems, like those in place in Canada and many European countries. It could also be considered a more bottom-up approach to needs assessments, while it also draws from top-down approaches and indicators of SMI from national epidemiological surveys like CCHS 1.2 in Canada. Both top-down and bottom-up approaches are required to sensibly estimates need[19] and produce estimates to inform planning of specialist, primary care, and public health services for treatment, rehabilitation, and prevention in a balanced mental health care system.

REFERENCES

1 Schinnar AP, Rothbard AB, Kanter R, et al. An empirical literature review of definitions of severe and persistent mental illness. *Am J Psychiatry* 1990;147:1602–8.

2 NIMH. *Towards a Model for a Comprehensive Community-based Mental Health System*. Washington, DC: National Institute of Mental Health, 1987.

3 Dewa CS, Rochefort DA, Rogers J, et al. Left behind by reform: The case for improving primary care and mental health system services for people with moderate mental illness. *Appl Health Econ Health Policy* 2003;2:43–54.

4 Shapiro S, Skinner EA, Kramer M, et al. Measuring need for mental health services in a general population. *Med Care* 1985;23:1033–43.

5 Regier DA, Burke JD, Jr., Manderscheid RW, et al. The chronically mentally ill in primary care. *Psychol Med* 1985;15:265–73.

6 Kessler RC, Berglund PA, Zhao S, et al. The 12-month prevalence and correlates of serious mental illness. In: Manderscheid RW, Sonnenschein MA, eds. *Mental Health, United States, 1996*. U.S. Department of Health and Human Services, Substance Abuse and Mental Health Services Administration, Center for Mental Health Services; DHHS Publ. No. (SMA)96-3098. Washington, DC: U.S. Government Printing Office.

7 Kessler RC, Koretz D, Merikangas K, et al. The epidemiology of adult mental disorders. In: Lubotsky LB, Petrila J, Hennessy KD, eds. *Mental Health Services: A Public Health Perspective*. Toronto: Oxford University Press, 2004:157–76.

8 Mechanic D. Is the prevalence of mental disorders a good measure of the need for services? *Health Aff (Millwood)* 2003;22:8–20.

9 Slade M, Powell R, Strathdee G. Current approaches to identifying the severely mentally ill. *Soc Psychiatry Psychiatr Epidemiol* 1997;32:177–84.

10 Bijl RV, de Graaf R, Hiripi E, et al. The prevalence of treated and untreated mental disorders in five countries. *Health Aff (Millwood)* 2003;22:122–33.

11 Ruggeri M, Leese M, Thornicroft G, et al. Definition and prevalence of severe and persistent mental illness. *Br J Psychiatry* 2000;177:149–55.

12 Narrow WE, Rae DS, Robins LN, et al. Revised prevalence estimates of mental disorders in the United States: Using a clinical significance criterion to reconcile 2 surveys' estimates. *Arch Gen Psychiatry* 2002;59:115–23.

13 Bachrach LL. Defining chronic mental illness: A concept paper. *Hosp Comm Psychiatry* 1988;39:383–8.

14 Barker A, Gregoire A. Defining severe mental illness. In: Gregoire A, ed. *Adult Severe Mental Illness*. London: Greenwich Medical Media Ltd., 2000:1–9.

15 Kovess V, Labarte S, Olivier JC. Modeles de soins et categories sociopro-fessionnelles a partir des donnees recueillies par le DIM du dispositif psychiatrique de la MGEN. *Encephale* 2001;27:205–11.

16 Kovess V, Lesage A, Boisguerin B, et al. *Planification et Évaluation des Besoins en Santé Mentale*. Paris: Flammarion, 2001.

17 Kirby MJL, Keon WJ. *Out of the Shadows at Last: Transforming Mental Health, Mental Illness and Addiction Services in Canada*. Ottawa: Final Report of the Standing Senate Committee on Social Affairs, Science and Technology, 2006.

18 Kirby MJL, Keon WJ. *Mental Health, Mental Illness and Addiction*. Ottawa: Interim Report of the Standing Senate Committee on Social Affairs, Science and Technology, 2004.

19 Wing JK, Brewin CR, Thornicroft G. Defining mental health needs. In: Thornicroft G, ed. *Measuring Mental Health Needs*. 2nd ed. London: The Royal College of Psychiatrists, 2001:1–21.

20 Brewin CR, Wing JK, Mangen SP, et al. Needs for care among the long-term mentally ill: A report from the Camberwell High Contact Survey. *Psychol Med* 1988;18:457–68.

21 Thornicroft G, Tansella M. *What Are the Arguments for Community-based Mental Health Care?* Copenhagen: World Health Organization, 2003.
22 Kessler RC, Merikangas KR, Berglund P, et al. Mild disorders should not be eliminated from the DSM-V. *Arch Gen Psychiatry* 2003;60:1117–22.
23 Andrews G, Henderson, S. *Unmet Need in Psychiatry.* Cambridge University Press, 2000.
24 Wing JK. Severe Mental Illness. [cited August 28, 2007]. Available at: http://hcna.radcliffe-oxford.com/mentalframe.htm.
25 Lesage AD, Bonsack C, Clerc D, et al. Alternatives to acute hospital psychiatric care in east-end Montreal. *Can J Psychiatry* 2002;47:49–55.
26 Lesage AD, Gelinas D, Robitaille D, et al. Toward benchmarks for tertiary care for adults with severe and persistent mental disorders. *Can J Psychiatry* 2003;48:485–92.
27 Reinharz D, Contandriopoulos AP, Lesage AD. Organizational analysis of deinstitutionalization in a psychiatric hospital. *Can J Psychiatry* 2000;45:539–43.
28 Vasiliadis HM, Briand C, Lesage A, et al. Health care resource use associated with integrated psychological treatment. *J Ment Health Policy Econ* 2006;9:201–7.
29 Amaddeo F, Beecham J, Bonizzato P, et al. The use of a case register to evaluate the costs of psychiatric care. *Acta Psychiatr Scand* 1997;95:189–98.
30 Smith P, Sheldon TA, Martin S. An index of need for psychiatric services based on in-patient utilisation. *Br J Psychiatry* 1996;169:308–16.
31 Lesage AD, Clerc D, Uribe I, et al. Estimating local-area needs for psychiatric care: A case study. *Br J Psychiatry* 1996;169:49–57.
32 Croudace TJ, Kayne R, Jones PB, et al. Non-linear relationship between an index of social deprivation, psychiatric admission prevalence and the incidence of psychosis. *Psychol Med* 2000;30:177–85.
33 Goeree R, Farahati F, Burke N, et al. The economic burden of schizophrenia in Canada in 2004. *Curr Med Res Opin* 2005;21:2017–28.
34 Blomqvist AG, Leger PT, Hoch JS. The cost of schizophrenia: Lessons from an international comparison. *J Ment Health Policy Econ* 2006;9:177–83.
35 Thornicroft G, Tansella M, Becker T, et al. The personal impact of schizophrenia in Europe. *Schizophr Res* 2004;69:125–32.
36 Thornicroft G TM. *The Mental Health Matrix. A Manual to Improve Services.* Cambridge: Cambridge University Press, 1999.
37 Carpentier N, Lesage A, Goulet J, et al. Burden of care of families not living with young schizophrenic relatives. *Hosp Community Psychiatry* 1992;43:38–43.

38 Warner R, de Girolamo G, Belelli G, et al. The quality of life of people
    with schizophrenia in Boulder, Colorado, and Bologna, Italy. *Schizophr
    Bull* 1998;24:559–68.

39 van Wijngaarden B, Schene A, Koeter M, et al. People with schizophrenia
    in five countries: Conceptual similarities and intercultural differences in
    family caregiving. *Schizophr Bull* 2003;29:573–86.

40 North CS, Eyrich KM, Pollio DE, et al. Are rates of psychiatric disorders
    in the homeless population changing? *Am J Pub Health* 2004;94:103–8.

41 Fryers T. Estimation of need on the basis of case register studies: British
    case register data. In: Hafner H, ed. *Estimating Needs for Mental Health
    Care: A Contribution of Epidemiology*. Berlin: Springer Verlag, 1979:52–63.

42 Sartorius N, Gulbinat W, Harrison G, et al. Long-term follow-up of schiz-
    ophrenia in 16 countries. A description of the International Study of
    Schizophrenia conducted by the World Health Organization. *Soc Psychia-
    try Psychiatr Epidemiol* 1996;31:249–58.

43 Harding CM, Brooks GW, Ashikaga T, et al. The Vermont longitudinal
    study of persons with severe mental illness. I: Methodology, study
    sample, and overall status 32 years later. *Am J Psychiatry* 1987;144:718–26.

44 an der Heiden W, Hafner H. The epidemiology of onset and course of
    schizophrenia. *Eur Arch Psychiatry Clin Neurosci* 2000;250:292–303.

45 Bromet EJ, Naz B, Fochtmann LJ, et al. Long-term diagnostic stability and
    outcome in recent first-episode cohort studies of schizophrenia. *Schizophr
    Bull* 2005;31:639–49.

46 Donabedian A. Evaluating the quality of medical care. *Milbank Mem Fund
    Q* 1966;44(suppl):166–206.

47 Holloway F, Carson J, Davis S. Rehabilitation in the United Kingdom:
    Research, policy, and practice. *Can J Psychiatry* 2002;47:628–34.

48 Slade M, Powell R, Rosen A, et al. Threshold Assessment Grid (TAG):
    The development of a valid and brief scale to assess the severity of
    mental illness. *Soc Psychiatry Psychiatr Epidemiol* 2000;35:78–85.

49 Parabiaghi A, Bonetto C, Ruggeri M, et al. Severe and persistent mental
    illness: A useful definition for prioritizing community-based mental
    health service interventions. *Soc Psychiatry Psychiatr Epidemiol*
    2006;41:457–63.

50 Bisson J, Lesage, AD, Bouchard, C. *Le Profil Clinique de la Clientèle des
    Cliniques Externes de l'Hôpital Louis-H. Lafontaine*. 2004. Available at:
    http://www.hlhl.qc.ca/ pdf/profil_clin_client_2004.pdf

51 Kessler RC, Merikangas KR, Wang PS. Prevalence, comorbidity, and
    service utilization for mood disorders in the United States at the begin-
    ning of the twenty-first century. *Annu Rev Clin Psychol* 2007;3:137–58.

52 Kessler RC, Demler O, Frank RG, et al. Prevalence and treatment of mental disorders, 1990 to 2003. *N Engl J Med* 2005;352:2515–23.

53 Kessler RC, Berglund PA, Glantz MD, et al. Estimating the prevalence and correlates of serious mental illness in community epidemiological surveys. In: Manderscheid RW, Henderson MJ, eds. *Mental Health, United States, 2002.* Rockville, MD: U.S. Department of Health and Human Services, Substance Abuse and Mental Health Services Administration, Center for Mental Health Services, 2002:155–64.

54 Lesage AD, Vasiliadis HM, Gagné MA, et al. *Prevalence of Mental Illnesses and Related Service Utilisation in Canada: An Analysis of the Canadian Community Health Survey.* Report prepared for the Canadian Collaborative Mental Health Initiative. Mississauga, Ontario, 2006. Available at: http://www.ccmhi.ca/en/products/documents/ 09_Prevalence_EN.pdf

55 Kessler RC, Barker PR, Colpe LJ, et al. Screening for serious mental illness in the general population. *Arch Gen Psychiatry* 2003;60:184–9.

56 van Os J, Hanssen M, Bijl RV, et al. Prevalence of psychotic disorder and community level of psychotic symptoms: an urban-rural comparison. *Arch Gen Psychiatry* 2001;58:663–8.

57 Faris RE, Dunham, W. *Mental Disorders in Urban Areas: An Ecological Study of Schizophrenia and Other Psychoses.* Chicago: University of Chicago Press, 1939.

58 Kates N, Krett E. Socio-economic factors and mental health problems: Can census-tract data predict referral patterns? *Can J Comm Ment Health* 1988;7:89–98.

59 Roberge M, Lesage, AD. *Modélisation des Besoins des Services de Santé Mentale de la Population de la Région de Montréal-Centre, V 2.3: Services de Santé Mentale.* Régie régionale de la santé et des services sociaux de Montréal-Centre, 2000.

60 Glover G, Arts G, Wooff D. A needs index for mental health care in England based on updatable data. *Soc Psychiatry Psychiatr Epidemiol* 2004;39:730–8.

61 Insel TR, Fenton WS. Psychiatric epidemiology: It's not just about counting anymore. *Arch Gen Psychiatry* 2005;62:590–2.

62 Goldberg D, Thornicroft, G. *Mental Health in Our Future Cities.* Maudsley Monograph 42. Published by Psychology Press: London, 1998.

9 The Epidemiology of Co-occurring Substance Use and Other Mental Disorders in Canada: Prevalence, Service Use, and Unmet Needs

BRIAN R. RUSH, KAREN A. URBANOSKI, DIEGO G. BASSANI,
SAULO CASTEL, AND T. CAMERON WILD

A wealth of population data measuring substance use, abuse, and mental health has recently emerged in Canada, allowing researchers to generate national prevalences of co-occurring substance use and mental disorders, and to examine a wide range of related questions and hypotheses about treatment needs and health service utilization. In this chapter, we provide a brief summary of the extant international literature on these topics, and summarize key findings from a comprehensive research program using the Canadian Community Health Survey (cycle 1.2) to explore the comorbidity of substance use and other mental disorders in Canada. In addition to prevalence estimates, our work examines sociodemographic profiles of individuals with co-occurring disorders, assesses regional differences, and provides an analysis of issues related to help-seeking, including service satisfaction and unmet needs for care.

Co-occurring Disorders: An Issue of Importance

The high rate of co-occurrence of substance use and other mental disorders in the community has been recognized for almost two decades, with the first such findings reported from the National Institutes of Health's Epidemiologic Catchment Area (ECA) study.[1] Since that time, this phenomenon has been replicated in numerous community-based population surveys conducted in the United States,[2–5] Canada,[6,7] Australia and New Zealand,[8,9] Europe,[10–14] and Latin America.[15] It is estimated that 1% to 2% of adults in the general population experience co-occurring mood or anxiety and substance use disorders in a 12-month period.[3,10,16] Although this percentage is small, it does amount to a large number of individuals when aggregated across the entire population. It is also instructive to consider the situation from the perspective of the subpopulation of individuals with either one of the disorders. For instance, synthesizing data from community-based population surveys internationally, a recent review estimated that between 7% to 45% of survey respondents with an alcohol use disorder and 9% to 56% of those with an illicit drug use disorder also have a 12-month comorbid mood or anxiety disorder.[17] Clinical studies of those in either substance abuse or mental health treatment centres have confirmed an even higher rate of overlap,[18–20] in part because the 'double trouble' of co-occurring disorders increases the likelihood of help-seeking.[21]

A large body of population and clinical research evidence is also available demonstrating that, compared to individuals with either type of disorder alone (i.e., 'pure' disorders), those with co-occurring substance use and other mental disorders have increased risks of experiencing a variety of negative consequences including suicide, arrests and incarceration, homelessness, family conflict, violent and disruptive behaviour, victimization, and physical health problems.[22–26] This research also documents higher use of health care services for individuals with comorbid disorders, including hospital and emergency services.[24,25,27–29] When presenting for treatment, people with comorbid disorders report greater psychiatric symptom severity, elevated distress, and diminished quality of life.[20,30] Finally, many studies have demonstrated negative effects of psychiatric comorbidity on substance abuse treatment outcomes,[31–37] including higher rates of relapse and readmission to treatment.[38] Attenuated treatment engagement and early dropout have been identified as key factors contributing to these negative outcomes.[36,39,40]

Despite the high degree of overlap of substance use and other mental disorders and its impact on a range of health and social outcomes, evidence indicates that mental health and addiction service providers consistently fail to detect comorbidity and, consequently, fail to develop integrated treatment and support plans.[41,42] Routine screening and assessment of mental disorders among clients in addiction treatment services, and vice versa, has been posited as a necessary first step in facilitating adequate treatment planning and positive treatment outcomes.[24,43–47] Similarly, it is widely acknowledged that the planning, funding, and administration of addiction and mental health service delivery systems have been too segregated.[24,28] This 'siloing' undermines detection of comorbid disorders among presenting patients and has slowed development of integrated care at the clinical level, despite promising evidence on the efficacy of an integrated clinical approach over services offered in parallel or consecutively.[48–51] Taken together, these findings have spurred interest in identifying and disseminating empirically supported treatments and best practice guidelines at both the service and system levels. Such efforts attempt to increase identification rates, improve outcomes through more integrated treatment, and reduce associated consequences and costs to individuals, families, and society as a whole.

Historically in Canada, the development of policies and the planning and delivery of services for people with substance use and/or other mental disorders has not adequately considered the rates of co-occurring versus pure substance use and other mental disorders in the general population and the degree of overlap in these populations.[24] Poor coordination of services across disparate service sectors mirrors the situation in the United States and many other developed countries. Bridging the gap between these historically divided service sectors requires the attention and commitment of policy makers and funders. These parties, in turn, require reliable and valid data on the level of need in the population. To date, efforts to disseminate best practice guidelines and system-level recommendations have been hampered by a paucity of Canadian and regional data on the prevalence and sociodemographic correlates of the co-occurrence of mental and substance use disorders. The aim of this chapter is to synthesize what has been gleaned from our program of secondary analyses of the Canadian Community Health Survey cycle 1.2 (CCHS 1.2) to fill this gap in knowledge.

Methods and Classification of Co-occurring Disorders

The CCHS is a cross-sectional population health survey conducted biennially by Statistics Canada. Cycle 1.2, conducted in 2002, focused on mental health and well-being and was the first attempt to generate national estimates of the burden of mental and substance use disorders in Canada ($n = 36,984$, response rate = 77%). A detailed description of the survey is available elsewhere[52] (see also chapter 5).

Mental disorders were defined according to a modified version of the World Mental Health Composite International Diagnostic Interview (WMH-CIDI),[53] which uses the diagnostic categories of the *DSM-*

IV.[54] The present work used survey data on the 12-month prevalence of major depressive episode, manic episode, panic disorder, social phobia, and agoraphobia.Ψ

Additional items probed into past-12-month alcohol and illicit drug use, problems, and dependence symptoms. Several illicit drugs were covered, including cannabis, cocaine and crack, speed and other amphetamines, ecstasy (MDMA), hallucinogens, glue or solvents, heroin, and steroids. Twelve-month dependence symptoms were assessed separately for alcohol, and for all illicit drugs combined (i.e., dependence on *specific* illicit drugs was not covered). In the present analyses, respondents who endorsed three or more of the alcohol or illicit drug dependence symptoms were classified as exhibiting *dependence*. Past-12-month drinkers or illicit drug users who reported one or two of the alcohol or illicit drug dependence symptoms were classified as *problem drinkers or problem users without dependence*. Three additional items assessed psychosocial consequences of alcohol use. Individuals who endorsed any of these three items (but who did not meet the criteria for dependence, as described) were similarly classified as *problem drinkers without dependence*. A corresponding set of items for the psychosocial consequences of illicit drug use was not included in the survey. Those who had used alcohol or illicit drugs in the past 12 months, but did not report consequences or dependence symptoms, were classified as *non-problem drinkers or users*. Finally, those who reported no use of alcohol or illicit drugs in the year prior to the survey were classified as *abstainers*. In summary, two four-level categorical variables were created to measure respondents' alcohol and other drug use and related problems in the 12-months preceding the survey: (1) abstainers; (2) non-problem drinkers or illicit drug users; (3) problem drinkers or illicit drug users without dependence; and (4) individuals with alcohol or illicit drug dependence. To ensure adequate sample size and to maximize reliability of parameter estimates, categories three and four were combined for some analyses, and are referred to as *alcohol use problems* and *illicit drug use problems*. Finally, a third four-level categorical variable was also created to represent 12-month *substance use and problems*, with alcohol and illicit drugs combined.

Prevalence and Correlates of Co-occurring Disorders

A total of 9.5% of the Canadian population met criteria for alcohol dependence (2.2%) or problem drinking (7.3%). A total of 3.0% of the population met criteria for illicit drug dependence (1.1%) or illicit drug problems (1.9%). Combining the two, an estimated 11% of the Canadian population experienced substance use problems in the 12 months prior to the survey, 8.0% meeting the criteria for problem use and 3.0% for dependence. In addition, 8.4% of Canadians met the criteria for a 12-month mental disorder, including 5.2% for any mood disorder and 4.7% for any anxiety disorder. Table 9.1 provides a detailed summary of these prevalence rates with projected estimates of the number of Canadians in each category. These projections assist in the interpretation of the rates of overlap in substance use and other mental disorders presented in subsequent sections.

In the following sections, prevalence rates of co-occurring disorders are calculated in two ways. First, the prevalence of co-occurring mental disorders *among those with alcohol or illicit drug use problems* is presented. While other population data are available for substance use and related problems,[55] these represent the first available estimates of co-occurring mental disorders among those with substance use problems at the national population level in Canada. Second, the prevalence of co-occurring mental disorders and substance use problems is presented for the entire Canadian population. These population-based rates will be of particular interest to public health practitioners and policy makers for examining broader population trends and subtle differences between individuals living with these disorders in the community. These population prevalence estimates are also used in the multivariate analyses of correlates and help-seeking patterns, presented in the following sections. In each case, 12-month rates are used, as opposed to lifetime rates, as these are assumed to more adequately reflect needs of individuals meeting criteria for disorders at the time of their participation in the survey. All estimates are weighted to the general adult population of Canada (15 years +).

Comorbidity among Those with Substance Use Problems

The rate of mood and anxiety disorders among those reporting substance use problems was 15.9%, approximately double that among those with no substance use problems (7.5%). In accordance with previous literature,[1,5,17,56] co-occurring mental disorders were more common among those with illicit drug use problems than those with alcohol use problems (26.3% vs. 14.3%). Also similar to previous work,[56] we identified a 'dose-response' relationship, whereby the

Table 9.1
National prevalence of pure and co-occurring substance use and other mental disorders, 95% confidence intervals (CI), and estimated population size.

	Prevalence[a]	(95% CI)	Projected population size
Pure disorders			
Alcohol			
Abstainers	23.0	(18.9;28.7)	5,707,893
Non-problem users	67.6	(61.5;73.1)	16,809,830
Problem users	7.3	(5.9;8.9)	1,803,753
Dependence	2.2	(1.9;2.6)	551,024
Illicit drugs			
Abstainers	88.4	(85.0;91.1)	22,021,966
Non-problem users	8.6	(6.6;11.2)	2,155,006
Problem users	1.9	(1.5;2.5)	477,125
Dependence	1.1	(0.8;1.5)	266,339
Any substance			
Abstainers	22.6	(17.8;28.3)	5,653,727
Non-problem users	66.4	(60.6;71.7)	16,583,384
Problem users	8.0	(6.6;9.7)	2,003,574
Dependence	3.0	(2.4;3.6)	738,595
Mental disorders (MD)			
Mood disorders	5.2	(5.0;5.6)	1,309,347
Anxiety disorders	4.6	(4.1;5.2)	1,161,952
Any mood/anxiety disorder	8.4	(8.0;8.8)	2,098,354
Co-occurring disorders			
Alcohol & MD	1.3	(1.1;1.7)	336,761
Drugs & MD	0.8	(0.6;1.0)	196,013
Any substance & MD	1.7	(1.4;2.2)	435,050

[a] Reported estimates are percentages (%)

prevalence of co-occurring mental disorders was higher among those with dependence versus less severe problems, or non-problematic use (figure 9.1). These findings are relevant for public health messaging around prevention of co-occurring disorders, as well as in treatment system development. For example, services targeted specifically at illicit drug treatment and/or more severe cases of addiction should be particularly proactive in both screening for mental disorders and the provision of integrated assessment and treatment options.

Another common finding in the international literature is that, among people with substance use disorders, the prevalence of mood and anxiety disorders is generally higher among women, while among those with mood and anxiety disorders, the prevalence of substance use disorders is higher for men.[2] These patterns mirror gender differences in the population rates of pure mental and substance use disorders,[57,58] and were replicated in the present analysis (figure 9.2). For instance, 22.0% of women with alcohol use problems met the criteria for a mood or anxiety disorder, compared to 11.6% of men. Fully one-third of women with drug use problems had another co-occurring mental disorder, compared to 23.6% of men.

Of the age groups examined in figure 9.3, the prevalence of co-occurring mental disorders among those with alcohol use problems was somewhat lower for the over age 55 group (9% compared to the other categories between 14% and 15%). Compared to alcohol use problems, the prevalence for illicit drug use problems was higher across all age groups for which reliable estimates are available. Combining across alcohol and illicit drug use problems, the prevalence of co-occurring mood and anxiety disorders varied from 15.6% of those aged 15–24 and 25–34 years, to 15.4% of 35–44 year olds, 15.7% of 45–54 year olds, and 10.0% of those aged 55 years and older.

Figure 9.4 presents regional differences across Canada in the prevalence of co-occurring mental disorders among those with past-year alcohol and illicit drug use problems. As with gender and age, the prevalence of a co-occurring mental disorder was consistently higher across all regions for those with illicit drug use problems compared to those with alcohol use problems. The prevalence of co-occurring mental disorders among those with alcohol use problems did not vary appreciably across the regions (i.e., from 13%–16%). Conversely, the prevalence of co-occurring disorders among those with illicit drug use problems is lower in Quebec (18%) and the Prairies (24%), relative to Atlantic Canada (31%), Ontario (30%), and British Columbia (34%). Combining across alcohol and drug use problems, the prevalence of mood and anxiety disorders among those with substance use problems was 16.0% in Atlantic Canada, 17.2% in British Columbia, and 18.0% in Ontario, with lower levels in Quebec (13.5%) and the Prairies (13.4%).

Figure 9.1 Odds of a past-year co-occurring mental disorder by level of substance use and related problems[a]

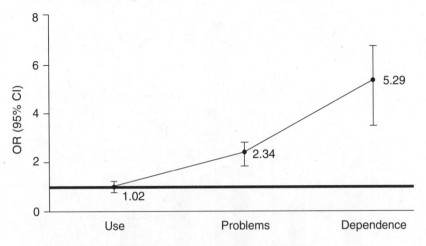

ᵃ Relative to those who were abstinent in the year prior to the survey

Figure 9.2 Prevalence of co-occurring mental disorders among those with alcohol and illlicit drug use problems, by gender

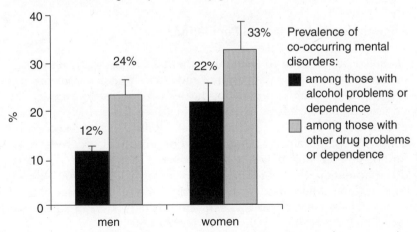

Figure 9.3 Prevalence of co-occurring mental disorders among those with alcohol and illlicit drug use problems, by age group

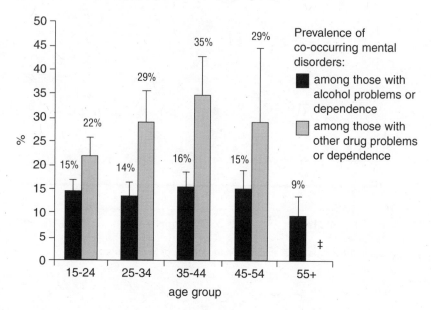

‡ Estimate suppressed due to small sample size (n < 30)

Comorbidity in the General Population

As noted, in addition to examining the rates of co-occurring mental disorders among those with alcohol and illicit drug use problems, it is also of interest from a population health perspective to examine the prevalence and correlates of co-occurring disorders in the population as a whole. In the total survey sample, the prevalence of co-occurring substance use problems and any mood or anxiety disorder was 1.4% for females, 2.1% for males, and 1.7% overall. Projecting to the Canadian population, this represents approximately 435,000 adults. Prevalence estimates decreased with age: from 3.8% of 15–24 year olds, to 2.6% of 25–34 year olds, 2.0% of 35–45 year olds, 1.1% of 45–54 year olds, and 0.2% of those 55 years and older.

We used multivariate multinomial logistic regression to explore the

Figure 9.4 Prevalence of co-occurring mental disorders among those with alcohol and illicit substance use problems, by region of Canada

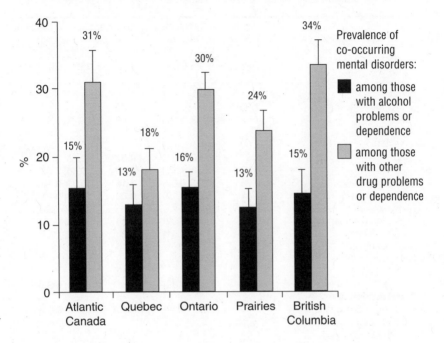

correlates of comorbidity in more detail and present a population-based profile of co-occurring disorders in a Canadian context. Table 9.2 presents results from the analysis estimating the odds of comorbidity relative to those with no disorders, adjusting for selected sociodemographic characteristics and other covariates associated with mental and substance use problems in bivariate analyses. These include gender, age, marital status, nationality of birth, social support, household income, employment, education, and geographic region.

Demographic Characteristics

Male gender was strongly associated with co-occurring disorders, for both alcohol and illicit drug use problems. This stands in contrast to the gender differences in comorbidity in the subset of individuals with substance use problems (see figure 9.2), and reflects population

Table 9.2

Multivariate associations between the demographic and socioeconomic variables and alcohol use problems and illicit drug use problems and other mental disorders[a]

	Alcohol use problems & other mental disorders		Illicit drug use problems & other mental disorders	
	OR	(99% CI)	OR	(99% CI)
Gender				
Women	1.00		1.00	
Men	1.74	(1.52; 1.97)	1.60	(1.18; 2.15)
Age				
15–24	1.00		1.00	
25–34	0.97	(0.40; 2.31)	0.97	(0.28; 3.38)
35–44	0.77	(0.36; 1.65)	0.70	(0.15; 3.09)
45–64	0.36	(0.21; 0.62)	0.16	(0.03; 0.77)
65 and over	0.01	(0.01; 0.10)	0.03	(0.02; 0.21)
Marital status				
Married/common-law	0.52	(0.44; 0.62)	0.36	(0.26; 0.50)
Widow/sep/div	1.92	(1.47; 2.51)	1.23	(0.94; 1.61)
Single/never married	1.00		1.00	
Nationality at birth				
Canadian	1.00		1.00	
Other	0.30	(0.23; 0.39)	0.31	(0.26; 0.36)
Social support (0 to 76)				
Per each 5 points in scale	0.79	(0.72; 0.88)	0.80	(0.75; 0.84)
Income adequacy				
Low	1.00		1.00	
Lower-middle	0.72	(0.57; 0.87)	0.58	(0.43; 0.75)
Upper-middle	0.76	(0.59; 0.95)	0.68	(0.39; 1.18)
High	1.13	(0.72; 1.79)	0.63	(0.39; 1.01)
Education				
< Secondary	1.00		1.00	
Secondary graduate	1.38	(1.11; 1.96)	0.93	(0.59; 1.47)
Some post-secondary	1.50	(1.29; 2.17)	0.99	(0.78; 1.26)
Post-secondary graduate	0.81	(0.67; 1.27)	0.73	(0.59; 0.91)
Working status				
Had job last week	1.00		1.00	
No job last week	0.73	(0.37; 1.45)	1.84	(1.47; 2.12)
Unable/permanently disabled	2.40	(1.30; 4.41)	6.27	(4.76; 7.85)
Geographic region[b]				
Atlantic Canada	1.18	(0.65; 2.15)	0.98	(0.30; 3.27)
Quebec	0.64	(0.55; 0.75)	0.73	(0.53; 1.03)
Ontario	1.07	(0.91; 1.27)	0.97	(0.69; 1.37)
Prairies	0.99	(0.76; 1.29)	0.88	(0.42; 1.84)
British Columbia	1.24	(1.05; 1.46)	1.61	(1.15; 2.26)

[a] Reference category: no disorders

[b] Rather than selecting one region to serve as the reference category (i.e., dummy coding), effect coding was used such that the reference category within this variable is the weighted national rate.

differences in the gender distribution of pure substance use disorders. This finding in particular, therefore, highlights the importance of selecting the appropriate method for calculating comorbidity rates, as the choice of denominators (i.e., the full population versus a specific disorder subgroup) can have implications for findings and interpretation.

The odds of co-occurring disorders decreased with increasing age, and were lowest among those who were married, relative to single individuals. Those who were widowed, separated, or divorced had elevated odds of co-occurring mental disorders and alcohol use problems. These findings are largely similar to those found in other jurisdictions.[17] Finally, the odds of co-occurring disorders were significantly lower among immigrants to Canada. A recent study using CCHS 1.2 data has shown a lower rate of substance use problems among immigrants to Canada[59] and other work has reported that the risk of mental disorders among immigrants varies by place of origin, and increases with length of time in Canada.[60] One may expect to find, therefore, lower rates of co-occurring disorders among those who have newly immigrated to Canada. This pattern is also consistent with U.S. studies assessing the relationship between immigration status and substance use and other mental disorders,[61,62] but stands in contrast to studies from many European countries, which report higher rates of disorders among immigrants from Eastern Europe, the Caribbean, and elsewhere.[63,64] Health and social disparities between country of origin and country of immigration, as well as variation in screening processes and criteria, may account for reported differences on the relationship between immigration status and substance use and other mental disorders separately. To our knowledge, the association between co-occurring disorders and immigration status has not been previously reported in a representative population sample.

Social Support

The CCHS 1.2 included the Medical Outcomes Study (MOS) Social Support Survey.[65] The scale assesses levels of emotional, informational, and tangible support, positive social interaction and affection (range 0–76, with higher scores indicating greater social support). The odds of co-occurring disorders, relative to no disorders, decreased by approximately 20% with each five-point increase in the scale. In other words, greater social support was associated with a lower odds of comorbidity.

Socioeconomic Status

The CCHS provided a measure of income adequacy, adjusted for household size.† Relative to those in the lowest income adequacy category, the odds of co-occurring disorders were lowest for the lower-middle income adequacy group. This held for both alcohol and illicit drug use problems. The odds of co-occurring disorders were also lower among those in the upper-middle income category for alcohol use problems. The association with education was more complex, however. Relative to those with less than secondary school education, those who had graduated high school or who had some post-secondary education had elevated odds of co-occurring mental disorders and alcohol use problems. In contrast, those who had completed post-secondary education had lower odds of co-occurring mental disorders and illicit drug use problems.

Relative to those who reported working in the past week, those who did not work because they were unable due to disability had elevated odds of co-occurring disorders, for both alcohol and illicit drug use problems. Those who reported having no job in the past week for other reasons also had an elevated odds of co-occurring mental disorders and illicit drug use problems. Others have also noted particularly elevated rates of past-week unemployment and days of restricted activity among those with co-occurring disorders.[66,67] It should be mentioned, however, that household population surveys such as the CCHS are not designed for the study of individuals suffering from chronic unemployment, homelessness, or extreme poverty. Furthermore, due to the cross-sectional nature of the survey, it is not possible to determine with these data whether comorbidity leads to increased unemployment and lower income adequacy, or vice versa. The mechanisms underlying these relationships are likely to be multifaceted and complex, with numerous intervening factors at both individual and societal levels.

Geographic Region

There was a significantly elevated rate of co-occurring mental disorders and illicit substance problems in British Columbia compared to the national rate, as well as an elevated rate of co-occurring alcohol use problems and mental disorders. The odds of co-occurring mental disorders and illicit drug use problems were lowest in Quebec, although not statistically different from the national rate. Quebec had significantly lower odds of alcohol use problems and other mental disorders. These findings largely mirror a recent study examining the geographical prevalence of substance problems across Canada, in which rates were significantly lower than the national rate in Quebec, but significantly elevated in the western provinces.[59]

These are the first estimates of co-occurring disorders at a regional level in Canada and they warrant further exploration. In particular, the lower rates of co-occurrence in Quebec leave open an important question about potential protective or moderating factors in this province. The notably higher rates of co-occurring illicit drug use problems and other mental disorders among individuals living in British Columbia may be due to provincial variability in lifestyle, as well as factors related to broader health care and social and legal policies. However, without further data, it is not possible to explore these issues in more depth.

Co-occurring Disorders and Help-Seeking

It is a ubiquitous finding in the international literature that only a minority of individuals with substance use and/or other mental disorders seek professional help for their problems.[9,11,12,68,69] Even after adjusting for illness severity, the proportion of those with a substance use disorder or mental disorder diagnosis who report service use varies from 50% to 65% .[9,69–72] Also, previous research has consistently found that those with co-occurring mental and substance use disorders are more likely than those with either disorder alone to seek help.[12,73–76]

Based on the CCHS 1.2 data, 9.4% of all Canadians sought help for mental health or addiction-related concerns in 2001 (for a more detailed presentation of these findings see).[77] This amounted to 39% of those who met the criteria for a 12-month disorder, ranging from 13.6% of those with pure substance dependence, 44.1% of those with a mood or anxiety disorder, and 50.6% of those with co-occurring disorders. Here, *service use* is defined as the past-year use of a comprehensive array of formal and informal sources of mental health and addiction-related care, including hospital services, visits to physicians, psychologists, social workers, and other trained professionals, as well as self-help and internet support groups, and telephone helplines. In considering the link between help-seeking and comorbidity, *substance dependence*, rather than substance use problems, is used because it is more closely associated with need and demand for health-care services.

The most commonly used source of care was general practitioners, reported by 6.2% of those with pure substance dependence, 31.6% of those with pure mood/anxiety disorders, and 34.6% of those with co-occurring disorders. Notably, 27% of those who had used services in the prior year saw *only* a general practitioner. This may be expected given the exclusion of individuals living in institutions, as well as the lack of survey coverage of psychotic disorders, which are more commonly treated by mental health specialists. Numerous other studies have noted the predominance of general medical care for mood and anxiety disorders in other jurisdictions and health care systems.[9,11,68,69,78,79]

Other commonly reported sources of care included psychiatrists (1.8% of those with pure substance dependence, 14.1% of those with pure mood/anxiety disorders, and 16.1% of those with co-occurring disorders), psychologists (2.3% of those with pure substance dependence, 10.0% of those with pure mood/anxiety disorders, and 11.0% of those with co-occurring disorders), and social workers (4.8% of those with pure substance dependence, 11.3% of those with pure mood/anxiety disorders, and 15.1% of those with co-occurring disorders).

The present findings clearly indicate that the likelihood of service use is elevated among those with a mental disorder, *with or without* co-occurring substance dependence. To examine this issue further, multivariate binary and multinomial logistic regressions were conducted to estimate the odds of any service use and of the number of services used in the year prior to the survey, adjusting for factors known to be associated with help-seeking, including diagnoses and comorbidity, gender, age, education, mental distress, and frequency and quantity of substance use (see table 9.3). Relative to those with no mental disorder, the odds of any service use were significantly elevated for those with any diagnosis and were highest among those with co-occurring disorders. The association between substance dependence and help-seeking, although statistically significant, was small relative to that of other mental disorders.

In addition, those with substance dependence reported greater psychological distress than those with no disorder, but lower levels than those with other mental disorders (data not shown, see).[77] Previous research has also noted a lower impact of addiction disorders on dis-

Table 9.3
Adjusted odds of service use by diagnostic group.

	Used any service[a]		Number of services used[b]			
			1 vs. 2		1 vs. 3+	
	AOR[c]	95% CI	AOR	95% CI	AOR	95% CI
No disorder	1.00		1.00		1.00	
Pure substance dependence	2.07**	1.49, 2.89	2.40*	1.12, 5.11	4.05**	2.12, 7.72
Pure mental disorders	4.68**	3.97, 5.52	2.27**	1.72, 2.99	2.88**	2.09, 3.96
Co-occurring disorders	5.21**	2.98, 9.11	1.31	0.70, 2.47	5.62**	2.99, 10.57

[a] analysis includes full sample (unweighted N=34747)
[b] analysis includes those who used services in the past year (unweighted N=3526)
[c] adjusted odds ratio; adjusted for gender, age, education, mental distress, and frequency and quantity of substance use
* p<.05; ** p<.001

ability,[8,75,80–82] perceived need for care,[80,83] and help-seeking,[69,70] relative to mood and anxiety disorders. The experience of substance-related problems in the general population may therefore play a relatively minor role in bringing people into care. Alternatively, it is possible that personal factors such as low motivation to change use or enter treatment, and societal factors such as social stigma and negative attitudes are barriers to seeking and receiving care for substance-related concerns.[84,85]

Among those who reported using services in the year prior to the survey, there was little variation in the numbers of different services used by diagnostic group: the mean number of services used was 1.8 among those with substance dependence, 2.0 among those with pure mood or anxiety disorders, and 2.3 among those with co-occurring disorders. However, those with co-occurring disorders had six times the odds of using three or more services relative to those with no disorder (table 9.3).

Satisfaction with Services

Respondents who reported using services in the past year were asked whether they were generally satisfied with these services and whether they were helpful. Satisfaction was fairly high in this sub-sample, with

71% of those with co-occurring disorders reporting satisfaction with the care they received, compared to 78% of those with pure substance dependence and 84% of those with pure mood or anxiety disorders. In addition, 65% of those with co-occurring disorders reported that the care they received had been helpful, in comparison to 72% and 79% of those with pure mental disorders and substance dependence, respectively. In other words, while the vast majority of all individuals with disorders who sought care reflected positively on the experience, satisfaction and perceived helpfulness was lower among those with co-occurring disorders. Satisfaction with care can affect compliance with prescribed interventions, treatment outcomes, and future patterns of help-seeking,[86,87] and is therefore a highly relevant aspect of the help-seeking process. Importantly, this finding may speak to system-level inadequacies in the management of co-occurring disorders.[84,85,88] It is also possible to speculate on the role of personal factors such as poor motivation or care preferences (e.g., dissatisfaction with a care plan that involves medications negatively viewed as substitutes for substances of abuse), as well as stigma and the attitudes of professionals on consumer satisfaction with the process of care;[84] however, this issue cannot be addressed specifically without a more in-depth consideration of additional real and perceived aspects of the adequacy of care.

Perceived Unmet Need

Other than objective considerations of need, such as diagnosis, numerous perceptual, attitudinal, predisposing, and enabling factors are known to influence decisions to seek health care.[89] Those who report a need for help but do not go on to seek services are of particular interest, as perceptions of unmet need may influence health outcomes, attitudes toward health care, and future help-seeking behaviours. Such perceptions are associated with many of the same factors associated with help-seeking, including comorbid diagnoses, mental health status, disability, and distress.[77,90–93] In health care systems such as Canada's, which attempts to limit financial barriers to care, it is of interest to examine why individuals who perceive a need for care do not seek help. A full understanding of the factors that underlie or contribute to unmet needs is essential in order to determine population need for mental health care, and to prevent the potentially negative health and economic outcomes associated with delays and failures to obtain this care.

The CCHS 1.2 assessed perceived unmet need for mental health or addiction-related care with the following question: 'During the past 12 months, was there ever a time when you felt that you needed help for your emotions, mental health or use of alcohol or drugs, but you didn't receive it?' Respondents who endorsed this item were asked to state the reasons why care was not obtained. Overall, approximately 4.5% of Canadians reported a perceived unmet need for mental health or addiction-related care in the year prior to the survey. This amounted to approximately 1 in 5 (22.0%) of those with mood/anxiety disorder or substance dependence. The prevalence of unmet need varied considerably across diagnostic subgroups, from a low of 13.4% among those with pure substance dependence, to fully half (50.7%) of those with co-occurring disorders (table 9.4). Relative to those with pure substance dependence, individuals with co-occurring disorders had just under seven times the odds of reporting a perceived unmet need for care.

Inasmuch as people experiencing co-occurring disorders are more likely to seek care, it remains possible that they may be more likely to encounter difficulties and, in turn, report perceived unmet need, simply as a result of their greater overall exposure to the health care system. To examine the relationship between perceived unmet need and co-occurring disorders in more detail, we therefore conducted a multivariate logistic regression analysis, taking into account past-year help-seeking and a number of additional measures that are known or expected to play a role in the help-seeking process. The last column in table 9.4 presents the odds of reporting perceived unmet need across diagnostic status, adjusted for gender, age, education, income adequacy, rural residence, self-rated mental health status, generalized distress, and past-year use of mental health and addiction-related care.

The elevated odds of perceived unmet need among those with co-occurring disorders persisted in the full model, although the adjusted odds ratio was reduced by approximately half (table 9.4). Among the other covariates examined, the odds of perceived unmet need were significantly greater among younger individuals, those who reported greater distress (OR = 1.06; 95% CI = 1.04–1.08) and poorer mental health status (OR = 0.80; 95% CI = 0.70–0.93), and those who had sought formal services (OR = 1.32; 95% CI = 1.01–1.72) and informal services (OR = 1.51; 95% CI = 1.05–2.19). Gender, education, income adequacy, and rural residence were not significantly associated with perceived unmet need in the full model.

Table 9.4
Perceived unmet need for mental health and addiction related services among those
with mood and anxiety disorders, and substance dependence.

	%	OR (95% CI)	AOR (95% CI)[a]
Any disorder	22.0%		
Pure substance dependence	13.4%	1.00	1.00
Pure mental disorder	20.8%	1.73 (1.26, 2.39)**	1.09 (0.76, 1.55)
Co-occurring disorders	50.7%	6.66 (4.22, 10.50)**	3.25 (1.96, 5.37)[b]

[a] adjusted odds ratio; adjusted for gender, age, education, income adequacy, rural residence, self-rated mental health status, generalized distress, and past-year health service use
[b] $p<0.001$

Results from these adjusted analyses suggest that the greater level of perceived unmet need for care among those with co-occurring disorders is not entirely accounted for by a greater likelihood of exposure to the health care system (or other factors such as those mentioned). Due to the cross-sectional nature of the CCHS data, it is not possible to determine whether the elevated distress level and poorer mental health status have contributed to a decreased ability to effectively mobilize existing resources, resulting in a perceived unmet need, or whether the perceived unmet need is itself contributing to increased distress levels. It is important to note that, after adjusting for these factors, those with co-occurring disorders still had over three-times the odds of reporting unmet need relative to their counterparts with either type of disorder alone. Clearly, the identification of other factors that may explain the higher perceived unmet need in this population is required. Socioeconomic factors and rural residence were not significant contributors to the explanation of perceived unmet need in these analyses. As the outcome of interest is perceptual in nature, it is likely that additional perceptual measures, such as former experiences with care, and beliefs and attitudes relating to mental health and mental health professionals, will play an important role. Other potential explanatory factors include motivation for behaviour change, especially with respect to substance dependence, the availability of social supports, and the presence of co-occurring physical disorders. To the extent that the latter influence help-seeking patterns and attitudes towards health and health care providers, they may also influence perceptions of need.

Reasons for Not Seeking Care

The different reasons for unmet need reported across the disorder groups provide interesting insight into consumer perceptions and experiences of the mental health and addiction treatment system (figure 9.5). Due to the small numbers of individuals in some of these categories, the majority of differences are not statistically significant, although some interesting trends are noted. A general preference to self-manage symptoms was commonly reported to explain unmet need across all three diagnostic groups. However, this preference was more commonly reported among those with pure substance dependence (40% versus 25–30%, $p > .05$). Those with pure substance dependence were also less likely than others to report that they did not know how to get help (10% versus 15%–16%, $p > .05$), but were more likely to state that they were afraid to ask for it (20% versus 15%–17%, $p > .05$). People with co-occurring disorders were more likely than others to report that they did not obtain care because they did not get around to it (29% versus 12%–16%, $p = .015$) or that care was unavailable when they needed it (17% versus 8%–9%, $p > .05$).

Relative to those with pure mental disorders or comorbid mental disorders and substance dependence, fewer of those with pure substance dependence did not know where to get help. This may be related to the high profile and availability of community-based self-help groups such as Alcoholics or Narcotics Anonymous. A stronger preference to self-manage symptoms or being afraid to ask for help among those with pure substance dependence may reflect greater stigmatization of the disorder and seeking care for substance-related concerns, or alternatively, low motivation and readiness to change substance-using behaviours.[94] In a previous study of perceived unmet needs, a diagnosis of substance use disorder increased the odds of reporting embarrassment as a barrier to seeking required care.[93]

The relatively higher prevalence of 'not getting around to seeking care' among those with co-occurring disorders may similarly reflect issues of stigma, embarrassment, or low motivation to change substance-using behaviours. Given that those with co-occurring disorders were more likely to have sought services in the year prior to the survey, and were more likely to be dissatisfied with these services, it is possible that satisfaction with the care received in prior treatment episodes is impacting on the individual's desire to seek further services. Other work has noted that individuals with multiple mental dis-

Figure 9.5 Self-reported reasons for perceived unmet need among those with substance dependence and other mental disorders and perceived unmet need

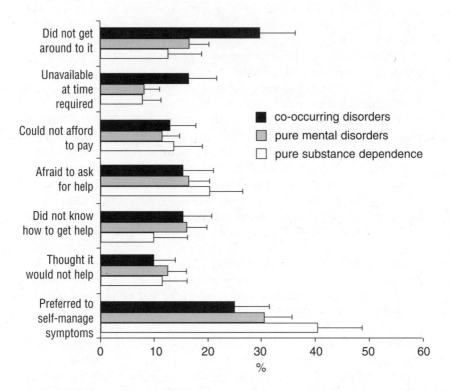

orders have more serious problems in several life areas,[9,56,95] potentially suggestive of greater challenges in managing illness burden and mobilizing available resources for help. The CCHS data do not allow for a direct analysis of these hypotheses, and therefore remains an important area for further work.

Those with co-occurring disorders were also more likely to report that care was unavailable when needed. While this might be due to factors at the individual level (for instance, a lack of knowledge about services), it may also indicate a lack of the preparedness of the health care system to deal with comorbid diagnoses. Systemic, structural, and attitudinal barriers to effective interventions with this subpopulation are commonly cited by clinicians and administrators.[84,85,96] Given the central role of general practitioners in treating those with mental health and addiction problems in Canada[77,78] and elsewhere,[9,11,69,79] the potential for shared care approaches with addiction and mental health professionals should be explored further.

Limitations

Importantly, the CCHS 1.2 survey used a modified version of the WMH-CIDI resulting in data that are *not* compromised by problems around the alcohol dependence items that exist in the original version, and which negatively affected most psychiatric epidemiological surveys that adopted that instrument.[97,98] However, the 'CCHS-modified' version of the WMH-CIDI may itself suffer from as yet unknown biases in disorder estimation. In particular, it did not assess dependence separately for each illicit substance that a respondent reported using, precluding the calculation of drug-specific dependence rates. In addition, it did not include any assessment of prescription drug use, a relevant limitation in light of the evidence of increasing rates of prescription opiate abuse such as OxyContin in many parts of Canada.[99,100]

The survey also omitted one *DSM-IV* criterion for alcohol abuse: recurrent alcohol-related legal problems. Using data from the 2002 U.S. National Survey on Drug Use and Health (NSDUH), post-hoc analysis determined that of all respondents meeting criteria for alcohol abuse in the absence of dependence, only 3.1% uniquely responded in the affirmative to this one criterion. Using these data and projecting to the total Canadian sample, our estimate of 7.3% prevalence of problem use without dependence would be increased by only about 0.2% if the criterion of recurrent alcohol-related legal problems had not been omitted, provided the two samples are comparable on relevant variables (this analysis is available from Brian Rush upon request). However, rates for some sub-groups such as young males may be more prone to underestimation. In contrast to this single criterion exclusion for alcohol abuse, all four criteria for illicit drug abuse were unfortunately excluded from the CCHS instrument.

The instrument also did not include diagnostic algorithms for several psychiatric disorders known to be highly comorbid with substance use disorders, including personality disorders and post-traumatic stress disorder.[56,101,102] In a recent study conducted in the United States, the 12-month prevalence of personality disorders was 14.8%, and the percentage of people with at least one personality disorder was 28.6% and 47.7% among those with alcohol use and drug use disorders, respectively.[101] The exclusion of psychotic disorders in the CCHS 1.2 survey will not have substantially attenuated the population prevalences of co-occurring disorders in this study, as these are fairly uncommon.[103] However, given the severity of psychotic disorders, the high rate of co-occurring substance use disorders, and the significant burden added by the co-occurrence,[24] their absence from the current description of co-occurring disorders in the Canadian population must be noted as a limitation for clinical or system planning purposes.

Finally, household population surveys such as the CCHS are unable to provide coverage of specific subgroups of the population that might be expected to exhibit higher rates of comorbidity. These groups, often hidden from population research, include the homeless, those living in institutions, and Aboriginal people living on reserves. An analysis from the recent OPICAN study found that approximately half of out-of-treatment, street-involved opiate users met criteria for major depression.[104] High levels of co-occurring substance use and other mental disorders have similarly been reported among Aboriginal people living on reserves.[105,106] This issue in particular warrants more in-depth assessment in the Canadian context.

Sample size and reliability concerns in the survey estimates precluded a systematic examination of the co-occurrence of alcohol and illicit drug use problems and more specific diagnoses. When made possible by sufficiently large base rates of the mental disorders, other studies based on CCHS 1.2 are filling in our knowledge for specific diagnostic combinations.[107–110] In this vein, however, we caution other investigators to carefully examine standard errors around their survey estimates and follow Statistics Canada guidelines for reporting and interpreting the associated prevalence rates.

The limitations inherent to the cross-sectional nature of the survey call for longitudinal surveys that would help elucidate the potentially modifiable risk factors for co-occurring mental disorders and substance use disorders, as well as the etiologic pathways to comorbidity. A focus on children and adolescents is critical in this regard.

Summary and Conclusions

Despite these limitations, the CCHS 1.2 is the first survey to systematically and comprehensively describe the prevalence and distribution of co-occurring mental disorders and substance use problems in the Canadian population. The work reported here contributes to a substantive body of knowledge on this topic internationally. It also provides pan-Canadian data for the first time – information that should prove valuable for program planning and policy development across the country.

Overall, 1.7% of Canadian residents, or about 435,000 people, experienced co-occurring mood or anxiety disorders and substance use problems during the year prior to the survey. Although roughly in line with population estimates reported elsewhere,[3,10,16] this prevalence estimate is no doubt an underestimation of the overall extent of co-occurring disorders in Canada given the exclusion of several mental disorders from the survey. While data are available establishing the societal cost of substance use and other mental disorders in Canada,[111,112] projections have not been made of the costs attributable to co-occurring disorders specifically. Based on available data demonstrating increased costs of health care associated with co-occurring, relative to pure, disorders,[29,113] the cumulative costs to Canadian society are likely substantial.

The Canadian data concur with previous work in that the rate of other mental disorders is higher among those with substance use problems than those without. Summarizing broadly across the various categories of mental disorders and across alcohol versus illicit drugs, we identified prevalence estimates that ranged from two to three times that of the subgroup with no disorders. Reliable cross-study comparisons are hampered by methodological differences; however, these estimates are at the lower end of the range of reported estimates from other countries.[17] As discussed, we believe this may have resulted from the exclusion of several disorders known to be highly comorbid with substance use disorders.[56,101,102]

The sociodemographic profile of Canadians experiencing co-occurring disorders reported here is the first to incorporate diagnostic data at the national population level. Such findings are important for the development and targeting of prevention and treatment programs. More than other analyses, the correlates of comorbidity highlight the importance of selecting the appropriate denominator for statistical analysis. As an illustration, when estimates of co-occurring mental disorders are calculated among people with substance use disorders (as we have done in this chapter), females predominate as they do in the general population.[57] When estimates of substance use disorders are calculated among people with other mental disorders (not shown in this chapter), males predominate, again reflecting population gender differences.[114,115] The nature and direction of associations are also likely to differ in clinical and population samples, due to differences in help-seeking and service utilization. Turning national prevalence data into policy relevant information, therefore, requires careful attention to the perspective brought to the data. Returning to the example of gender, however, regardless of perspective, women and men differ in terms of prevalence, course, and treatment outcome for co-occurring disorders,[116] reinforcing the need for a gendered perspective to clinical, policy work, and research in this area.

While these data draw attention to the overlap between mental disorders and substance use disorders in the general population, it should also be recognized that the majority of people with substance use problems do *not* have co-occurring mood or anxiety disorders, and vice versa. The significant, but not overwhelming, degree of overlap cautions us to also maintain a focus, as appropriate, on the large majority of people presenting with pure disorders. That said, the rates of overlap in some subgroups are indeed substantial; for example, close to one-third of women with illicit drug use problems met the criteria for a co-occurring mood or anxiety disorder. Furthermore, these rates of co-occurrence are based on the general population and are much lower than what has been observed in clinical populations.[18-20] Both population and clinical perspectives need to be brought to bear in establishing the relative priority for policies and programs for people with co-occurring disorders, and the present analyses set the stage for more in-depth Canadian interdisciplinary work on this topic.

Data on the prevalence and correlates of comorbidity provide important context for our assessment of service utilization, satisfaction with care, and perceived unmet needs in this population. A higher proportion of people with co-occurring disorders seek care and use an array of community services and health professionals, most notably primary care physicians. Interestingly, the use of services appears to be driven more by mental disorders than by substance use problems. However, those with co-occurring disorders express lower satisfaction with services, and are up to three times more likely to report unmet needs compared to those with pure disorders. These findings warrant further exploration of the associations between need, demand, and optimal treatment planning and delivery.

Taken together, these data confirm that the subgroup of the general population in Canada experiencing both substance use and mental disorders are worthy of special consideration in the planning of mental health and substance abuse services. Recently launched national efforts to improve Canada's substance abuse treatment services (www.nationalframework-cadrenational.ca), as well as the newly announced Mental Health Commission,[117] should work to ensure adequate attention is directed towards these individuals. Given the role played by primary care physicians in treatment, efforts to integrate primary health care and mental health and substance abuse services[118] also need to anticipate and plan for the needs of this sub-population.[73,77]

NOTES AND REFERENCES

Ψ   Problem gambling was also assessed and the co-occurrence of problem gambling, other mental disorders and substance use disorders is addressed in a separate paper available from the authors.

†   Respondents were divided into 4 income categories as follows: *low income adequacy* for a total household income of < $15,000 if 1–2 people, < $20,000 if 3–4 people, or <$30,000 if 5+ people; *lower-middle* if $15,000–$29,999 if 1–2 people, $20,000–39,999 if 3–4 people, or $30,000–$59,999 if 5+; *upper-middle* if $30,000–$59,999 if 1–2 people, $40,000–$79,999 if 3–4 people, or $60,000–$79,999 if 5+ people; and *high* if > $60,000 if 1–2 people or $80,000 if 3+ people (Source: Statistics Canada, CCHS cycle 1.2 Derived Variable Specifications).

1   Regier DA, Farmer ME, Rae DS, et al. Comorbidity of mental disorders with alcohol and other drug abuse. Results from the Epidemiologic Catchment Area (ECA) Study. *J Am Med Assoc* 1990;264:2511–8.

2   Kessler RC, Crum RM, Warner LA, et al. Lifetime co-occurrence of DSM-III-R alcohol abuse and dependence with other psychiatric disorders in the National Comorbidity Survey. *Arch Gen Psychiatry* 1997;54: 313–21.

3   Grant BF, Stinson FS, Dawson DA, et al. Prevalence and co-occurrence of substance use disorders and independent mood and anxiety disorders: Results from the National Epidemiologic Survey on Alcohol and Related Conditions. *Arch Gen Psychiatry* 2004;61:807–16.

4   Kessler RC, Chiu WT, Demler O, et al. Prevalence, severity, and comor-

bidity of 12-month DSM-IV disorders in the National Comorbidity
Survey Replication. *Arch Gen Psychiatry* 2005;62:617–27.

5 Kessler RC, Nelson CB, McGonagle KA, et al. The epidemiology of co-
occurring addictive and mental disorders: Implications for prevention
and service utilization. *Am J Orthopsychiatry* 1996;66:17–31.

6 Bland RC, Orn H, Newman SC. Lifetime prevalence of psychiatric disorders in Edmonton. *Acta Psychiatr Scand* 1988;Suppl 338:24–32.

7 Ross HE. DSM-III-R alcohol abuse and dependence and psychiatric
comorbidity in Ontario: Results from the Mental Health Supplement to
the Ontario Health Survey. *Drug Alcohol Depend* 1995;39:111–28.

8 Scott KM, McGee MA, Oakley Browne MA, et al. Mental disorder comorbidity in Te Rau Hinengaro: the New Zealand Mental Health Survey.
Aust N Z J Psychiatry 2006;40:875–81.

9 Andrews G, Henderson S, Hall W. Prevalence, comorbidity, disability
and service utilisation. Overview of the Australian National Mental
Health Survey. *Br J Psychiatry* 2001;178:145–53.

10 Pirkola SP, Isometsa E, Suvisaari J, et al. DSM-IV mood-, anxiety- and
alcohol use disorders and their comorbidity in the Finnish general population – results from the Health 2000 Study. *Soc Psychiatry Psychiatr Epidemiol* 2005;40:1–10.

11 Bijl RV, Ravelli A. Psychiatric morbidity, service use, and need for care in
the general population: Results of The Netherlands Mental Health
Survey and Incidence Study. *Am J Pub Health* 2000;90:602–7.

12 Jacobi F, Wittchen H-U, Holting C, et al. Prevalence, co-morbidity and
correlates of mental disorders in the general population: Results from the
German Health Interview and Examination Survey (GHS). *Psychol Med*
2004;34:597–611.

13 Farrell M, Howes S, Taylor C, et al. Substance misuse and psychiatric
comorbidity: An overview of the OPCS National Psychiatric Morbidity
Survey. *Addict Behav* 1998;23:909–18.

14 Bromet EJ, Gluzman SF, Paniotto VI, et al. Epidemiology of psychiatric
and alcohol disorders in Ukraine: Findings from the Ukraine World
Mental Health survey. *Soc Psychiatry Psychiatr Epidemiol* 2005;40:681–90.

15 Vicente B, Kohn R, Rioseco P, et al. Lifetime and 12-month prevalence of
DSM-III-R disorders in the Chile psychiatric prevalence study. *Am J Psychiatry* 2006;163:1362–70.

16 De Graaf R, Bijl RV, Smit F, et al. Risk factors for 12-month comorbidity of
mood, anxiety, and substance use disorders: Findings from the Netherlands Mental Health Survey and Incidence Study. *Am J Psychiatry*
2002;159:620–9.

17 Jane-Llopis E, Matytsina I. Mental health and alcohol, drugs and tobacco: A review of the comorbidity between mental disorders and the use of alcohol, tobacco and illicit drugs. *Drug Alcohol Rev* 2006;25: 515–36.

18 Castel S, Rush B, Urbanoski K, et al. Overlap of clusters of psychiatric symptoms among clients of a comprehensive addiction treatment service. *Psychol Addict Behav* 2006;20:28–35.

19 Chan Y-F, Dennis ML, Funk RR. Prevalence and comorbidity co-occurrence of major internalizing and externalizing disorders among adolescents and adults presenting to substance abuse treatment. *J Subst Abuse Treat* 2008;34:14–24.

20 Urbanoski K, Cairney J, Adlaf E, et al. Substance abuse and quality of life among severely mentally ill consumers: A longitudinal modeling analysis. *Soc Psychiatry Psychiatr Epidemiol* 2007;42:810–8.

21 Berkson J. Limitations of the application of the 4-fold table analyses to hospital data. *Biometrics* 1946;2:47–53.

22 Bellack AS, Gearon JS. Substance abuse treatment for people with schizophrenia. *Addict Behav* 1998;23:749–66.

23 Havassy BE, Arns PG. Relationship of cocaine and other substance dependence to well-being of high-risk psychiatric patients. *Psychiatr Serv* 1998;49:935–40.

24 Health Canada. *Best Practices: Concurrent Mental Health and Substance Use Disorders*. Ottawa, ON: Health Canada, 2002.

25 RachBeisel J, Scott J, Dixon L. Co-occurring severe mental illness and substance use disorders: A review of recent research. *Psychiatr Serv* 1999;50:1427–34.

26 Russo J, Roy-Byrne P, Reeder D, et al. Longitudinal assessment of quality of life in acute psychiatric inpatients: Reliability and validity. *J Nerv Ment Dis* 1997;185:166–75.

27 Carey MP, Carey KB, Meisler AW. Psychiatric symptoms in mentally ill chemical abusers. *J Nerv Ment Dis* 1991;179:136–8.

28 Curran GM, Sullivan G, Williams K, et al. Emergency department use of persons with comorbid psychiatric and substance abuse disorders. *Ann Emerg Med* 2003;41:659–67.

29 McGovern MP, Clark RE, Samnaliev M. Co-occurring psychiatric and substance use disorders: A multistate feasibility study of the quadrant model. *Psychiatric Serv* 2007;58:949–54.

30 Rush BR, Scott CK, Dennis ML, et al. The interaction of co-occurring psychiatric problems and recovery management checkup. *Eval Rev* 2008;32:7–38.

31 Rounsaville BJ, Kosten TR, Weissman MM, et al. Prognostic significance

of psychopathology in treated opiate addicts. A 2.5-year follow-up study. *Arch Gen Psychiatry* 1986;43:739–45.

32 McLellan AT, Luborsky L, Woody GE, et al. Predicting response to alcohol and drug abuse treatments: Role of psychiatric severity. *Arch Gen Psychiatry* 1983;40:620–5.

33 Rounsaville BJ, Tierney T, Crits-Christoph K, et al. Predictors of outcome in treatment of opiate addicts: Evidence for the multidimensional nature of addicts' problems. *Compr Psychiatry* 1982;23:462–78.

34 Weisner C, Matzger H, Kaskutas LA. How important is treatment? One-year outcomes of treated and untreated alcohol-dependent individuals. *Addiction* 2003;98:901–911.

35 Kranzler HR, Del Boca FK, Rounsaville BJ. Comorbid psychiatric diagnosis predicts three-year outcomes in alcoholics: A posttreatment natural history study. *J Stud Alcohol* 1996;57:619–26.

36 Carroll KM, Power ME, Bryant K, et al. One-year follow-up status of treatment-seeking cocaine abusers. Psychopathology and dependence severity as predictors of outcome. *J Nerv Ment Dis* 1993;181:71–9.

37 Project MATCH Research Group. Matching alcoholism treatments to client heterogeneity: Project MATCH posttreatment drinking outcomes. *J Stud Alcohol* 1997;58:7–29.

38 Moos RH, Mertens JR, Brennan PL. Rates and predictors of four-year readmission among late-middle-aged and older substance abuse patients. *J Stud Alcohol* 1994;55:561–70.

39 Booth MC, Cook CAL, Blow FC. Comorbid mental disorders in patients with AMA discharges from alcoholism treatment. *Hosp Community Psychiatry* 1992;43:730–1.

40 Hanson M, Kramer TH, Gross W. Outpatient treatment of adults with coexisting substance use and mental disorders. *J Subst Abuse Treat* 1990;7:109–16.

41 Ananth J, Vandewater S, Kamal M, et al. Missed diagnosis of substance abuse in psychiatric patients. *Hosp Community Psychiatry* 1989;40:297–301.

42 Barnaby B, Drummond C, McCloud A, et al. Substance misuse in psychiatric inpatients: Comparison of a screening questionnaire survey with case notes. *Br Med J* 2003;327:783–4.

43 Rush BR. On the screening and assessment of mental disorders among clients seeking help from specialized substance abuse treatment services: An international symposium [Editorial]. *Int J Ment Health Addict* 2008;6:1–6.

44 Substance Abuse and Mental Health Services Administration, *Report to Congress on the Prevention and Treatment of Co-occurring Substance Abuse Disorders and Mental Disorders*. Substance Abuse and Mental Health Services Administration: Rockville, MD, 2002.

45 Center for Substance Abuse Treatment. *Assessment and Treatment of Patients with Coexisting Mental Illness and Alcohol and Other Drug Abuse. Treatment Improvement Protocol (TIP) Series 42, DHHS Publication No. (SMA) 95-3061.* Substance Abuse and Mental Health Services Administration: Rockville, MD, 1994.

46 Sacks S. Brief overview of screening and assessment for co-occurring disorders. *Int J Ment Health Addict* 2008;6:7–19.

47 Center for Substance Abuse Treatment, *Substance Abuse Treatment for Persons with Co-occurring Disorders. Treatment Improvement Protocol (TIP) Series, 42.* Substance Abuse Mental Health Services Administration: Rockville, MD, 2005..

48 O'Brien CP, Charney DS, Lewis L, et al. Priority actions to improve the care of persons with co-occurring substance abuse and other mental disorders: A call to action. *Biol Psychiatry* 2004;56:703–13.

49 Bellack AS, Bennett ME, Gearon JS, et al. (2006). A randomized clinical trial of a new behavioral treatment for drug abuse in people with severe and persistent mental illness. *Arch Gen Psychiatry* 2006;63:426–32.

50 Drake RE, Mueser KT, Brunette MF, et al. A review of treatments for people with severe mental illnesses and co-occurring substance use disorders. *Psychiatr Rehab J* 2004;27:360–74.

51 Grella CE, Stein JA. Impact of program services on treatment outcomes of patients with comorbid mental and substance use disorders. *Psychiatric Serv* 2006;57:1007–15.

52 Gravel R, Béland Y. The Canadian Community Health Survey: Mental health and well-being. *Can J Psychiatry* 2005;50:573–9.

53 Kessler RC, Ustun TB. The World Mental Health (WMH) Survey Initiative Version of the World Health Organization (WHO) Composite International Diagnostic Interview (CIDI). *Int J Methods Psychiatr Res* 2004;13:93–121.

54 American Psychiatric Association. (1994). *Diagnostic and Statistical Manual of Mental Disorders* (4th ed). Washington, DC, American Psychiatric Association, 1994.

55 Adlaf EM, Begin P, Sawka E, *Canadian Addiction Survey (CAS): A National Survey of Canadian's Use of Alcohol and Other Drugs: Prevalence of Use and Related Harms: Detailed Report.* Canadian Centre on Substance Abuse: Ottawa, 2005.

56 Merikangas KR, Mehta RL, Molnar BE, et al. Comorbidity of substance use disorders with mood and anxiety disorders: Results of the International Consortium in Psychiatric Epidemiology. *Addict Behav* 1998;23:893–907.

57 Kessler RC, McGonagle KA, Zhao S, et al. Lifetime and 12-month preva-

lence of DSM-III-R psychiatric disorders in the United States. Results from the National Comorbidity Survey. *Arch Gen Psychiatry* 1994; 51:8–19.

58 Offord DR, Boyle MH, Campbell D, et al. One-year prevalence of psychiatric disorder in Ontarians 15 to 64 years of age. *Can J Psychiatry* 1996;41:559–63.

59 Veldhuizen S, Urbanoski K, Cairney J. Geographical variation in the prevalence of problematic substance use in Canada. *Can J Psychiatry* 2007;52:426–33.

60 Beiser M. The health of immigrants and refugees in Canada. *Can J Pub Health* 2005;96(suppl 2):S30–44.

61 Grant BF, Stinson FS, Hasin DS, et al. Immigration and lifetime prevalence of DSM-IV psychiatric disorders among Mexican Americans and non-Hispanic whites in the United States: Results from the National Epidemiologic Survey on Alcohol and Related Conditions. *Arch Gen Psychiatry* 2004;61:1226–33.

62 Alegria M, Mulvaney-Day N, Torres M, et al. Prevalence of psychiatric disorders across Latino subgroups in the United States. *Am J Pub Health* 2007;97:68–75.

63 Blomstedt Y, Johansson SE, Sundquist J.. Mental health of immigrants from the former Soviet Bloc: A future problem for primary health care in the enlarged European Union? A cross-sectional study. *BMC Pub Health* 2007;7:27.

64 Claassen D, Ascoli M, Berhe T, et al. Research on mental disorders and their care in immigrant populations: A review of publications from Germany, Italy and the UK. *Eur Psychiatry* 2005;20:540–9.

65 Sherbourne CD, Stewart AL. The MOS social support survey. *Soc Sci Med* 1991;32:705–14.

66 Ettner S, Frank R, Kessler R. The impact of psychiatric disorder on labor market outcomes. *Ind Labor Relat Rev* 1997;51:64–81.

67 El-Guebaly N, Currie S, Williams J, et al. Association of mood, anxiety, and substance use disorders with occupational status and disability in a community sample. *Psychiatr Serv* 2007;58:659–67.

68 Wang PS, Lane M, Olfson M, et al. Twelve-month use of mental health services in the United States: Results from the National Comorbidity Survey Replication. *Arch Gen Psychiatry* 2005;62:629–40.

69 Oakley Browne MA, Wells JE, McGee MA. Twelve-month and lifetime health service use in Te Rau Hinengaro: The New Zealand Mental Health Survey. *Aust N Z J Psychiatry* 2006;40:855–64.

70 Harris KM, Edlund MJ. Use of mental health care and substance abuse

treatment among adults with co-occurring disorders. *Psychiatric Serv* 2005;56:954–9.

71 Regier DA, Shapiro S, Kessler LG, et al. Epidemiology and health service resource allocation policy for alcohol, drug abuse, and mental disorders. *Pub Health Rep* 1984;99:483–92.

72 WHO World Mental Health Survey Consortium. Prevalence, severity, and unmet need for treatment of mental disorders in the World Health Organization World Mental Health Surveys. *J Am Med Assoc* 2004;291:2581–90.

73 Regier DA, Narrow WE, Rae DS, et al. The de facto US mental and addictive disorders service system. Epidemiologic Catchment Area prospective 1-year prevalence rates of disorders and services. *Arch Gen Psychiatry* 1993;50:85–94.

74 Bland RC, Newman SC, Orn H. Help-seeking for psychiatric disorders. *Can J Psychiatry* 1997;42:935–42.

75 Ross HE, Lin E, Cunningham J. Mental health service use: A comparison of treated and untreated individuals with substance use disorders in Ontario. *Can J Psychiatry* 1999;44:570–7.

76 Wu LT, Kouzis AC, Leaf PJ. Influence of comorbid alcohol and psychiatric disorders on utilization of mental health services in the National Comorbidity Survey. *Am J Psychiatry* 1999;156:1230–6.

77 Urbanoski KA, Rush BR, Wild TC, et al. Use of mental health care services by Canadians with co-occurring substance dependence and mental disorders. *Psychiatric Serv* 2007;58:962–9.

78 Parikh SV, Lin E, Lesage AD. Mental health treatment in Ontario: Selected comparisons between the primary care and specialty sectors. *Can J Psychiatry* 1997;42:929–34.

79 Wang PS, Demler O, Olfson M, et al. Changing profiles of service sectors used for mental health care in the United States. *Am J Psychiatry* 2006;163:1187–98.

80 Meadows G, Burgess P, Bobevski I, et al. Perceived need for mental health care: Influences of diagnosis, demography and disability. *Psychol Med* 2002;32:299–309.

81 Bijl RV, Ravelli A. Current and residual functional disability associated with psychopathology: Findings from the Netherlands Mental Health Survey and Incidence Study (NEMESIS). *Psychol Med* 2000;30:657–68.

82 Goering P, Lin E, Campbell D, et al. Psychiatric disability in Ontario. *Can J Psychiatry* 1996;41:564–71.

83 Mojtabai R, Olfson M, Mechanic D. Perceived need and help-seeking in adults with mood, anxiety, or substance use disorders. *Arch Gen Psychiatry* 2002;59:77–84.

84 Todd FC, Sellman JD, Robertson PJ. Barriers to optimal care for patients with coexisting substance use and mental health disorders. *Aust N Z J Psychiatry* 2002;36:792–9.
85 Young NK, Grella CE. Mental health and substance abuse treatment services for dually diagnosed clients: Results of a statewide survey of county administrators. *J Behav Health Serv Res* 1998;25:83–92.
86 Ware JE, Jr., Davies AR. Behavioral consequences of consumer dissatisfaction with medical care. *Eval Program Plann* 1983;6:291–7.
87 Lebow JL. Research assessing consumer satisfaction with mental health treatment: A review of findings. *Eval Program Plann* 1983;6:211–36.
88 Ducharme LJ, Knudsen HK, Roman PM. Availability of integrated care for co-occurring substance abuse and psychiatric conditions. *Community Ment Health J* 2006;42:363–75.
89 Andersen RM. Revisiting the behavioral model and access to medical care: Does it matter? *J Health Soc Behav* 1995;36:1–10.
90 Wang J. Perceived barriers to mental health service use among individuals with mental disorders in the Canadian general population. *Med Care* 2006;44:192–5.
91 Craske MG, Edlund MJ, Sullivan G, et al. Perceived unmet need for mental health treatment and barriers to care among patients with panic disorder. *Psychiatr Serv* 2005;56:988–94.
92 Sareen J, Cox BJ, Afifi TO, et al. Perceived need for mental health treatment in a nationally representative Canadian sample. *Can J Psychiatry* 2005;50:643–51.
93 Sareen J, Jagdeo A, Cox BJ, et al. Perceived barriers to mental health service utilization in the United States, Ontario, and the Netherlands. *Psychiatr Serv* 2007;58:357–64.
94 Wu LT, Pilowsky DJ, Schlenger WE, et al. Alcohol use disorders and the use of treatment services among college-age young adults. *Psychiatr Serv* 2007;58:192–200.
95 Gamma A, Angst J. Concurrent psychiatric comorbidity and multimorbidity in a community study: Gender differences and quality of life. *Eur Arch Psychiatry Clin Neurosci* 2001;251(suppl 2):II43–6.
96 Tracy SW, Trafton JA, Weingardt KR, et al. How are substance use disorders addressed in VA psychiatric and primary care settings? Results of a national survey. *Psychiatr Serv* 2007;58:266–9.
97 Grant BF, Compton WM, Crowley TJ, et al. Errors in assessing DSM-IV substance use disorders. *Arch Gen Psychiatry* 2007;64:379–80; author reply 381–2.

98 Cottler LB. Drug use disorders in the National Comorbidity Survey: Have we come a long way? *Arch Gen Psychiatry* 2007;64:380–1; author reply 381–2.

99 Fischer B, Rehm J. Illicit opioid use in the 21st century: Witnessing a paradigm shift? *Addiction* 2007;102:499–501.

100 Fischer B, Rehm J, Patra J, et al. Changes in illicit opioid use across Canada. *Can Med Assoc J* 2006;175:1385.

101 Grant BF, Stinson FS, Dawson DA, et al. Co-occurrence of 12-month alcohol and drug use disorders and personality disorders in the United States: Results from the National Epidemiologic Survey on Alcohol and Related Conditions. *Arch Gen Psychiatry* 2004;61:361–8.

102 Brady K, Killeen T, Saladin ME, et al., *Clinical and Research Reports: Comorbid Substance Abuse and Posttraumatic Stress Disorder. Rep. #3(2).* The American Academy of Psychiatrists in Alcoholism and Addictions: South Carolina, 1994.

103 Perala J, Suvisaari J, Saarni SI, et al. Lifetime prevalence of psychotic and bipolar I disorders in a general population. *Arch Gen Psychiatry* 2007;64:19–28.

104 Wild TC, El-Guebaly N, Fischer B, et al. (2005). Comorbid depression among untreated illicit opiate users: Results from a multisite Canadian study. *Can J Psychiatry* 2005;50:512–8.

105 Westermeyer J, Neider J, Westermeyer M. Substance use and other psychiatric disorders among 100 American Indian patients. *Cult Med Psychiatry* 1992;16:519–29.

106 Duran B, Sanders M, Skipper B, et al. Prevalence and correlates of mental disorders among Native American women in primary care. *Am J Pub Health* 2004;94:71–7.

107 McIntyre RS, McElroy SL, Konarski JZ, et al. Problem gambling in bipolar disorder: Results from the Canadian Community Health Survey. *J Affec Dis* 2007;102:27–34.

108 El-Guebaly N, Patten SB, Currie S, et al. Epidemiological associations between gambling behavior, substance use and mood and anxiety disorders. *J Gambl Stud* 2006;22:275–87.

109 Currie SR, Patten SB, Williams JV, et al. Comorbidity of major depression with substance use disorders. *Can J Psychiatry* 2005;50:660–6.

110 Schaffer A, Cairney J, Cheung A, et al. Community survey of bipolar disorder in Canada: Lifetime prevalence and illness characteristics. *Can J Psychiatry* 2006;51:9–16.

111 Gnam W, Sarnocinska-Hart A, Mustard C, et al. *The Economic Costs of*

204   B.R. Rush, K.A. Urbanoski, D.G. Bassani, S. Castel, and T.C. Wild

    Mental Disorders and Alcohol, Tobacco, and Illicit Drug Abuse in Ontario,
    2000: A Cost-of-Illness Study. Centre for Addiction and Mental Health:
    Toronto, ON, 2006.
112 Rehm J, Baliunas D, Brochu S, et al., *The Cost of Substance Abuse in*
    Canada 2002. CCSA – CCLAT: Ottawa, ON, 2006.
113 Dickey B, Azeni H. Persons with dual diagnoses of substance abuse and
    major mental illness: Their excess costs of psychiatric care. *Am J Pub*
    Health 1996;86:973–7.
114 Hasin DS, Stinson FS, Ogburn E, et al. Prevalence, correlates, disability,
    and comorbidity of DSM-IV alcohol abuse and dependence in the
    United States: Results from the National Epidemiologic Survey on
    Alcohol and Related Conditions. *Arch Gen Psychiatry* 2007;64:830–42.
115 Somers JM, Goldner EM, Waraich P, et al. Prevalence studies of sub-
    stance-related disorders: A systematic review of the literature. *Can J Psy-*
    chiatry 2004;49:373–84.
116 Zilberman ML, Tavares H, Blume SB, et al. Substance use disorders: Sex
    differences and psychiatric comorbidities. *Can J Psychiatry* 2003;48:5–13.
117 Kirby MJL. *Out of the Shadows at Last – Transforming Mental Health,*
    Mental Illness and Addiction Services in Canada. The Standing Senate Com-
    mittee on Social Affairs, Science and Technology: Ottawa, ON, 2006.
118 Somers JM. Screening for co-occurring disorders and the promotion of
    collaborative care. *Int J Ment Health Addict* 2008;6:141–4.

10 Perspectives on Child Psychiatric Disorder in Canada

MICHAEL H. BOYLE AND KATHOLIKI GEORGIADES

Child psychiatric disorder involves maladaptive processes in cognitive, affective, physiological, and/or behavioural domains of functioning, or in the ways in which these domains are integrated.[1-3] These maladaptive processes emerge over time as the child interacts with the environment. The most common approaches to the classification of childhood disorder are: (1) 'categorical' classification systems such as the American Psychiatric Association's (APA) *Diagnostic and Statistical Manual of Mental Disorders* (*DSM*),[4] and (2) empirically based 'dimensional' classification systems arising from multivariate statistical analyses of children's behaviour such as the Child Behavior Checklist.[5]

The *DSM* includes commissioned literature reviews and clinical consensus on the nature of psychiatric disorder; it takes a categorical approach to disorder in which individuals either meet or do not meet specific criteria. The criteria that separate one disorder from another are symptoms hypothesized to form a meaningful and distinctive cluster. The *DSM* identifies the number of symptoms at or above which a child is to be classified as exhibiting a disorder.[6] In addition to specific symptoms, children must also show signs of personal suffering, delayed development, impaired social relations, or school achievement below their potential. While symptom groupings are used to distinguish different types of child disorder, the presence of distress or impairment is a common prerequisite for being classified with child psychiatric disorder in general.

The dimensional approach to classification characterizes childhood disorder as a continuum of behavioural responses possessed to varying degrees by all children. It assumes that 'classes' of disorder are independent dimensions that give rise to a group of associated behaviours. These behaviours can be identified through statistical analysis. Behaviours exhibiting strong associations with one another are grouped together to represent these independent dimensions. In this approach, parents, teachers of children in school, and children themselves, if older than 8 years of age, are asked about the occurrence of problem behaviours (symptoms) within a specific period of time. There may be a variety of ways to record responses. For example, behaviours might be classified as absent (0) or present (1). Behaviours identified as present might be further divided on a continuum of severity or intensity (e.g., 1, sometimes present; 2, always present). These individual behaviours are grouped empirically according to the dimension of behavioural abnormality they represent and responses are added together to produce a count or scale score. The dimensional approach is not based on theoretical assumptions about the diagnostic meaningfulness of behavioural clusters. The goal of this approach is descriptive. The dimensions may be converted to 'categories' by applying cut-off scores derived from normative (general population) data or by titrating scores to locate optimal thresholds against alternative (clinical) classifications.[7]

Although the two approaches to classifying childhood psychiatric disorder rely on different methods and reflect different traditions, they have much in common.[8] Indeed, strong correspondence exists between the dimensions of psychopathology recovered from empirical analyses and many of the disorders identified in clinical consensus exercises. Furthermore, within corresponding dimensions and categories, the behavioural indicators (dimensions) and symptom criteria (categories of disorder) are very closely aligned. Finally, in the study of child psychiatric epidemiology, both approaches to classification have been used to estimate the prevalence and associated features of specific types of disorder. In response to the dominance of clinical conceptualizations of disorder in child epidemiological research, we focus on the classification system that has emerged from the DSM.

DSM Classification of Disorder

In DSM-IV,[4] there are three classes of psychiatric disorder applicable to children: (1) developmental and learning disorders, including mental retardation, pervasive developmental disorders such as autism, specific problems related to reading and math, and communication difficulties; (2) disorders that are usually first diagnosed in infancy, childhood, or adolescence, such as attention-deficit/hyperactivity disorder, disruptive behaviour disorders, attachment disorders, and separation anxiety disorders. Traditionally, these disorders have been thought of as first occurring in childhood, or as exclusive to childhood, and have specific criteria for children that are distinct from those used to define adult disorders; and (3) disorders that can be diagnosed in children and adolescents but are not listed in *DSM-IV* as distinct disorders that first occur in childhood or that require criteria that are different from those used for adults (i.e., mood disorders, anxiety disorders, eating disorders). The reliance on adult criteria has obvious limitations because it does not place children's symptoms into a clear developmental or social context.[9]

Childhood psychiatric disorders such as autism spectrum disorder that affect fewer than three children per 1,000 are very difficult to study in general populations.[10] Our methods for classifying rare conditions are too unreliable. Identifying one child correctly invariably leads to identifying many children incorrectly (false positives). As a result, our knowledge about child psychiatric disorder in the general population focuses on the 'common' forms of disorder. In *DSM-IV*, these disorders fall into two broad groupings: behavioural and emotional.[11] Behavioural disorders include: conduct disorder (CD: a persistent pattern of extreme antisocial behaviour in which the rights of others and age-appropriate social norms are violated), oppositional-defiant disorder (ODD: a behavioural pattern of persistent disobedience, defiance, negativism, and provocation), and attention-deficit/hyperactivity disorder (ADHD: a behavioural syndrome that includes over-activity, inattention, and/or impulsiveness). The emotional disorders include two major groupings: the mood disorders and the anxiety disorders. The former include major depressive disorder (MDD) and dysthymia defined using the same criteria for adults as children. Among the anxiety disorders, only separation anxiety disorder (SAD: developmentally inappropriate and excessive anxiety concerning separation from home or from those to whom the individual is attached) remains in the childhood section of the *DSM-IV*.[11]

Assessments of emotional and behavioural problems of childhood can be obtained by personal interview[12] or through a checklist completed by the respondent on his or her own. The personal interview includes extensive questioning by trained interviewers while the checklist approach is usually self-completed and involves short descriptive phrases.

Scope of Child Psychiatric Disorder in Canada – Prevalence Estimates

Substantial variation exists in prevalence estimates of child psychiatric disorder, depending on the conditions selected for study, the instruments used in classification, and the sample participating in assessments.[13] Arguably, the 'best' overall prevalence estimates of child psychiatric disorder applicable to Canadian children come from a review by Waddell and colleagues.[14,15] In selecting studies for review, the authors imposed a number of criteria to optimize their validity (quality of instruments and data collection) and applicability to Canadian children (sample representativeness and study location). Six studies met criteria for inclusion. Adapted from Waddell and colleagues,[15] table 10.1 shows the pooled prevalence estimates for specific types of child psychiatric disorder exceeding 0.5 per 100 in the general population.

The estimates in table 10.1 suggest the following. One, the prevalence of child psychiatric disorder is high. At any given time, about 14% of children will meet criteria: this estimate translates into more than 800,000 Canadian children. Two, anxiety is the most common disorder affecting children (6.4%). Although attention-deficit/hyperactivity disorder, conduct disorder, and depression occur less frequently, they still affect from 3.5 to 4.8% of the population. Three, there are relatively wide 95% confidence intervals around each category of disorder (e.g., 11.4%–17.6% for any disorder), reflecting substantial study-to-study variability in these estimates.

Child Psychiatric Disorder in Canada – Importance

Population-based prevalence estimates such as those in table 10.1 provide information on the scope of child psychiatric disorder. To understand its importance as a public health problem, we must also consider its impact on individual life quality; its burden to society in terms of geographic, temporal, and socioeconomic distribution, as well as cost; and the extent to which it is under societal control. These considerations can be framed as questions. (1) What is the individual loss of functioning, time course, and outcomes associated with child psychiatric disorder? (2) Are there differences among regions and provinces in levels of child psychiatric disorder? (3) Are levels of child psychiatric disorder increasing, decreasing, or about the same as they

Table 10.1
Prevalence of children's mental disorders and population affected in Canada.[a]

Disorder	Estimated % prevalence[b]	95% CI[b]	Age	Population in '000s affected[c]
Any anxiety [d,e,f,g]	6.4	4.2–9.2	5–17	340
Attention-deficit hyperactivity disorder [d,e,f,g,h,i]	4.8	2.7–7.3	4–17	272
Conduct disorder [d,e,f,g,h,i]	4.2	2.4–6.5	4–17	238
Any depressive disorder [d,e,f,g,i]	3.5	1.0–7.1	5–17	186
Substance abuse [d,e]	0.8	0.5–1.3	9–17	30
Any disorder [d,e,f,g,h,i]	14.3	11.4–17.6	4–17	811

[a] Adapted from Waddell et al.[14,15]
[b] For methods used to pool estimates and derive confidence intervals, refer to Waddell et al.[14]
[c] Estimated prevalence multiplied by estimated population
[d] NIMH Methods for the Epidemiology of Child and Adolescent Mental Disorders Study[55]
[e] Great Smoky Mountains Study[56]
[f] Quebec Child Mental Health Survey[57]
[g] British Child Mental Health Survey[58]
[h] Ontario Child Health Study[59]
[i] Virginia Twin Study of Adolescent Behavioral Development[60]

were ten years ago? (4) Is there evidence that child psychiatric disorder is concentrated in certain segments of the population? (5) To what extent is child psychiatric disorder consuming societal resources? (6) Are programmatic responses meeting the public health needs posed by child psychiatric disorder?

In an attempt to address these questions, we provide new information drawn from two Canadian studies: the Ontario Child Health Study (OCHS)[7,16,17] and the National Longitudinal Survey of Children and Youth (NLSCY).[18] The OCHS was a community survey done in 1983, with follow-ups in 1987 and 2001, of 3294 children, aged 4 to 16 years , living in 1869 families. The objective of the OCHS was to investigate the distribution, determinants, and long-term course of child health problems, including psychiatric disorder. The NLSCY is a large-scale prospective study of Canadian children aged 0 to 11 years old at study inception in 1994. The objective of the NLSCY was to create a national database on the characteristics and life experiences of children and youth in Canada as they grow from infancy to adulthood; it collects assessment data on participants every two years and has integrated several prospective and cross-sectional samples throughout its course.

In its study of child psychiatric disorder, the OCHS focused on conduct disorder, attention deficit disorder (ADD), and emotional disorder (an amalgam of depression and anxiety) among children aged 4–16 years old in 1983. Parents, teachers, and adolescents (aged 12–16 years) completed problem behaviour rating scales aligned with *DSM* symptom criteria. The problem behaviours used to classify each disorder had responses coded (0) never or not true, (1) sometimes or somewhat true, and (2) often or very true that were added together to form separate, respondent-specific scale scores representing the three disorders. Optimal cut-offs for classifying these disorders were obtained in a separate study of 196 children and adolescents.[7,19] In this separate study, parent and teacher scale scores (children aged 4–11 years) and parent and adolescent scale scores (adolescents aged 12–16 years) were titrated in stepwise fashion against clinical classifications of disorder provided by child psychiatrists. The resulting thresholds were applied to scale scores obtained from respondents in the OCHS to classify child disorder. The NLSCY administered a subset of OCHS items to parents of children aged 4–11 years old. With no independent basis for identifying thresholds in the NLSCY, mean scores derived from 20 OCHS items are used here to represent levels of psychopathology.

*Question 1: Impact of Child Psychiatric Disorder on Individual
            Life Quality*

The impact of child psychiatric disorder on individual life quality is marked by concurrent distress and impairment as well as long-term functional loss. Using data from the OCHS, levels of need for professional help with emotional-behavioural problems and impaired interpersonal functioning and/or poor school achievement among children classified with disorder in 1983 are contrasted with children reported to have one or more chronic health problems (long-term chronic illnesses or medical conditions). A chronic health problem in the OCHS was parent reported and consisted of one or more illnesses/conditions of at least six months duration drawn from a list of 22 separate categories that included problems of vision, hearing and speech, paralysis, deformity, pain, and chronic diseases such as asthma and epilepsy.[20,21]

Further to this, we examine continuity of child psychiatric disorder versus chronic health problems from 1983 to 1987 and examine their association with functional outcomes in 2001.

The first three columns of table 10.2 show the per cent of children and adolescents classified with child psychiatric disorder (by parent/teacher reports for children aged 6–11 years and parent/youth reports for adolescents aged 12–16 years) versus chronic health problems in 1983 that are reported by the same respondents to be: (1) in need of professional help for emotional-behavioural problems (or to have received help in the past 6 months); and (2) doing poorly in school and/or to have had problems in the past six months getting along with peers, teachers, or family members. Among children classified with one or more of conduct disorder, ADD, and/or emotional disorder, about 40% are judged to need professional help for emotional-behavioural problems and another 25% to have a social or school impairment (table 10.2). Analogous estimates for children classified with chronic health problems are substantially lower: about 19% are reported to need professional help and about 8% to have impairment. Need for professional help and levels of impairment are comparable between the two major groupings of disorder (conduct/ADD versus emotional) (table 10.2). The last column in table 10.2 exhibits continuity of classifications from 1983 to 1987. Among those classified with child psychiatric disorder in 1983, about 33% are classified again in 1987 (table 10.3). This contrasts with 54% of those classified with chronic health problems. There is stronger evidence of continuity among children classified with conduct/ADD (41%) versus emotional disorder (14%).

Table 10.3 examines mean levels and standardized differences in functional outcomes assessed in 2001 for children classified with psychiatric disorder versus chronic health problems in 1983. Those in 1983 classified with child psychiatric disorder versus without child psychiatric disorder achieved 1.5 years less of education (15.5–14.0). This difference represents a standardized 'effect' of –0.72. In contrast, children classified with chronic health problems exhibited a loss of 0.6 years of education – a standardized 'loss' of –0.29. In all comparisons – years of education achieved, household income, health status assessed by the SF-12,[22] and life satisfaction (a composite variable derived from nine items that include health, education, job/main activity, finances, housing, neighbourhood, spouse/partner/being single, and relationship with family and friends) – children classified with psychiatric dis-

Table 10.2
Per cent of OCHS children aged 6–16 years classified with psychiatric disorder versus chronic health problems by the proportion reported to need professional help or exhibit impairment in 1983 and proportion of OCHS children aged 6–12 years reclassified with psychiatric disorder versus a chronic health problem between 1983 and 1987.

1983 classification	Proportion in 1983 (n=2186)			Proportion 1987 (n=951)
	Needs help[a]	Impairment	Neither	Reclassified
Any psychiatric disorder:				
% pres/abs (12.1/87.9)	.40/.06	.25/.08	.36/.86	.33/.10[b]
Conduct/ADD:				
% pres/abs (8.5/91.5)	.40/.08	.25/.09	.34/.84	.41/.07[b]
Emotional:				
% pres/abs (5.7/94.3)	.47/.08	.22/.09	.30/.83	.14/.05[b]
Any chronic health problems:				
% pres/abs (17.5/82.5)	.19/.08	.08/.11	.74/.81	.54/.18[b]

[a] With/without impairment
[b] $p < 0.001$

order did worse than children classified with chronic health problems. Among children classified with psychiatric disorder, educational losses were stronger among children with conduct/ADD, while household income and health losses were stronger among children with emotional disorder (table 10.3).

Questions 2 to 4: Societal Burden – Geographic, Temporal, and Socioeconomic Distributions

The societal burden of child psychiatric disorder is shaped not only by its scope (prevalence) and adverse impact on the individual but also by geographic, temporal, and socioeconomic patterns of occurrence in the population. Prevalence differences between geographic areas and/or population sub-groups may represent sociodemographic health inequalities that need to be addressed. Temporal trends consider the extent to which health problems are getting better or worse over time: negative trends indicative of increasing levels of child emotional-behavioural problems would represent an important call to action at the societal level.

Table 10.3
OCHS children aged 6–16 years classified with psychiatric disorder versus chronic health problems in 1983: mean levels and standardized differences (Δ) in 2001 functional outcomes.

| | Mean levels in 2001 for present/absent in 1983 (standardized difference, Δ)[d] | | | |
	Years education	Hhld income $000	Health SF12	Life satisfaction
1983 classification	Pres/abs (Δ)	Pres/abs (Δ)	Pres/abs (Δ)	Pres/abs (Δ)
Any psychiatric disorder	14.0/15.5 (−.72)[c]	64.1/72.5 (−.17)[a]	38.8/40.7 (−.33)[c]	30.6/32.8 (−.45)[c]
Conduct/ADD	13.6/15.4 (−.86)[c]	65.3/72.1 (−.13)	39.0/40.6 (−.31)[c]	30.6/32.7 (−.43)[c]
Emotional disorder	14.1/15.4 (−.62)[c]	60.5/72.3 (−.23)[c]	38.4/40.6 (−.44)[c]	30.2/32.7 (−.51)[b]
Any chronic health problem	14.8/15.4 (−.29)[a]	70.5/71.8 (−.03)	39.5/40.7 (−.23)[b]	31.9/32.7 (−.16)[b]

[a] $p < 0.05$
[b] $p < 0.01$
[c] $p < 0.001$
[d] Mean difference divided by the standard deviation of the outcome (standardized difference).

Table 10.4 shows levels of parent-reported emotional-behavioural problems among children 4–11 years old over four cycles of the NLSCY by regions of Canada. In 1994, mean levels of child emotional-behavioural problems assessed by parents went from 7.10 (Atlantic) to 8.17 (Quebec). These mean levels represent standardized differences of −.081 (Atlantic) and +.104 (Quebec) when Canada serves as the reference. Contrasting levels of emotional-behavioural problems across regions reveal some differences. For example, levels are higher in Quebec than the rest of Canada in 1994, but in 1996, levels are higher in Ontario than the rest of Canada. Over time, these cross-sectional comparisons suggest only one consistent finding: the Atlantic region has lower mean levels. Furthermore, changes in levels of emotional-behavioural problems over time within regions and Canada show no evidence of temporal trends: the estimates for Canada overall are almost identical at each cycle.

Table 10.4
Mean levels of emotional-behavioural problems by region and standardized difference from Canada average (Δ) in the NLSCY based on parent report for children aged 4–11 years from 1994 to 2000.

Region	%[b]	1994 (n=13,926)[a] mean	Δ[c]	1996 (n=9707) mean	Δ	1998 (n=15,366) mean	Δ	2000 (n=13,320) mean	Δ
Atlantic	7.7	7.10[e]	−.081	6.74[e,f]	−.131	6.97[d]	−.107	6.97[d]	−.088
Quebec	23.1	8.17[d]	+.104	7.28[e]	−.037	7.51[e]	−.012	7.96[e,f]	+.093
Ontario	38.3	7.32[e]	−.043	7.86[d]	+.065	7.73[e]	+.026	7.09[g,h]	−.066
West	30.7	7.54[e]	−.005	7.37[e,g]	−.021	7.58[e]	.000	7.63[e,i]	+.033
Canada (sd)	100.0	7.57	(5.77)	7.49	(5.73)	7.58	(5.68)	7.45	(5.48)

[a] Sample size for cycle
[b] Average per cent of total sample for each region across all cycles
[c] Mean difference between region and Canada divided by the standard deviation for Canada (standardized difference) within each cycle.
Statistically significant differences between regions within cycle at $p < 0.05$ exist for [d] versus [e]; [f] versus [g]; and [h] versus [i]

Although only small regional differences exist in levels of child emotional-behavioural problems, there is some evidence to suggest that differences between smaller areas are comparatively larger. In taking up residence in particular communities, selection mechanisms will lead families with similar sociodemographic characteristics to converge. Evidence from the NLSCY indicates that between-neighbourhood differences (enumeration areas) account for about 7%–8% of the variability in levels of child emotional-behavioural problems.[23] Furthermore, about 25%–30% of the variability in these problems is associated with between-family differences.

Strong associations exist between family socioeconomic disadvantage and poor health. These associations are illustrated in table 10.5, which shows levels of emotional-behavioural problems in 1994 for children aged 4–11 years by family income and family structure. Several points emerge: (1) levels of child emotional-behavioural problems are higher for children living in poor families: mean levels are 8.1 versus 6.6 for families below the poverty line versus above it; (2) there are large differences between single- and two-parent families in reported levels of child problem behaviour irrespective of income, and

Table 10.5
Levels of parent assessed emotional-behavioural problems for children aged 4–11 · years in the 1994 NLSCY by family poverty and structure

Family characteristics	[Number of children] (% in family)	Emotional-behavioural problems (mean)
Income < poverty line	[532,528]	8.1
Lone-parent family	(49.8%)	9.1
Two-parent family	(50.2%)	7.1
Income > poverty line	[2,541,246]	6.6
Lone-parent family	(9.3%)	8.1
Two-parent family	(90.7%)	6.4

these differences are similar within income categories; and (3) given that the overall proportion of children in single-parent families is 17.4%, the per cent in single-parent families exposed to incomes below the poverty line is extraordinarily high at 49.8%.

Question 5: Societal Burden – Direct and Indirect Costs

The direct economic costs for prevention and treatment associated with child psychiatric disorder in Canada are very difficult to estimate. These costs would accrue across political jurisdictions (federal, provincial, municipal), across sectors (public and private), within sectors (health, education, social welfare, and judicial), and between programs (treatment, prevention). We are unaware of any attempt in Canada to estimate these costs. Narrowing the scan to organizations with a special interest in children's mental health and child welfare provides some perspective on recent trends in expenditures. In Ontario, for example, total net expenditures among Children's Aid Societies increased from $751 million in 2000/2001 to $1.221 billion in 2005/2006; a 62.5% increase.[24] In the United States, a recent study of adolescents participating in the FAST TRACK project placed the average annual public cost associated with conduct disorder at $14,000 per child compared to $2300 for youth without conduct disorder.[25]

There is strong evidence to indicate that psychiatric disorder and conditions related to psychiatric disorder among adults are associated with substantial costs to society. In 1996, the World Health Organization developed an approach to quantify the burden of different diseases in commensurate units called disability-adjusted life years (DALYs). These units integrate premature death (years lost) with functional impairment (years of life with disability). In developed countries, eight of the ten leading causes of DALYs among 15–44 year olds were psychiatric disorders or closely aligned conditions (major depressive disorder, schizophrenia, bipolar disorder, obsessive compulsive disorder, alcohol use, self-inflicted injuries, drug use, and violence).[26] Furthermore, there is evidence to suggest that a substantial portion of psychiatric disorder identified in adulthood has a childhood origin.[27]

Question 6: Effectiveness of Programmatic Responses to Child Psychiatric Disorder

Programs to improve the mental health of our children fall along a continuum.[28,29] At one extreme are clinical services provided to individual children referred to health professionals for care (treatment approaches). At the other extreme are universal programs intended to improve the life skills and capabilities of children through enrichment (prevention programs). In the middle are programs directed to children and families believed to be 'at risk' for poorer mental health. The definition of risk can refer to child behaviour that elicits some concern and/or to stressful family circumstances, such as poverty, that may undermine child mental health. The boundary between universal and targeted approaches becomes blurry in programs set up in 'disadvantaged' neighbourhoods to serve all residents. Locating the program in a particular community is consistent with the idea of 'targeting,' while opening the program up to all residents in the community is consistent with the idea of 'universal.'

There are differences in program objectives and intended beneficiaries associated with this continuum. Clinical programs focus on the resolution of mental health problems among the few; universal programs aim to build competency among the many. Targeted programs may address individual deficits or strengths and serve small or large numbers of individuals, depending on their objectives and scope. A rational planning model to increase mental health and reduce psychiatric disorder among children would call for balance among these approaches to optimize impact and minimize cost. In attempting to locate this balance, the critical questions for programs associated with each approach are the same: On average, what effects do they have on the mental health of children they serve? How many children do they benefit? And what does it cost to serve each child?

There has been little apparent progress in rationalizing societal responses to the needs posed by children's mental health in general and child psychiatric disorder in particular. The dominant role of treatment services in Canada is a formidable obstacle to seeking, let alone achieving, a balanced societal response. In 2002, Canada spent less than $300 per capita on public health, compared with total health expenditures of about $3900 per capita.[15] If the overall health care system allocations apply to children's mental health, then treatment services will be consuming up to 90% of expenditures. A change in this distribution is difficult to visualize. Treatment services have the urgency of responding to immediate expressions of need and distress, and preoccupation with treatment is continuing to grow among the public and in government, fuelled by concerns over access to care, wait times, and burgeoning costs. Although exceptions exist, prevention services rarely command the same public response.

Discussion

Child psychiatric disorder is an important public health problem in Canada. Waddell and colleagues[14,15] argue that it may affect as many as 14.1% of Canadian children. Taking into account parent and teacher perceptions of need, along with the pervasiveness of impairment and continuity in disorder, we estimate that the per cent of children with clinically meaningful psychiatric disorder might be closer to 5%–8%. Placing levels of child psychiatric disorder at this level in Canada would still identify from 305,000 to 488,000 children and adolescents aged 5 to 19 years in need of care – far beyond the capacity of specialized mental health services.

Individual and Societal Burden of Child Psychiatric Disorder in Canada

The individual and societal burden of child psychiatric disorder may exceed the collective impact of most other chronic health problems. Being classified with child psychiatric disorder is associated in early adulthood with substantial losses in education, household income, personal health, and life satisfaction. In comparison with children classified with chronic health problems, these losses are as much as two to three times greater among children classified with psychiatric disorder. Further to this, using disability life years (DALYs) as a measure of adverse life impact, it has been estimated that eight of the ten leading causes of DALYs among 15–44 year olds in developed countries were psychiatric disorders or closely aligned conditions.[26]

There is some evidence to indicate that mean levels of emotional-behavioural problems are consistently lower in Atlantic Canada. However, the differences between Atlantic Canada and the other regions are small and variable over time, and no obvious explanation exists for their occurrence. In smaller geographical areas, there is reliable evidence of spatial clustering. Between-neighbourhood differences account for about 7%–8% of the variability in levels of emotional behavioural problems. It is well known that selection mechanisms sort families into neighbourhoods based on their social, economic, and cultural fit. The extent to which developmental influences are due to places (contextual effects) versus residents (compositional effects) is an important question that needs to be addressed in future research.

Problems linked with poor mental health are believed to have risen over the past 50 years,[30] and a recent report from the United Kingdom, based on information from three different studies between 1974 and 1999, concluded that there has been an increase in conduct problems reported by parents of 15–16 year olds.[31] However, studies of secular trends from the United States[32] and the Netherlands[33] have been mixed, and data applicable to Canada provide no evidence that levels of emotional-behavioural problems have changed from 1994 to 2000. Obtaining valid estimates of secular trends entails numerous methodological challenges of sampling and measurement. Although 1994 to 2000 spans a relatively short period of time for trends to occur, it is important to note that in the NLSCY: (1) the methods of assessment were identical at each cycle, and (2) the samples were nationally representative and large enough to generate very precise estimates.

In addition to material disadvantage, the less well off in our society shoulder an unfair burden of ill health. In Canada, as in most countries, there are marked socioeconomic gradients in levels of child emotional-behavioural problems.[34] This report highlighted the strong links between household poverty, family structure (single-parent status), and levels of child emotional-behavioural problems. Similar associations exist for inadequate housing.[35] The socioeconomic patterning of child mental health is a fundamental problem that calls out to be addressed in a country committed to health equity.

Issues in the Conceptualization of Child Psychiatric Disorder

The study of child psychiatric disorder as an epidemiological phenomenon in the general population is fraught with many challenges. The *DSM* created a system of classification based on categorical structures to facilitate clinical practice and communication, not to represent the underlying nature of psychopathology.[36] Despite some advances in the instruments used to classify child psychiatric disorder in general populations,[37] there remain a number of important methodological challenges.[6,38,39,40,41] Child psychiatry has no criterion measures of disorder; symptom clusters are limited to emotional (affective) and behavioural response patterns – cognitive and physiological domains have yet to be incorporated into child psychiatric nosology; symptom thresholds for classifying different types of psychiatric disorder are arbitrary – the result of clinical consensus – and there is no consensus on the integration of assessment data collected from multiple respondents. Finally, relatively small changes in assessment approach, for example, to question/item wording, to response options, and to methods of data collection can systematically alter patterns of response and lead to the identification of different numbers and configurations of children with disorder.

The challenges to classifying child psychiatric disorder today are evocative of the same problems identified twenty years ago,[42] and there is no indication that these issues will be resolved in the near future. Standardized methods and conventional criteria for classifying child psychiatric disorder help to reduce variability in prevalence estimates, but do nothing to resolve core issues. The concept of psychiatric disorder combined with categorical approaches to classifying children emphasizes disjunctions between normal and abnormal. This approach has been critically important to advocacy by providing a foundation to discuss child mental health needs in the population. Unfortunately, it has also reinforced the primacy of treatment interventions in meeting these needs. There is no evidence that the childhood disorders studied in the general population conform to the categorical representations outlined in the *DSM-IV*. Arguably, child mental health problems exist on a continuum of response. At present, resource allocations for children's mental health are devoted to a relatively small segment of the child population with elevated symptoms and the family wherewithal to access specialized services.

Adequacy of Programmatic Responses to Child Psychiatric Disorder

Is there a need to reassess our programmatic responses to child psychiatric disorder? The continued dominance of treatment models needs to be reviewed for the following reasons. One, treating patients one at a time is labour intensive and expensive. Current estimates of needs based on the prevalence of child psychiatric disorder encompass far more children than can be seen by professionals.[29] Two, help for children in need of children's mental health services depends on referral. Referral takes time and is accompanied by prolonged distress. Furthermore, not all referred children will need or can benefit from services, resulting in the poor targeting of specialized services.[38] Three, there is substantial measurement error and elasticity in the classification of child psychiatric disorder. This raises intractable problems in assessing: (1) the coverage provided by treatment services (extent to which specialized services can meet children's mental health needs in the population); and (2) the ability of specialized services to distinguish between referrals who need and can benefit from services and those who cannot.[38] Four, concern exists about the effectiveness of 'usual clinical care' available in children's mental health settings. Although there are numerous, structured, manual-guided treatment interventions that have proven to be effective,[43,44] existing evidence suggests that there is little or no benefit associated with usual clinical care.[45,46]

Strategies to improve children's mental health (and to reduce child psychiatric disorder) need to consider a mix of effective prevention/ intervention programs. Integrated models have been proposed that call for a continuum of programs responsive to the type and level of child mental health problems in the population.[29,47] Unfortunately, nothing is known about the appropriate mix of strategies. We can only speculate about the relationship between case-based and population-based strategies to address child mental health needs. Prevention programs that leverage population changes in risk exposure may (or may not) offer returns to child mental health in the form of overall symptom reductions that exceed the leverage available to specialized treatment services.[48] In parallel with evidenced-based treatments, there are a number of universal and high risk prevention programs for youth that have demonstrated significant long-term benefits.[49,50] Attempts to discern the appropriate mix of programs must begin with interventions of demonstrated effectiveness and develop research strategies for monitoring secular changes in children's mental health at the population level.

Addressing Child Mental Health Needs in the Future

The new conceptualizations of psychiatric disorder that accompanied the *DSM* in the 1980s, along with the development of standardized approaches to assessment and classification, provided the foundation for a new discipline, child psychiatric epidemiology. Community studies in Canada that emerged from this discipline raised important societal concerns about the high levels and adverse impact of child mental health problems, about socioeconomic inequalities in the distribution of these problems, and about the inability of specialized mental health services to address the public health needs associated with these problems.

Governments at all levels of Canada have been responsive to these concerns. In the past ten to fifteen years, there have been unprecedented increases in the allocation of resources to specialized services (child welfare and children's mental health) and to early years programs intended to improve developmental outcomes among children at risk.[51] These resource increases are most welcome and the emerging programs are motivated undoubtedly by a genuine concern for enhancing child development. Unfortunately, there is little evidence that these programs are effective[52] and a number of factors exist that make it very difficult to produce evidence of their usefulness. One, program administrators are preoccupied with 'rolling them out' – ensuring that resources are allocated and spent. This may reflect concerns about the budgetary process – unspent money being clawed back – and/or the vulnerability of these initiatives to changes of government. Two, rather than viewing program evaluation as an integral part of program development, it is perceived as an activity to be contracted out after programs are established. This invariably leads to weak evaluation studies that provide minimally useful information about program effects. Three, evaluation efforts focus almost exclusively on process indicators under the assumption that, if the programs are being used, they must be useful. Four, in many programs, there is an ideological predisposition to place undue trust in 'local expertise' and undue mistrust in academic expertise for developing and evaluating program content. Field experience is a critical component of program development and implementation but academic knowledge about developmental influences and evaluation methods are critical to achieving standards of evidence.

Many of these factors are applicable to the Community Action Program for Children. It began in the 1990s as part of the federal government's first early development initiative, whereby community organizations receive funding to develop programs aimed at improving developmental outcomes among high risk children aged 0–6 years. Although there is no empirical evidence of positive developmental effects,[53] it is a popular, expensive, well established program.[54]

In our view, moving forward in the development and implementation of effective interventions for children's mental health will require partnerships between government sponsors, community organizations responsible for programs, and academic specialists with both substantive and methodological expertise. Traditionally, developmental research and program evaluation have been a central focus and responsibility of the academic community. However, the federal government is now playing a much larger role in these activities, and the resources available to the government for both developmental research (e.g., NLSCY) and new programs (e.g., Early Development Initiative) go far beyond the scale of developmental research and program evaluation studies that have been carried out in academic settings. These new research and program initiatives need to be informed by diverse stakeholders fully committed to generating evidence of effectiveness. Our children should expect no less than programs that create equal opportunities for developmental success through the early life course.

NOTES AND REFERENCES

Michael Boyle is supported by a Canada Research Chair in the Social Determinants of Child Health. During this work, Katholiki Georgiades was supported by a post-doctoral fellowship from the Social Sciences and Humanities Research Council.

1 Garber J. Classification of childhood psychopathology: A developmental perspective. *Child Dev* 1984;55:30–48.
2 Lease, CA, Ollendick TH. Development and psychopathology. In: Bellack AS, Hersen M, eds. *Psychopathology in Adulthood*. New York: Allyn and Bacon, 1993:89–103.

3 Sroufe LA, Rutter M. The domain of developmental psychopathology. *Child Dev* 1984;55:17–29.

4 American Psychiatric Association. *Diagnostic and Statistical Manual of Mental Disorders.* 4th ed. Washington DC: Author, 1994.

5 Achenbach TM, Edelbrock CS. Behavioral problems and competencies reported by parents of normal and disturbed children aged four through sixteen. *Monogr Soc Res Child Dev* 1981;46:1–82.

6 Boyle MH, Offord DR, Racine Y, et al. Identifying thresholds for classifying childhood psychiatric disorder: Issues and prospects. *J Am Acad Child Adolesc Psychiatry* 1996;35:1440–8.

7 Boyle MH, Offord DR, Hofmann HF, et al. Ontario Child Health Study: I. Methodology. *Arch Gen Psychiatry* 1987;44:826–31.

8 Kasius MC, Ferdinand, RF, van den Berg H, et al. Associations between different diagnostic approaches for child and adolescent psychopathology. *J Child Psychol Psychiatry* 1997;38:625–32.

9 Cummings EM, Davies PT, Campbell SB. *Developmental Psychopathology and Family Process.* New York: Guilford Press, 2000.

10 Williams JG, Higgins JPT, Brayne CEG. Systematic review of prevalence studies of autism spectrum disorders. *Arch Dis Child* 2007;91:8–15.

11 Volkmar FR, Schwab-Stone M. Annotation: Childhood disorders in DSM-IV. *J Child Psychol Psychiatry* 1996;37:779–84.

12 McClellan JM, Werry JS. Research diagnostic interviews for children and adolescents. *J Am Acad Child Adolesc Psychiatry* 2000;39:19–27.

13 Roberts RE, Attkisson CC, Rosenblatt A. Prevalence of psychopathology among children and adolescents. *Am J Psychiatry* 1998;155:715–25.

14 Waddell C, Offord DR, Shepherd CA, et al. Child psychiatric epidemiology and Canadian public policy-making: The state of the science and the art of the possible. *Can J Psychiatry* 2002;47:825–32.

15 Waddell C, McEwan K, Shepherd CA, et al. A public health strategy to improve the mental health of Canadian children. *Can J Psychiatry* 2005;50:226–33.

16 Boyle MH, Georgiades K, Racine Y, et al. Neighborhood and family influences on educational attainment: Results from the Ontario Child Health Study Follow-up 2001. *Child Dev* 2007;78:168–89.

17 Offord DR, Boyle MH, Szatmari P, et al. Ontario Child Health Study: II. Six-month prevalence of disorder and rates of service utilization. *Arch Gen Psychiatry* 1987;44:832–6.

18 Special Surveys Division. *Special Surveys. National Longitudinal Survey of Children and Youth: User's Handbook and Microdata Guide.* Ottawa: Statistics Canada and Human Resources Development Canada, 1996.

19 Boyle MH, Offord DR, Racine YA, et al. Evaluation of the original Ontario Child Health Study Scales. *Can J Psychiatry* 1993;38:397–405.

20 Cadman DT, Boyle MH, Offord DR, et al. Chronic illness and functional limitations in Ontario children: Findings of the Ontario Child Health Study. *Can Med Assoc J* 1986;135:761–7.

21 Cadman DT, Boyle MH, Szatmari P, et al. Chronic illness, disability and mental health: Findings of the Ontario Child Health Study. *Pediatrics* 1987;79:805–13.

22 Ware JE, Kosinski M, Keller SD. A 12-item short form health survey: Construction of scales and preliminary tests of reliability and validity. *Med Care* 1996;34:220–33.

23 Boyle MH, Lipman EL. Do places matter? Socioeconomic disadvantage and child problem behavior in Canada. *J Consult Clin Psychol* 2002;70:378–89.

24 Ontario Association of Children's Aid Societies. *CAS Facts April 1, 2005 – March 31, 2006*. Available at http://www.oacas.org/aboutoacas/annual-report.htm.

25 Foster EM, Jones DE, Conduct Problems Prevention Research Group. The high costs of aggression: Public expenditures resulting from conduct disorder. *Am J Pub Health* 2005;95:1767–72.

26 Murray CJL, Lopez AD. *The Global Burden of Disease, Vol 1*. Geneva: World Health Organization, 1996.

27 Kessler R, Berglund P, Demler O, et al. Lifetime prevalence and age of onset distributions of DSM-IV disorders in the National Co-morbidity Survey Replication. *Arch Gen Psychiatry* 2005;62:593–602.

28 Institute of Medicine. *Reducing Risks for Mental Disorders: Frontiers for Preventive Intervention Research*. Washington, DC: National Academy Press, 1994.

29 Offord DR, Kraemer HC, Kazdin AE, et al. Lowering the burden of suffering from child psychiatric disorder: Trade-offs among clinical, targeted, and universal interventions. *J Am Acad Child Adolesc Psychiatry* 1998;37:686–94.

30 Rutter M, Smith DJ. *Psychosocial Disorders in Young People: Time Trends and Their Causes*. Chichester: John Wiley and Sons, 1995.

31 Collishaw S, Maughan B, Goodman R, et al. Time trends in adolescent mental health. *J Child Psychol Psychiatry* 2004;45:1350–62.

32 Achenbach TM, Dumenci L, Rescorla LA. Are American children's problems getting worse? A 23-year comparison. *J Abnorm Child Psychol* 2003;31:1–11.

33 Verhulst FC, van der Ende J, Rietbergen A. Ten-year time trends of psy-

chopathology in Dutch children and adolescents: No evidence for strong trends. *Acta Psychiatr Scand* 1997;96:7–13.

34 Bradley RH, Corwyn RF. Socioeconomic status and child development. *Annu Rev Psychol* 2002;53:371–99.

35 Boyle MH. Home ownership and the emotional and behavioral problems of children and adolescents. *Child Dev* 2002;73:883–92.

36 Clark LA, Watson D, Reynolds S. Diagnosis and classification of psychopathology: Challenges to the current system and future directions. *Annu Rev Psychol* 1995;46:121–53.

37 Costello EJ, Egger H, Angold A. 10-year research update review: The epidemiology of child and adolescent psychiatric disorders: I. Methods and public health burden. *J Am Acad Child Adolesc Psychiatry* 2005;44:972–86.

38 Boyle MH. Children's mental health issues. In: Johnson L, Barnhorst D, eds. *Children, Families and Public Policy in the 90's*. Toronto: Thompson Educational Publishing Inc., 1991:73–104.

39 Boyle MH, Offord DR, Racine YA, et al. Interviews versus checklists: Adequacy for classifying childhood psychiatric disorder based on parent reports. *Arch Gen Psychiatry* 1997;54:793–9.

40 Offord, DR, Boyle MH, Racine YA, et al. Integrating assessment data from multiple informants. *J Am Acad Child Adolesc Psychiatry* 1996;35:1078–85.

41 Pickles A, Angold A. Natural categories or fundamental dimensions: On carving nature at the joints and the rearticulation of psychopathology. *Dev Psychopathol* 2003;15:529–51.

42 Rutter M, Tuma AH, Lann IS, eds. *Assessment and Diagnosis in Child Psychopathology*. London: The Guilford Press, 1988.

43 Weisz JR, Weiss B, Han SS, et al. Effects of psychotherapy with children and adolescents revisited: A meta-analysis of treatment outcome studies. *Psychol Bull* 1995;117:450–68.

44 Weisz JR, Jensen-Doss A, Hawley KM. Evidence-based youth psychotherapies versus usual clinical care. *Am Psychol* 2006;61:671–89.

45 Weisz JR. *Psychotherapy for Children and Adolescents: Evidence-based Treatments and Case Examples*. Cambridge, UK: Cambridge University Press, 2004.

46 Weisz JR, Jensen AL. Child and adolescent psychotherapy in research and practice contexts: Review of the evidence and suggestions for improving the field. *Eur Child Adolesc Psychiatry* 2001;10:12–8.

47 Weisz JR, Sandler IN, Durlak JA, et al. Promoting and protecting youth mental health through evidence-based prevention and treatment. *Am Psychol* 2005;60:628–48.

48 Zuberbier OA, Boyle MH. *A Population Approach To Preventing Mental Disorders in Canadian Children.* Working paper. Hamilton Ontario: Offord Centre for Child Studies, McMaster University and Hamilton Health Sciences Corporation, 2007.

49 Durlak JA, Wells AM. Primary prevention mental health programs for children and adolescents: A meta-analytic review. *Am J Community Psychol* 1997;25:115–52.

50 Durlak JA, Wells AM. Evaluation of indicated preventive intervention (secondary prevention) mental health programs for children and adolescents. *Am J Community Psychol* 1998;26:775–802.

51 Government of Canada. *Federal/Provincial/Territorial Early Childhood Development Agreement: Report on Government of Canada Activities and Expenditures 2001-02.* (Cat. No. H21-183/2001E). Ottawa: Minister of Public Works and Government Services, 2001.

52 McLennan JD, MacMillan HL, Jamieson E. Canada's programs to prevent mental health problems in children: The research-practice gap. *CMAJ* 2004;171:1069–71.

53 Boyle MH, Willms DW. Impact evaluation of a national community-based program for children at risk in Canada. *Can Public Policy* 2002;28:461–82.

54 Health Canada. *Growing Up with CAPC.* Accessed April 7, 2007. Available at: http://www.phac-aspc.gc.ca/dca-dea/publications/pdf/capc-growingup_e.pdf

55 Shaffer D, Fisher P, Dulcan MK, et. al. The NIMH Diagnostic Interview Schedule for Children Version 2.3 (DISC-2.3): Description, acceptability, prevalence rates, and performance in the MECA study. *J Am Acad Child Adolesc Psychiatry* 1996;35:865–77.

56 Costello EJ, Angold AA, Burns BJ, et. al. (1996). The Great Smoky Mountains Study of Youth: Goals, design, methods, and the prevalence of DSM-III-R disorders. *Arch Gen Psychiatry* 1996;53:1129–36.

57 Breton JJ, Bergeron L, Valla JP, et al. Quebec Child Mental Health Survey: Prevalence of DSM-III-R mental disorders. *J Child Psychol Psychiatry* 1999;40:375–84.

58 Meltzer H, Gatward R, Goodman R, et al. *Mental Health of Children and Adolescents in Great Britain.* London: Her Majesty's Stationary Office, 2000.

59 Offord DR, Boyle MH, Fleming JE, et al. Ontario Child Health Study: Summary of selected results. *Can J Psychiatry* 1989;34:483–91.

60 Simonoff E, Pickles A, Meyer JM, et. al. The Virginia Twin Study of Adolescent Behavioral Development: Influences of age, sex, and impairment on rates of disorder. *Arch Gen Psychiatry* 1997;54:801–8.

11 Psychiatric Disorder in Later Life: A Canadian Perspective

LAURIE M. CORNA, LAURA GAGE, JOHN CAIRNEY, AND
DAVID L. STREINER

Introduction and Overview

Like so many other areas of Canadian psychiatric epidemiology, researchers have only just begun to explore psychiatric disorders and impairment in later life. Recent interest has been fuelled by the release of the Canadian Community Health Survey (CCHS 1.2), the first national survey of psychiatric disorders in Canada. For the first time, the prevalence of five major disorders (major depressive disorder, bipolar disorder, social phobia, agoraphobia, panic disorder), as well as substance abuse/dependence can be estimated in a large, representative sample of Canadians, which includes older adults. Prior to this survey, only a few studies (the Edmonton Study[1] and the Ontario Mental Health Supplement[2]) were available to examine the prevalence and correlates of psychiatric disorders in old age. Therefore, to date we have only limited information for this subset of the population in Canada.

In this chapter, we review some major conceptual and methodological issues in the study of aging and psychiatric disorders, especially in relation to depression, which has received the most attention from epidemiologists. Next, we review the prevalence of several major psychiatric disorders in old age in Canada, including known risk markers or correlates and psychiatric comorbidity. A brief discussion of mental health care service use is followed by a review of where future research in this area may be most fruitfully orientated.

Background: Mental Illness in an Aging Population

The epidemiology of psychiatric disorders among older adults is a relatively new area in psychiatric epidemiology, which is likely related to changing demographics.[3] Canada, like Britain and the United States, has been characterized as an 'aging' society because the relative proportion of adults over 65 years has increased substantially relative to other age groups and is expected to continue to increase. By the year 2026, it is estimated that one in five Canadians will be 65 and older.[4] Concerns regarding the social, economic, and health impacts of an aging society abound in the academic literature. In particular, much research has been devoted to health care issues germane to older adults, both with respect to quality of life, well-being, and the capacity of the current health care resources to meet the growing needs of an aging population.

With respect to mental health issues, one of the recurring debates in the literature concerns the question of whether the prevalence of mental illness declines or increases with age. The challenges associated with measuring psychological or psychiatric disorder(s) makes the answer to this question complex. Depression serves as a useful illustration. Studies that have used measures of depressive symptomatology have documented a U-shaped relationship between age and depression with the lowest prevalence among 45 to 50 year-olds.[5,6] These studies suggested that depression is a highly prevalent and important health concern among young adults (20 to 24) and the very old (80 and older).

However, a different pattern of findings emerges when we consider the findings from studies that used *DSM* criteria to determine the prevalence of disorders. Several studies, including the Epidemiologic Catchment Area study (ECA), have documented a negative linear relationship between age and depression with the lowest reported prevalence estimates among those over the age of 65.[7,8] Using a large, representative sample of Canadians aged 15 and older, Wade and Cairney[9] reported a reversed J-shaped relationship between age and depression across successively older age cohorts. Here, the prevalence of depression declined until about age 75, followed by a modest upturn. It may be the case that these discrepancies between studies reflect real differences in the manifestation of depressive illness in old age. Older adults may be more likely than younger adults to have sub-syndromal or minor depression rather than major depressive disorder.[10,11] However, there are other possible explanations that may account for the low prevalence estimates of *DSM* disorders among older adults.

Prevalence Estimates and Explanations for Age-Related Differences in Psychiatric Disorders in Older Adults

Most studies that use *DSM* criteria for caseness report a lower prevalence of psychiatric disorders among community dwelling older adults (aged 65 and older) than among younger age groups (18–64).[8,12] For example, pooled data from all sites in the ECA studies showed that the prevalence of any disorder (1-month estimates) among older adults to be 12.3% compared with 17% in adults aged 18–24.[8] With the exception of severe cognitive impairment, where the prevalence estimates were highest among older adults, this general pattern was evident for all disorders examined in the ECA study (major depressive disorder, panic disorder, etc.). Indeed, the most prevalent disorders in old age (65+) in the ECA data were anxiety, cognitive impairment, phobia, and dysthymia (5.5%, 4.9%, 4.8%, 1.8% respectively). Bland et al. reported similar findings from the Edmonton study. With the exception of cognitive impairment, both 6-month and lifetime prevalence estimates of disorder were consistently lower among respondents ages 65 and older as compared to the whole population (all ages).[12,13] For example, the 6-month prevalence of any disorder was 10.9% among older adults compared to 17.1% for all adults in the study.

At the time of their publication, these findings were contrary to the consensus that mental health problems were highly prevalent among older adults.[14] In particular, the relatively low prevalence for major depressive episode of 0.9% was surprising,[8] as many of the experiences associated with aging (e.g., loss of loved ones, the onset of chronic physical health problems, and the loss of valued social roles) were also associated with increased risk for psychopathology, especially depression.[3,5] Yet, despite greater exposure to these negative occurrences, older adults were less likely than younger adults to suffer from psychiatric disorders. Moreover, these findings were inconsistent with other data that showed high use of psychotropic medication among the elderly, a proxy measure for the presence of psychiatric disorder.[11]

In the period following the publication of the ECA data, epidemiologists interested in aging and mental health increasingly focused their attention on potential explanations to account for these rather surprising findings. Hocking and her colleagues[3] identified two explanations to explain low prevalence estimates in older adults. The first explanation was methodological in nature and concerned symptom reporting. They suggested that it was not that psychiatric disorders were less common in later life per se, but that older adults were less likely to report symptoms than younger adults, more likely to forget symptoms, and/or more likely to express psychological mood or behavioural symptoms in somatic terms. Closely related to reporting is the issue of who is being captured when conventional sampling techniques are employed. Older adults with psychiatric disorders may be less likely to participate in community surveys, or may be excluded from the sampling frame altogether because of institutionalization.

While not dismissing the probable contribution of methodological and sampling issues in explaining the low rates of psychiatric disorder in later life, most epidemiologists interested in aging and mental health treated the findings as real, not artefactual, and believed the explanation for the pattern of results may be accounted for by period and/or cohort effects.[3,15] Proponents of the cohort interpretation argued that individuals born prior to 1920 (aged 65 and older at the time of the ECA survey) were psychologically heartier than individuals born after (or much earlier) than that time period, although no specific causal mechanism was identified. In this view, older adults reported lower rates of disorder because they had always been healthier than younger cohorts. Increasing suicide trends in successively older age cohorts have been used to support this hypothesis.[3]

A second, and more compelling explanation for lower rates of disorders among older adults is the cohort-period effect hypothesis because an actual causal mechanism was implicated. Here, a cohort-period effect hypothesis suggested that older adults at the time of the ECA survey shared several significant historical events (the Great Depression, the Second World War) that had a profound impact on psychological development. In particular, many individuals who lived through these periods endured significant economic and social hardships. However, these same individuals also experienced significant improvements to their economic and social circumstances during the post–World War II period. Conversely, younger adults (e.g., the 'baby boom' generation), not having experienced such dramatic changes in their standard of living, were simply not as adept at handling adversities as the generation preceding them. Additionally, the 'baby boom' generation had set high expectations for themselves in terms of a material standard of living and, as a result of growing up during a population boom, have had to compete for fewer social and economic resources. Together, these effects explain the higher prevalence estimates of psychiatric disorders observed in younger cohorts, as opposed to older cohorts.

Another potential explanation is that age differences in the prevalence of psychiatric disorders are the result of true aging effects. That is, psychiatric disorders are less common in older adults because psychological well-being improves with age. As we noted earlier, this is at odds with some gerontological and psychological theories of aging that focus on what is lost as people age (e.g., physical health, social roles, friends, and loved ones) and how this affects psychological well-being.[5,16–20] However, stage theories of human development and theoretical perspectives on successful aging, which have also been influential in gerontology and the psychology of aging, support the notion that positive mental well-being accompanies aging.[21–27] For example, Levinson et al.[27] portray aging as a process of maturational unfolding. With age comes greater maturity and acceptance as individuals either learn to master their environments, or learn to accept limitations and change, and hence perceive situations in a more positive light than younger adults. Adaptation theory would also suggest that individuals demonstrate fairly consistent levels of well-being or happiness despite experiences of adversity.[28]

While slightly less optimistic, a second variant of an aging effect explanation is the healthy survivor or selection explanation. This account suggests that the prevalence of psychiatric disorder is lower in later life because only the healthiest members of a given cohort actually survive to old age, and are thus overrepresented in older populations. This particular explanation has been used to account for narrowing socioeconomic status (SES) gaps in physical health with age[29] although there is no reason it cannot also be applied to psychiatric outcomes (see, e.g.,[30]). Finally, we must also consider the influence of biological explanations for the lower prevalence of disorders later in life. That is, the expression of symptoms among older adults may be qualitatively different in some respects compared to the manifestation of the same condition among younger adults. For example, changes in neurotransmitters with age may decrease the reporting of anxiety symptoms and disorders.[31,32]

Impact of ECA Study on Subsequent Research

Regardless of the explanation, the findings of the ECA and other studies that used the Diagnostic Interview Schedule (DIS) conducted throughout the 1980s have had a significant impact on subsequent psychiatric epidemiologic investigations. Most notably, many post-ECA community studies have focused exclusively on younger adults (under age 55) because prevalence estimates for disorders among older adults were so low (e.g., the National Co-morbidity Study[33]). Yet, if period and/or cohort explanations are correct, age differences in psychiatric disorders are apt to change as younger cohorts, such as the baby boom generation, move into retirement. For example, the cohort hypothesis would predict that estimates of psychiatric disorders should increase relative to the ECA estimates as the baby boomers move into old age. Alternatively, if the aging effect or adaptation hypotheses (survivor effect or otherwise) are correct, then prevalence estimates for disorders should remain comparable to those observed for older adults in the ECA data. In other words, there should be continuity in prevalence estimates across studies collected in different time periods. In either case, there are only two means by which the adequacy of either hypothesis can be ascertained: (1) longitudinal data spanning decades in order to capture the transition from early adulthood to advanced old age; or (2) cross sectional data collected across different periods where we can examine representative samples from the same age cohorts in different time periods (e.g., data collected in 1980 compared with data collected in 2000). Until the CCHS 1.2, the lack of data on older adults in more contemporary surveys has made examination of these questions impossible.

Studying Age Differences in Psychiatric Disorders in a Canadian Context

In Canada, there have been limited data with which to estimate psychiatric disorder among older adults living in the community. For example, large-scale community mental health surveys in Canada have been geographically specific (the Ontario Mental Health Supplement,[2] the Edmonton Study,[1] and the Montreal Area Catchment study[34]). Moreover, these particular surveys are also limited by their respective sample sizes (Edmonton: $n = 3,258$; Ontario: $n = 11,000$; Montreal: $n = 893$), making accurate estimation of the prevalence of disorders and service use among older adults problematic. In the Ontario Mental Health Supplement, for example, there were only 1837 respondents over the age of 65[2] and the number of adults 65 years and older in the Edmonton study was even smaller (n = 358).[1] Moreover, the data for both of these studies were collected not long after ECA data in the United States (between 1983 and 1990), making it more difficult to investigate the cohort effects discussed. Finally, other more recent surveys such as the Toronto Co-morbidity Study, followed the lead of the NCS study and only sampled adults under the age of 55.[35] Other data sources based on probability samples of the whole population (e.g., National Population Health Survey and the General Social Surveys), while large, included limited measures of psychopathology (e.g., NPHS: 12-month major depressive episode only). This absence of population level data concerning mental health and psychological disorders, especially among those over the age of 55, has resulted in a number of questions with conflicting answers, such as whether the rates of depression and suicidal ideation increase or decrease with age. Indeed, studies using smaller samples have indicated both trends. The availability of the CCHS 1.2 and its inclusion of older adults provided researchers with a unique opportunity to examine age-related differences in psychiatric disorders and address some of the competing explanations within a Canadian context.

Comorbid Disorders among Older Adults

In addition to the limited amount of research that has examined prevalence estimates for specific disorders among older adults, an even smaller number of studies have examined patterns of comorbidity among older adults. As noted, this may be due to the general belief that psychiatric disorders were less common in later life, based upon the results of studies such as the ECA, and/or because epidemiologic studies on psychiatric disorders in later life have tended to focus on depression and dementia.[36] Yet, studies employing both clinical[37,38] and general population samples demonstrate that comorbidity among psychiatric disorders is not uncommon, even in community samples.[39-42] Indeed, approximately 50% of all lifetime disorders in the general population occur in individuals who have a history of some additional psychiatric disorder.[33,43] Consistent with research on younger adults, the results of these studies suggest substantial co-morbidity, particularly with anxiety disorders and major depressive disorder. Yet, until now, the opportunity to estimate prevalence and patterns of comorbidity in a large sample of older Canadians was non-existent.

Prevalence and Correlates of Major Psychiatric Disorders in Old Age in Canada

Data from the CCHS 1.2 allow us to look at the prevalence and correlates of both 12-month and lifetime mood and anxiety disorders using *DSM-IV* diagnostic criteria among a large, representative sample of Canadians aged 55 years and older, and to compare these estimates with results from other large epidemiological surveys. In this sample, the most common disorder among respondents 55+ years was major depressive disorder (2.92%), followed by social phobia (1.32%), panic disorder (0.84%), agoraphobia (0.61%), and bipolar disorder (0.26%). Overall, the prevalence of psychiatric disorders is low in this population and tends to decline among successively older age groups (see figure 11. 1).

In the sections that follow, we review the epidemiology of five major psychiatric disorders (major depression, bipolar disorder, social phobia, panic disorder, and agoraphobia), substance use, psychiatric comorbidity, and mental health service utilization among older adults based on data from the CCHS 1.2. Where possible, we draw comparisons from our findings with existing epidemiological data for each disorder. Our decision to include adults aged 55 years and older was based on a number of considerations. First, since many large scale epidemiological studies have not included adults over the age of 54, investigation of this age group is important and provides a broader picture of mental health in the second part of the life course. Second, although age 65 is commonly thought to mark retirement age, it is increasingly common for individuals to either retire early, or work well beyond this age. Finally, this broader age range afforded a larger sample with which to study psychiatric disorders.

Major Depression

Major depressive disorder (MD) is characterized by a period of time lasting no less than two weeks during which there is depressed mood and/or loss of interest or pleasure in nearly all activities, and during which additional symptoms are present (symptoms include changes in appetite or weight, sleep, and psychomotor activity, decreased energy, feelings of worthlessness, difficulty thinking, concentrating, or making decisions, recurrent thoughts of death, or suicidal ideation).[44] As mentioned, the prevalence of depression and depressive symptoms among

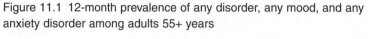

Figure 11.1 12-month prevalence of any disorder, any mood, and any anxiety disorder among adults 55+ years

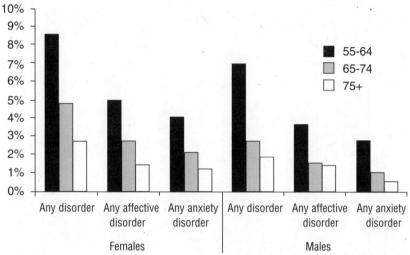

the elderly has been assessed using a number of measurement strategies. Prevalence estimates are typically lowest among older adults compared to any other age group in studies where researchers have employed *DSM* criteria. Conversely, results from studies that use depression scales designed for use with older adults or measures that evaluate depressive symptoms typically report higher rates of depression or depressive symptomatology in older age groups than the rates estimated using *DSM* criteria.[45,46]

Indeed, one of the central debates in the gerontological literature with respect to depression concerns whether or not the prevalence of depression increases or decreases with age. Where depressive symptomatology is concerned, a number of studies have indicated a curvilinear relationship between age and depressive symptoms, with the highest reported levels of symptoms occurring among young adults and the among the very old.[5,6] Using data from the Canadian National Population Health Survey, the highest levels of depressive symptoms were observed among younger adults followed by a decline in prevalence through mid-life, and a slightly increased prevalence again among the oldest old.[9] However, when MD is assessed, published estimates suggest that the rates are lowest among older adults.[3,7,12,13]

Table 11.1
Psychiatric disorder prevalence estimates among older adults across major epidemiological studies

Disorder	Canadian Community Health Survey 1.2[a]	Epidemiologic Catchment Area[b] Male/Female	National Comorbidity Study-Replication (NCS-R)[c]	Edmonton Study[d]	Ontario Mental Health Supplement[e] Male/Female
Major Depression					
6-Month	—	0.1–0.5/1.0–1.6	—	1.2	—
12-Month	2.92	—	—	—	—/4.2
Lifetime	9.02	0.8–1.8	10.6	4.1	—
Bipolar Disorder					
6-Month	—	0/0	—	0	—
12-Month	0.17	—	—	—	—
Lifetime	0.89	0.0–0.1	1.0	0	—
Social Phobia					
6-Month	—	0.1–1.5/0.3–1.9	—	3.0 (All phobias)	—
12-Month	1.32	—	—	—	2.3/5.9
Lifetime	4.94	—	6.6	0.4	—
Panic Disorder					
6-Month	—	0/0.1–0.4	—	0.3	—
12-Month	0.84	—	—	—	—
Lifetime	2.54	0.1–0.2	2.0	0.3	—

Table 11.1 (continued)

Disorder	Canadian Community Health Survey 1.2[a]	Epidemiologic Catchment Area[b] Male/Female	National Comorbidity Study-Replication (NCS-R)[c]	Edmonton Study[d]	Ontario Mental Health Supplement[e] Male/Female
Agoraphobia					
6-Month	—	0–3.3/1.0–5.5	—	3.0 (All phobias)	—
12-Month	0.61	—	—	—	—
Lifetime	1.38	1.2–7.5	1.0	2.5	—

[a] Adults 55+ years
[b] Adults 65+years from New Haven, Conn, Baltimore, and St. Louis (6-month[7]: lifetime[43])
[c] Adults 60+ years[47]
[d] Adults 65+ years[1,12,13]
[e] Adults 45–65 years[2]

Results from the CCHS 1.2 also showed the lowest rates of MD amongst older adults compared to all other age groups. The prevalence of MD among adults 55 and older was 2.92% (95% CI = 2.48–3.37), and as expected, we observed lower prevalence rates across each successively older age group in our sample (55–64, 65–74, 75+), with the lowest rates among those ages 75 and older (1.69%, 95% CI = 1.00–2.38) (unpublished data). The 12-month estimates from the CCHS 1.2 (2.92%) was somewhat higher than the 6-month prevalence estimates reported by Myers et al.[7] of between 0.1% and 1.6% from the ECA data and the reported 6-month prevalence of 1.2% among adults 65 years and older in the Edmonton study. However, the lifetime estimate of 9.02% in the CCHS 1.2 was similar to that reported by Kessler et al.[47] of 10.6% for adults 60 years and older.

In the CCHS 1.2, we did not observe a significant gender difference in the prevalence of depression that is commonly observed among younger cohorts. Using logistic regression, we looked at the effects of a number of sociodemographic markers for major depressive disorder. When all potential sociodemographic risk markers were considered simultaneously, being female and widowed or divorced were associated with an increased risk of meeting the criteria for MD compared to their male and married counterparts (female OR: 1.54, 95% CI = 1.10–2.14; widow OR: 2.17, 95% CI = 1.28–3.67; divorced OR: 2.41, 95% CI = 1.62–3.58). Education and geographic location of residence were not significantly associated with MD in this sample. Interestingly, when potential risk markers were considered individually, respondents in the low-income group had a significantly greater risk of reporting MD, yet in the adjusted model, there was no effect of income. Additionally, while we did not observe a significant effect of gender in the unadjusted model, gender was a significant predictor when other factors were considered together. It appears that the failure to consider multiple risk markers for depression simultaneously would have underestimated the importance of being female for risk of MD. The findings were fairly consistent with previous work with respect to the association of age, gender, and marital status with major depression,[3,11,48] although neither education nor income was significantly associated with depression in the adjusted model in this sample.

In both the unadjusted and adjusted models, the presence of other chronic health problems and limitations in activities of daily living were associated with an increased risk of depression. This is consistent with previous work that suggests a close relationship between mental and physical health problems in later life.[45] What is less clear, however, is the temporal ordering of relationship between the onset of a depressive episode and health problems.

Bipolar Disorder

Bipolar disorder (BD) is characterized by a distinct period of time during which there is an exaggerated or abnormally and persistently elevated, expansive or irritable mood, with or without a history of depression.[44] Some of the symptoms associated with a manic episode include the flight of ideas or racing thoughts, inflated self-esteem, decreased need for sleep, talkativeness, and irritability.

The estimated prevalence of BD among older adults residing in the community was 0–0.5% across fives sites of the ECA study using *DSM-III* criteria,[49] 0.2% among adults aged 55–64 in Edmonton, and 0% among those 65 years and older.[1] Using *DSM-IV* criteria, an HMO (health maintenance organization) sample from the United States reported the 12-month prevalence estimate to be 0.25% among adults 65 years and older.[50] In the CCHS 1.2, the 12-month and lifetime estimates were 0.17% (95% CI = 0.01–0.42) and 0.89% (95% CI = 0.66–1.12), respectively. All but one of these 12-month cases occurred in respondents who were between the ages 55 and 64 years and BD appeared more common among men than women, although this difference was not statistically significant. Although previous work has indicated a significant gender difference, with a higher prevalence among women,[51] the low number of respondents who met the criteria for BD limited our ability to test such effects.

While BD is more commonly associated with younger adults, a first episode in later life is not uncommon,[52] and although definitions of late onset vary in the published literature, late onset is generally defined as occurring at 50 years or older.[53] In the CCHS 1.2, nearly one-third of respondents who met the criteria for BD reported first onset after the age of 50, which is higher than many estimates of late onset bipolar disorder reported in the literature.[51] Unfortunately, the low prevalence of this disorder among older adults in the CCHS 1.2 (only 22 cases) precluded a more thorough analysis of the sociodemographic risk markers for BD in this population.

Social Phobia

Social phobia (SP), also referred to as social anxiety disorder, is characterized by a marked fear of embarrassment in common social situations. The distress experienced by individuals with SP typically leads to avoidance of social activities, resulting in substantial impairment in role functioning (e.g., intimate relationships, work performance), as well as a reduced quality of life.[54–56] Due to substantial changes to the diagnostic criteria for social phobia that occurred with the release of the *DSM-III-R*, the usefulness of the earlier epidemiological studies of the 1980s became limited with respect to our understanding of the prevalence and correlates of social phobia as it is presently understood.[57] For example, lifetime prevalence estimates in studies before the release of the *DSM-III-R* of 1%–4% were substantially lower than the reported lifetime prevalence rates of between 7% and 12% estimated using *DSM-III-R* or *DSM-IV* criteria.[13] Moreover, of the more contemporary studies, many excluded respondents over the age of 65 years,[58–60] combined prevalence estimates for SP with those for specific phobia or anxiety disorders in general,[36,57,61] or reported only a lifetime prevalence estimate of the disorder.[47]

In the CCHS 1.2, the 12-month and lifetimes estimates of SP in our sample were 1.32% (95% CI = 1.08–1.59) and 4.94% (95% CI = 4.40–5.48) respectively. [62] Consistent with our findings for mood disorders, the prevalence of both 12-month and lifetime SP declined significantly across each successively older age group (55–64, 65–74, 75+). Comparing these estimates to other contemporary findings suggested that estimates of SP are slightly lower in the CCHS. For example, using data from the Ontario Mental Health Survey, Stein and Kean[60] reported 12-month and lifetime estimates of 4.1% and 10%, respectively, for adults ages 45 to 64, and in the NCS-R survey, Kessler et al.[47] reported a lifetime prevalence of 6.6% for adults aged 60 and older. Although lifetime SP in the CCHS was slightly lower than these contemporary lifetime estimates, the samples were slightly different, and overall, our estimate of 4.94% was more consistent with other *DSM-III-R* and *DSM-IV* estimates than with prevalence estimates using *DSM-III* criteria. While we lack comparative 12-month estimates, our estimated 12-month prevalence of 1.34% among older adults would suggest that social phobia is not a rare disorder in later life.

More than half of all respondents who qualified for SP reported onset in the first 14 years of life; indeed, the mean age of onset was 16.9

years in the whole sample, and fewer than 10% of respondents with SP reported onset after the age of 54 years. Since one of the major changes to the diagnostic criteria for SP from *DSM-III* to *DSM-III-R* included an increase in the number of phobic situations assessed, we also examined the number of situations endorsed and whether the number or type of situations feared was different between younger (< 55 years) and older adults. The pattern of situations endorsed was remarkably similar and the number of phobic situations reported did not differ by age, either between the older and younger cohorts, or within the group of older adults.[62]

In terms of sociodemographic risk markers for 12-month SP, the predicted probability of meeting the criteria for SP decreased with increasing age, and respondents who reported French as their first language and those who also met the criteria for another *DSM-IV* disorder in the same 12-month period were at an increased risk for SP. Unlike previous work that has assessed sociodemographic risk markers for SP in the general population,[58] gender, marital status, and income were not significant predictors in this population. Since the prevalence of SP is typically greater among females,[58,63] we investigated further whether the failure to find a significant gender effect was due to restricting the sample to adults over the age of 54 years. We also tested whether or not gender differences converge with increasing age. Indeed, we did find that gender was highly significant in the multivariate model among younger adults (< 55 years). We also found that, using the entire sample (ages 15 years and older), there was a significant age by gender interaction, suggesting that the prevalence of SP is highest among women earlier in life, and this gender gap closes with increasing age.

Panic Disorder

Panic disorder (PD) is characterized by recurrent, unexpected panic attacks, followed by at least one month of persistent concern about having another attack, concern about the implications of the panic attacks, or a significant change in behaviour that is directly related to the attacks.[44] The definition of PD has also been modified in recent decades. For example, the primacy of agoraphobia and PD, where they occur together, was reversed in *DSM-III-R* ('agoraphobia with panic attacks' in *DSM-III* was replaced by 'panic disorder with agoraphobia'), and the requirement of a minimum frequency of panic attacks (three attacks in three weeks in *DSM-III*, four in four weeks in *DSM-III-R*) was removed in *DSM-IV*. In addition, the list of potential symptoms was also expanded in *DSM-III-R* to include nausea or abdominal distress.[64]

Due to these changes in diagnostic criteria and the absence of contemporary data with which to estimate PD, our understanding of PD among older adults has been limited. While some of the existing research on PD has excluded older adults altogether, others have not reported prevalence estimates by age group, thereby limiting their contribution to our understanding of PD in the second half of the life course.[33,65–67] Using *DSM-III* criteria, Beekman et al.[36] reported 12-month estimates for the youngest (55–64 years: 0.8%), middle (65–74 years: 1.7%) and oldest old (75–85 years: 0.5%) from the Amsterdam Longitudinal Study of Aging. Six-month and lifetime estimates of 0.3% and 1.2% respectively, were reported among adults aged 65 years and older in Edmonton, Canada,[1] and estimates from the ECA study sites using *DSM-III* criteria reported six-month prevalence estimates of between 0.1% and 0.4% among adults aged 65 years and older.[7] Finally, using *DSM-IV* criteria, Kessler et al.[47] estimated lifetime prevalence of PD for adults aged 60 and older at 2.0%, but did not provide 6-month or 12-month estimates for this age group. In the CCHS 1.2, 12-month and lifetime prevalence estimates among adults 55 and older were 0.84% (95% CI = 0.65–0.99) and 2.54% (95% CI = 2.16–2.74) respectively and 23% of respondents with PD reported onset after the age of 55.[68]

The findings with respect to sociodemographic risk markers for 12-month PD among this population have also been mixed. While some studies indicate that low education and low income are risk markers for PD or anxiety disorders in general,[36,66] many studies have not assessed measures of socioeconomic position as correlates of PD.[69] In unadjusted logistic regression models in the CCHS 1.2, the odds of reporting of PD decreased with age and were lower among widowed respondents and those speaking either both or neither official language. Low-income respondents reported nearly a four-fold risk of being diagnosed with PD compared to those in the high-income group. In a subsequent model, where we adjusted for the effects of other physical and mental health problems, the effect of being in the low-income group was no longer significant, suggesting that respondents in poorer health tend to cluster in the lower income group. Reporting any limitations in ADLs/IADLs significantly increased the odds of meeting the criteria for PD, although reporting any chronic health problems was not a significant correlate of PD in this sample. In both models, gender was not significantly associated with PD.[68]

Agoraphobia

Agoraphobia (AP) is characterized by anxiety about being in situations from which escape might be difficult or embarrassing, or in which help might not be available in the event of a panic attack or panic-like symptoms. This anxiety typically results in a pervasive avoidance of a number of situations, including but not limited to being outside the home, being home alone, being in a crowd of people, travelling in an automobile, or being on a bridge or in an elevator.[44] There is considerable variation in prevalence estimates of AP in the published literature. Six-month estimates of the disorder among older adults ranged from 0.5%–5.5% in the ECA studies,[32] and were estimated to be 2.3% and 2.2% among adults 55–64 and 65+ years respectively in the Edmonton study.[70] One-month estimates of AP in the Guy's/Age Concern study were even higher at 7.8% and 7.9% among those 65+ years.[71] The observed variation in published estimates is likely a result of the various diagnostic tools and systems of classification employed in these studies. For example, the Guy's/Age Concern study[72] may have misdiagnosed social phobia as AP based on the wording of their Anxiety Disorder Scale and, as a result, overestimated the rates of AP.[32] Both the ECA studies and the Edmonton study used the DIS, which required fear and avoidance of only one situation, although the avoidance of only one situation may have represented a simple phobia rather than AP, also resulting in the overestimation of true rates of the disorder.

Of the more contemporary estimates, the NCS-R study reported a lifetime estimate of AP without panic of 1.0% among adults 60 and older, but did not provide corresponding 6-month or 12-month estimates for this same age group.[47] In the CCHS 1.2, 12-month and lifetime estimates of AP were 0.61% (95% CI = 0.40–0.82) and 1.38 (95% CI = 1.10–1.65), with only 30% of adults reporting their first episode after the age of 54 years.[73]

While little is known about the sociodemographic risk markers for AP in the elderly, several risk factors for AP in the general population have been identified. These include being female, of lower socioeconomic position and reporting visible minority status.[74] We examined the importance of these factors as potential risk markers for 12-month AP, as well as the influence of age, marital status, urbanicity, language first spoken and still understood, physical health problems, and psychiatric comorbidities.[73] Age was negatively associated with AP (OR = 0.94, 95% CI = 0.89–0.99), and the predicted probability of meeting the criteria for AP was higher among women (OR = 2.29, 95% CI = 1.01–5.23) and the previously married (OR = 2.88, 95% CI = 1.12–7.42) compared to men or married respondents, respectively. Level of education, household income adequacy, and language first spoken were not significantly associated with meeting the criteria for 12-month AP.

The observed decline in AP with age is consistent with other studies that report a decline in phobias and in other anxiety disorders. Potential explanations for these observed changes with age include age-related changes in neurotransmitters, age-related changes in cognitive style, disorder-rated mortality, selection effects, and cohort explanations.[32,75]

Substance Use/Abuse

Alcohol and illicit drug abuse and dependence are more commonly conceived of as problems of younger adults, as rates of problematic substance use tend to decline with increasing age. However, as the baby boom cohort continues to age, rates of substance abuse (and need for treatment) are expected to increase by the year 2020.[76]

Findings from earlier epidemiological surveys, such as the ECA and the Edmonton study, suggested that the prevalence of alcohol and drug abuse and dependence was fairly low among older adults. For example, across three sites of the ECA study, 6-month estimates of alcohol abuse or dependence were less than 1% for females 65 and older, and between 3.0% and 3.7% among their male counterparts.[7] In these same data, the 6-month prevalence of drug abuse or dependence among those 65+ was 0% for males and 0.2% for females. Similarly, in the Edmonton study, 1.4% of respondents over the age of 65 met the criteria for 6-month alcohol abuse or dependence, and 0% reported drug abuse or dependence.[1,77]

More contemporary estimates using *DSM-IV* criteria are similarly low in this population. Grant et al.,[78] using data from the National Epidemiologic Survey on Alcohol and Related Conditions, estimated the prevalence of alcohol abuse and dependence among those 65 and older to be 1.21% and 0.24% respectively. Slightly higher estimates were found in the Canadian Study of Health and Aging, with a prevalence of definite alcohol abuse of 8.9% among adults 65+. This estimate was obtained using the Cambridge Exam for Mental Disorders of the Elderly (CAMDEX) and *DSM* criteria combined.[79]

In the CCHS 1.2, the prevalence of substance use is very low. Only two respondents met the criteria for *DSM-IV* illicit drug dependence, and 0.5% reported having used any illicit drugs (including cannabis) in the past year. Prevalence estimates are similarly low for alcohol use; only 49 respondents met the criteria for probable cases for alcohol dependence. Such low numbers precluded a more thorough analysis of the sociodemographic correlates of substance use/dependence in this population.

Comorbidity

Very few recent population-based studies have examined psychiatric comorbidity in later life, despite the frequency with which comorbid conditions occur[39,41,42] and the impact they have on prognosis. Drawing on data from the Longitudinal Study of Aging data from Amsterdam, Beekman et al.[36] estimated comorbidity in their sample of adults aged 55 years and older, and found that 47.5% of respondents with major depression also reported one or more anxiety disorders and 26.1% of those with anxiety also met the criteria for major depression. Multiple anxiety disorders were somewhat less common, occurring in 18% of the cases. Using a clinical sample, Lenze et al.[41] reported that 28% of participants aged 60 and older with major depression also had generalized anxiety disorder (GAD), and that 23% of depressed older adults also met the criteria for another anxiety disorder (other than GAD). Lindesay et al.,[72] reporting on data from the Guy's/Age Concern survey, found that among individuals with phobia, 39% were also depressed, compared to only 11% among non-phobics. Comorbid anxiety with bipolar disorder has also been reported. Among veterans 60 years and older, comorbid anxiety was evident in 23% of those with bipolar disorder.[80]

There are a number of limitations inherent in these published estimates that confine our current understanding of comorbidity in late life. First, estimates of comorbidity based on clinical samples likely produce rates that are much higher than those typically observed in community dwelling populations.[75] Second, in some of the mentioned studies, *DSM-III* criteria were used, and given the substantial changes made to the diagnostic criteria between earlier versions of the *DSM* and the *DSM-IV*, extrapolation of these findings to the updated criteria for disorder is problematic. Closely related to this point, studies that used the DIS to measure disorder are no longer comparable with more widely used instruments such as the UM-CIDI[81] and WMH-CIDI,[82] where modifications, especially regarding stem questions and entry into specific modules for disorders, have been made. These changes have resulted in notable differences in prevalence estimates for disorder in community samples.[33] Finally, neither of the Canadian epidemiological data sources (the Edmonton study and the Ontario Mental Health Supplement) estimated psychiatric comorbidity among older adults.

In the CCHS 1.2, over 4% of adults 55 years and older met the criteria for at least one 12-month disorder, and 0.8% met the criteria for two or more 12-month disorders. Among respondents with major depression, 23% reported a comorbid anxiety disorder, of which social phobia was the most common (14.5%, 95% CI = 8.5–20.6). Not surprisingly, 31.0% (95% CI = 20.0–42.0) of respondents who qualified for a diagnosis of social phobia also met the criteria for depression. Major depression was also the most frequently reported comorbid disorder among respondents with agoraphobia (25.1%, 95% CI = 9.9–40.4), as well as among respondents with panic disorder (29.5, 95% CI = 14.4–44.5).[83] The estimate of comorbid depression and anxiety disorders in the CCHS 1.2 is identical to that found in a recent study of 182 treatment-seeking depressed older adults conducted in the United States (23%),[41] and very close to the percentage of recently depressed individuals who also reported an anxiety disorder (22%) in a smaller, community-based sample in France.[42] However, this number is much lower than estimates of comorbidity reported in the Amsterdam study (47.5%).[39] This discrepancy can be at least partially accounted for by the exclusion of dysthymia and several other prevalent anxiety disorders, such as GAD, PTSD, specific phobia, and OCD in the CCHS, all of which are frequently comorbid with major depression.

Not surprisingly, meeting the criteria for multiple disorders was also associated with substantially greater impairment than reporting one or no disorders. Respondents with comorbid disorders reported significantly higher levels of psychological distress, limitations in activities of daily living and a higher number of disability days due to mental health reasons in the past two weeks than respondents who reported only one disorder. The average self-rated mental health score among respondents with multiple disorders was over 1.5 points lower (on a 5-point scale) than the average score for respondents with no disorder. These findings suggest that meeting the criteria for multiple disorders is especially detrimental for overall well-being and quality of life.[83]

Revisiting the Relationship between Prevalence of Disorder and Age

The data presented here and their comparison with earlier epidemiological studies allow us to return to the question of whether the lower rates of psychiatric disorder observed among older adults can be attributed to true aging effects, cohort effects, or selection effects. The relative consistency of lower rates of all psychiatric disorders among older adults in the CCHS 1.2 compared with their younger counterparts, and the consistency of these patterns in both contemporary studies and epidemiological work from twenty to thirty years ago, does indeed provide evidence against a period or cohort explanation. It is likely that a combination of measurement, aging and selection effects are operative. As Hocking et al.[3] suggested, advanced age may be associated with poorer recall of symptoms or the misattribution of mental health symptoms to physical health problems. It is also possible that *DSM* criteria are not sensitive to the types and severity of symptoms among older adults, resulting in an underestimation of disorder in this age group.[31] The observation of higher depressive symptomatology in older adults, despite lower rates of disorder, would tend to support this assertion. The assessment of a true aging effect is difficult in the absence of longitudinal data that assesses psychiatric disorder over a number of years.

Mental Health Service Use among Older Canadians

Questions about the type and frequency of contact with health care professionals for mental health reasons included in the CCHS 1.2 afforded the opportunity to investigate mental health service use among this subset of the population. Inquiry into the factors associated with mental health care use is important for a number of reasons. First, although the prevalence of most psychiatric disorders is lower in older adults compared to their younger counterparts, older adults are also less likely to seek out mental health care services.[84,85] Second, there is also a concern that physicians, especially general practitioners, tend to miss mental health problems in their older patients altogether, or mis-attribute them to other conditions or circumstances.[86] For example, symptoms of depression may be attributed to either the presence of a physical illness or dismissed as simply part of the normal aging process. From a population health perspective, it is important to understand whether certain groups who could benefit from mental health services (e.g., older women, widowed individuals, low SES groups) are more or less likely than other groups to access care. In Canada, where access is universal and therefore less influenced by non-need factors such as income or gender, it is critical to examine the correlates of use in this population.

In this part of the analysis, we focused exclusively on respondents who met the criteria for at least one 12-month psychiatric disorder. This decision was based on our interest in the factors associated with use above and beyond need. Of the 455 respondents aged 55 and older who met the criteria for at least one *DSM-IV* disorder, 37% reported accessing at least one type of service in the past 12 months. Of those who sought out at least one type of service, 23% reported accessing specialty mental health care (psychiatrist, psychologist, social worker), 31% reported accessing general mental health care (family doctor, nurse) and only 4% reported accessing another type of mental health care provider (religious advisor or alternative therapist). Although there are few comparative data on mental health service use among older adults, these mental health service use estimates are fairly consistent with other published estimates of service contact in the general population, in both Canada and the United States. For example, using data on the general population from the NCS-R, Wang et al.[87] reported that 41% of respondents who met 12-month caseness for any *DSM-IV* disorder received some type of treatment in the past year, and similarly, Lefebvre et al.[88] reported that 42% of respondents with at least one current disorder accessed mental health services in the previous year in Montreal. Using the full age range of the CCHS 1.2, Vasilliadis et al.[89] reported that 33.7% to 44% of respondents with *DSM-IV* disorders received mental health care in the previous 12 months.

Previous research on mental health service use in the general population has also identified a number of sociodemographic and need factors associated with accessing services. Being female, widowed, separated or divorced, and reporting higher income (in the United States) were all predictive of mental health service use.[84,88,90,91] Not surprisingly, need factors such as the presence of one or more psychiatric disorders was also significantly associated with greater service use.[89–91] The findings with respect to age are mixed – while some studies report that older adults are less likely to access services,[87,92] others do not find a significant effect for age.[88,92] Among older adults in the CCHS 1.2 who met the criteria for at least one current disorder, only one need-related factor – psychological distress – was predictive of any type of service use, suggesting equity of access. The absence of any statistically significant sociodemographic predictors of use may be partly related to the low number of older adults with a current disorder, as well as the possibility that the importance of sociodemographic factors as predictors of service use diminishes with age. Further research addressing this issue among samples of older adults is necessary to confirm the findings reported here.

Limitations of the CCHS 1.2 and Directions for Future Research

The results from the CCHS 1.2 presented in this chapter must be considered in the context of the limitations in the data. First, with respect to data collection, data were not collected among individuals residing in long-term care facilities, which may have resulted in the underestimation of the rate of all disorders considered here. Second, although all interviewers were trained in the administration of questions and diagnostic tools, such as the WMH-CIDI, the data collection relied on self-report, and a clinical assessment was not conducted. Third, there are a number of psychiatric disorders excluded from these data, many of which may be particularly important to our understanding of geriatric psychiatry. These include generalized anxiety disorder (GAD), dementia, and other measures of cognitive impairment. This is a serious limitation in that their omission not only inhibits our understanding of their prevalence among older adults, but also the degree to which they may be comorbid with disorders that were measured, such as depression.

Furthermore, a number of other variables of potential interest to the research presented here, such as comprehensive measures of stressors, and other psychosocial resources such as mastery and self-esteem, were not included in the CCHS 1.2. These variables represent another set of potentially important correlates of disorder in this population that still remain to be investigated.

NOTES AND REFERENCES

Dr. Cairney was supported by a Canada Research Chair in Psychiatric Epidemiology, funded by the Canadian Institutes for Health Research, at the time of the writing of this chapter.

1 Bland RC, Newman SC, Orn H. Prevalence of psychiatric disorders in the elderly in Edmonton. *Acta Psychiatr Scand* 1988;77(suppl 338):57–63.
2 Offord DR, Boyle MH, Campbell D, et al. One-year prevalence of psychiatric disorder in Ontarians 15–64 years of age. *Can J Psychiatry* 1996;41:559–63.
3 Hocking LB, Koenig HG, Blazer DG. Epidemiology and geriatric psychiatry. In: Tsuang MT, Tohen M, Zahner GEP, eds. *Textbook in Psychiatric Epidemiology*. New York: Wiley-Liss, 1995:437–52.
4 Health Canada, Division of Aging and Seniors [Internet]. [cited 2007]; Available at: http: //www.hc-sc.gc.ca/seniors-aines.
5 Mirowsky J, Ross CE. Age and depression. *J Health Soc Behav* 1992;33:187–205.
6 Kessler RC, Foster C, Webster PS, et al. The relationship between age and depressive symptoms in two national surveys. *Psychol Aging* 1992;7:119–26.
7 Myers JK, Weissman MM, Tischler GL, et al. Six-month prevalence of psychiatric disorders in three communities. *Arch Gen Psychiatry* 1984;41:959–67.
8 Regier DA, Boyd JH, Burke JD Jr, et al. One-month prevalence of mental disorders in the United States. *Arch Gen Psychiatry* 1988;45:977–86.
9 Wade TJ, Cairney J. Age and depression in a nationally representative sample of Canadians: A preliminary look at the National Population Health Survey. *Can J Public Health.* 1997;88:297–302.
10 Blazer DG. Clinical features of depression in old age: A case for minor depression. *Curr Opin Psychiatry* 1991;4:596–9.
11 Blazer DG, Hughes DC, George LK. The epidemiology of depression in an elderly community population. *Gerontologist* 1987;27:281–7.
12 Bland RC, Newman SC, Orn H. Period prevalence of psychiatric disorders in Edmonton. *Acta Psychiatr Scand* 1988;77(suppl 338):33–42.
13 Bland RC, Orn H, Newman SC. Lifetime prevalence of psychiatric disorders in Edmonton. *Acta Psychiatr Scand* 1988;77(suppl 338):24–32.
14 Goldstrum ID, Burns BJ, Kessler LG, et al. Mental health services use by elderly adults in a primary care setting. *J Gerontol* 1987;17:147–53.
15 Blazer DG. Depression in the elderly. *New Engl J Med* 1989;320:164–66.

16 Cumming E, Henry WF. *Growing Old: The Process of Disengagement*. New York, NY: Basic Books, 1961.

17 Rosow I. Status and role change through the life cycle. In: Binstock RH, Shanas E, eds. *Handbook of Aging and the Social Sciences*. 2nd ed. New York: Van Nostrand Reinhold, 1985:457–82.

18 Mirowsky J. Age and the sense of control. *Soc Psychol Q* 1995;58:31–43.

19 Rodin J. Aging and health: Effects of the sense of control. *Science* 1986;233:1271–6.

20 Cockerham WC. *The Aging Society*. Upper Saddle River, NJ: Prentice Hall, 1997.

21 Baltes PB, Baltes MM. Psychological perspectives on successful aging: The model of selective optimization with compensation. In: Baltes PB, Baltes MM, eds. *Successful Aging: Perspectives from the Behavioral Sciences*. Cambridge: Cambridge University Press, 1990:1–34.

22 Buhler C. The curve of life as studies in biographics. *J App Psychol* 1935;19:405–9.

23 Dannefer D. Adult development and social theory: A paradigmatic reappraisal. *Am Sociol Rev* 1984;49:100–6.

24 Erickson E. *Childhood and Society*. New York: Norton, 1963.

25 Erickson E. *The Life Cycle Completed*. New York: Norton, 1982.

26 Jung CG. *Psyche and Symbol*. New York: Anchor, 1958.

27 Levinson DJ, Darrow CN, Klein EB, et al. *Seasons of a Man's Life*. New York: Knopf, 1978.

28 Albrecht GL, Devlieger PJ. The disability paradox: High quality of life against all odds. *Soc Sci Med* 1999;48:977–88.

29 House JS, Lepkowski JM, Kinney AM, et al. The social stratification of aging and health. *J Health Soc Behav* 1994;35:213–34.

30 Cairney J. Age, socioeconomic status and the stress process [unpublished PhD dissertation]. London, ON: University of Western Ontario, 2002.

31 Flint AJ, Koszycki D, Vaccarino FJ, et al. Effect of aging on cholecystokinin-induced panic. *Am J Psychiatry* 1998;155:283–5.

32 Krasucki C, Howard R, Mann A. The relationship between anxiety disorders and age. *Int J Geriatr Psychiatry* 1998;13:79–99.

33 Kessler RC, McGonagle KA, Zhao S, et al. Lifetime and 12-month prevalence of DSM-III-R psychiatric disorders in the United States: Results from the National Comorbidity Survey. *Arch Gen Psychiatry* 1994;51:8–19.

34 Fournier L, Lesage AD, Toupin J, et al. Telephone surveys as an alternative for estimating prevalence of mental disorders and service utilization: A Montreal catchment area study. *Can J Psychiatry* 1997;42:737–43.

35 Turner, RJ, Wheaton B, Lloyd DA. The epidemiology of social stress. *Am Sociol Rev* 1995;60:104–25.

36 Beekman ATF, Bremmer MA, Deeg DJH, et al. Anxiety disorders in later life: A report from the Longitudinal Aging Study Amsterdam. *Int J Geriatr Psychiatry* 1998;13:717–26.

37 Ross HE, Glaser FB, Germanson T. The prevalence of psychiatric disorders in patients with alcohol and other drug problems. *Arch Gen Psychiatry* 1988;45:1023–31.

38 Wolf AW, Schubert DSP, Petterson MB, et al. Associations among major psychiatric diagnoses. *J Consult Clinical Psychol* 1988;56:292–4.

39 Beekman ATF, de Beurs E, van Balkom AJLM, et al. Anxiety and depression in later-life: Co-occurrence and communality of risk factors. *Am J Psychiatry* 2000;157:89–95.

40 Flint AJ. Epidemiology and comorbidity of anxiety disorders in the elderly. *Am J Psychiatry* 1994;151:640–9.

41 Lenze EJ, Mulsant BH, Shear MK, et al. Comorbid anxiety disorders in depressed elderly patients. *Am J Psychiatry* 2000;157:722–8.

42 Ritchie K, Artero S, Beluche I, et al. Prevalence of DSM-IV psychiatric disorder in the French elderly population. *Br J Psychiatry* 2003;184:147–52.

43 Robins LN, Locke BZ, Regier DA. *An Overview of Psychiatric Disorders: The Epidemiologic Catchment Area Study*. New York: Free Press, 1991:328–66.

44 American Psychiatric Association. *Diagnostic and Statistical Manual*. 4th ed. Washington: American Psychiatric Association, 2002.

45 Roberts RE, Kaplan GA, Shema SJ, et al. Does growing old increase the risk for depression? *Am J Psychiatry* 1997;154:1384–90.

46 Snowdon J. The prevalence of depression in old age. *Int J Geriatr Psychiatry* 1990;5:141–4.

47 Kessler RC, Berglund P, Demler O, et al. Lifetime prevalence and age-of-onset distributions of DSM-IV disorders in the National Comorbidity Survey Replication. *Arch Gen Psychiatry* 2005;62:593–602.

48 Regier DA, Farmer ME, Rae DS, et al. Comorbidity of mental disorders with alcohol and other drug abuse. Results from the Epidemiologic Catchment Area (ECA) Study. *JAMA* 1990;264:2511–8.

49 Weissman MM, Leaf PJ, Bruce ML, et al. The epidemiology of dysthymia in five communities: Rates, risks, comorbidity, and treatment. *Am J Psychiatry* 1988;145:815–9.

50 Unutzer J, Simon G, Pabiniak C, et al. The treated prevalence of bipolar disorder in a large staff-model HMO. *Psychiatr Serv* 1998;49:1072–8.

51 Depp CA, Jeste DV. Bipolar disorder in older adults: A critical review. *Bipolar Disord* 2004;6:343–67.

52 Stone K. Mania in the elderly. *Br J Psychiatry* 1989;155:220–4.

53 Van Gerpen MW, Johnson JE, Winstead DK. Mania in the geriatric population. *Am J Geriatr Psychiatry* 1999;7:188–202.

54 Kessler RC. The impairments caused by social phobia in the general population: Implications for intervention. *Acta Psychiatr Scand* 2003;108(suppl. 417):19–27.

55 Lipsitz JD, Schneier FR. Social phobia: Epidemiology and cost of illness. *Pharmacoeconomics* 2000;18:23–32.

56 Mendlowicz MV, Stein MB. Quality of life in individuals with anxiety disorders. *Am J Psychiatry* 2000;157:669–82.

57 Wittchen H-U, Fehm L. Epidemiology and natural course of social fears and social phobia. *Acta Psychiatr Scand* 2003;108(suppl. 417):4–18.

58 Magee WJ, Eaton WW, Wittchen HU, et al. Agoraphobia, simple phobia and social phobia in the National Comorbidity Survey. *Arch of Gen Psychiatry* 1996;53:159–68.

59 Pelissolo A, André C, Moutard-Martin F, et al. Social phobia in the community: Relationship between diagnostic threshold and prevalence. *Eur Psychiatry* 2000;15:25–8.

60 Stein MB, Kean YM. Disability and quality of life in social phobia: Epidemiologic findings. *Am J Psychiatry* 2000;157:1606–13.

61 Andrade L, Walters EE, Gentil V, et al. Prevalence of ICD-10 mental disorders in a catchment area in the city of Sao Paulo, Brazil. *Soc Psychiatry Psychiatr Epidemiol* 2002;37:316–25.

62 Cairney J, McCabe L, Veldhuizen S, et al. Epidemiology of social phobia in later life. *Am J Geriatr Psychiatry* 2007;15:224–33.

63 Schneier FR, Johnson J, Hornig CD, et al. Social phobia: Comorbidity and morbidity in an epidemiologic sample. *Arch Gen Psychiatry* 1992;49: 282–8.

64 Horwath E, Cohen RS, Weissman MM. Epidemiology of depressive and anxiety disorders. In: Tsuang MT, Tohen M, eds. *Textbook in Psychiatric Epidemiology*. 2nd ed. New York: Wiley-Liss & Sons, 2002:289–425.

65 Carlbring P, Gustafsson H, Ekselius L, et al. 12-month prevalence of panic disorder with or without agoraphobia in the Swedish general population. *Soc Psychiatry Psychiatr Epidemiol* 2002;37:207–11.

66 Eaton WW, Kessler RC, Wittchen H-U, et al. Panic and panic disorder in the United States. *Am J Psychiatry* 1994;151:413–20.

67 Goodwin RD, Faravelli C, Rosi S, et al. The epidemiology of panic disorder and agoraphobia in Europe. *Eur Neuropsychopharmacol* 2005;15:435–43.

68 Corna LM, Cairney J, Herrmann N, et al. Panic disorder in later life: Results from a national survey of Canadians. *Int Psychogeriatr* 2007;19:1084–96.

69 Wittchen H-U, Essau CA. Epidemiology of panic disorder: Progress and unresolved issues. *J Psychiatr Res* 1993;27:47–68.
70 Dick CL, Sowa B, Bland RC, et al. Phobic disorders. *Acta Psychiatr Scand Suppl* 1994;376:36–44.
71 Manela M, Katona C, Livingston G. How common are the anxiety disorders in old age? *Int J Geriatr Psychiatry* 1996;11:65–70.
72 Lindesay J, Briggs K, Murphy E. The Guy's/Age Concern survey: Prevalence rates of cognitive impairment, depression and anxiety in an urban elderly community. *Br J Psychiatry* 1989;155:317–29.
73 McCabe L, Cairney J, Veldhuizen S, et al. Prevalence and correlates of agoraphobia in older adults. *Am J Geriatr Psychiatry* 2006;14:515–22.
74 Weissman MM. Epidemiology of panic disorder and agoraphobia. *Psychiatr Med* 1990;8:3–13.
75 Flint AJ. Epidemiology and comorbidity of anxiety disorders in later life: Implications for treatment. *Clin Neurosci* 1997;4:31–6.
76 Gfroerer J, Penne M, Pemberton M, et al. Substance abuse treatment need among older adults in 2020: The impact of the aging baby-boom cohort. *Drug Alcohol Depend* 2003;69:127–35.
77 Russell JM, Newman SC, Bland RC. Drug abuse and dependence. *Acta Psychiatr Scand Suppl* 1994;376:54–62.
78 Grant BF, Dawson DA, Stinson FS, et al. The 12-month prevalence and trends in DSM-IV alcohol abuse and dependence: United States, 1991–1992 and 2001–2002. *Drug Alcohol Depend* 2004;74:223–34.
79 Thomas VS, Rockwood KJ. Alcohol abuse, cognitive impairment, and mortality among older people. *J Am Geriatr Soc* 2001;49:415–20.
80 Sajatovic M, Kales HC. Diagnosis and management of bipolar disorder with comorbid anxiety in the elderly. *J Clin Psychiatry* 2006;67(suppl 1):21–7.
81 Kessler RC, Wittchen H-U, Abelson JM, et al. Methodological studies of the Composite International Diagnostic Interview (CIDI) in the US National Comorbidity Survey. *Int J Methods Psychiatr Res* 1998;7:33–55.
82 Kessler RC, Üstün TB. The World Mental Health (WMH) survey initiative version of the World Health Organization (WHO) Composite International Diagnostic Interview (CIDI). *Int J Methods Psychiatr Res* 2004;13:93–121.
83 Cairney J, Corna LM, Veldhuizen S, et al. Comorbid depression and anxiety in later life: Patterns of association, subjective well-being and impairment. *Am J Geriatr Psychiatry* 2007;16:201–8.
84 Sareen J, Cox BJ, Afifi TO, et al. Mental health service use in a nationally representative Canadian Survey. *Can J Psychiatry* 2005;50:753–61.

85 Shapiro S, Skinner EA, Kessler LG, et al. Utilization of health and mental health services. *Arch Gen Psychiatry* 1984;41:971–8.

86 Krause N. Mental disorder in late life. In: Aneshensel CS, Phelan JC, eds. *Handbook of the Sociology of Mental Health*. New York: Kluwer Academic, 1999:183–208.

87 Wang PS; Lane M, Olfson M, et al. Twelve-month use of mental health services in the United States. *Arch Gen Psychiatry* 2005;62:629–40.

88 Lefebvre J, Lesage A, Cyr M, et al. Factors related to utilization of services for mental health reasons in Montreal, Canada. *Soc Psychiatry Psychiatr Epidemiol* 1998;33:291–8.

89 Vasiliadis H-M, Lesage A, Adair C, et al. Service use for mental health reasons: Cross-provincial differences in rates, determinants, and equity of access. *Can J Psychiatry* 2005;50:614–9.

90 Wang PS, Berglund P, Kessler RC. Recent care of common mental disorders in the United States. *J Gen Intern Med* 2000;15:284–92.

91 Lin E, Goering P, Offord DR, et al. The use of mental health services in Ontario: Epidemiologic findings. *Can J Psychiatry* 1996;41:572–7.

92 Bland RC, Newman SC, Orn H. Help-seeking for psychiatric disorder. *Can J Psychiatry* 1997;42:935–42.

PART FOUR

Special Topics

12 Gender and Depression

SARAH ROMANS AND LORI E. ROSS

The last fifty years have witnessed a concerted effort by psychiatric epidemiologists in many parts of the world to determine the rates of various psychiatric disorders in the community. We now know that mental disorders are more prevalent and begin earlier in life than had previously been assumed.[1] Canada has been one of the developed countries which had made a significant contribution to this new knowledge. One productive area in this work has been the attention paid to gender, with the ensuing interest in both the psychosocial and biological aspects of gender as possible locations for etiological factors for the high prevalence of psychiatric disorders of depression and anxiety.

One of the most replicated findings in psychiatric epidemiology is that of the greater prevalence of depressive and anxiety disorders in women when compared to men. In this chapter, we have set ourselves two goals that arise from this general research direction. First, we aimed to determine the strength of the evidence attesting to a female excess of depression and anxiety over the fifty years, with particular emphasis on several recent large scale national studies, noting in passing what plausible explanations have been advanced. We selected only studies with true random samples, in order to deal with generalizable results. The second goal was to examine informative subpopulations of women which have received special attention. These analyses potentially provide insights into the gender phenomenon. Both these goals are traditional uses of epidemiology, leading to hypothesis generation for later testing. In the search for the causes of health and disease, studying groups with high and low rates of the disorders of interest is useful.[2]

Methodology

Comprehensive literature searches were carried out with EMbase, Medline, and Unindexed Medline from 1970 to the present, using filters to identify national surveys. Citations and abstracts were examined to identify studies with random sampling methodology. These were then grouped according to total population and subpopulation categories. After removal of duplicates, we reviewed abstracts to exclude articles based on additional criteria. Papers were omitted if they did not report data from a national survey; there now exist in the literature a number of national survey studies and as a result of their size and quality, they provide optimal results. Reports that did not stratify by gender/sex, data that did not separate out bipolar and psychotic disorders, or which lacked an adequate description of the study methods were also omitted. The results are presented in table 12.1, which gives prevalence for depression in women, with men being the comparison group. It also includes one comprehensive report of a multinational study of primary care attenders, notable for its scope.[3] Table 12.2 reports prevalence estimates for depression in a number of specific subgroups of women, which have received particular attention in the literature. The most common reason for exclusion of articles for this table was failure to report gender/sex-stratified data. Results for 12 months and lifetime have been tabulated, and where these were not given in the original publication, figures from one and six months are tabulated.

Many of the large national surveys have generated several papers; in this case, we chose the publication(s) most informative for the two goals of this exercise. However, in the interests of space, two study clusters are reported only once, these are (1) the European Study of the Epidemiology of Mental Disorders (ESEMED), including six European countries – Belgium, France, Germany, Italy, the Netherlands, and Spain,[4] and (2) the International Consortium of Psychiatry Epidemiology studies.[5] ESEMED is itself part of the WHO World Mental Health Survey Initiative.

The Early History of Psychiatric Epidemiology

One of the earliest scientific reports attesting to this female predominance in depressive and anxiety disorders comes from the so-called first generation of psychiatric epidemiology, from the ground-breaking Canadian Stirling County study of Alexander Leighton and colleagues

Table 12.1
Prevalence for depression in women

Reference	Survey	Location	Age range	Definition	Time period	Sample size	Subgroup	Men (%)	Women (%)	Ratio W: M
79	Australian National Survey of Mental Health and Well Being	Australia	18+	CIDI-A (includes dysthymia)	12-month	10,641	Total	4.2	7.4	1.7
							18–24	3.0	11.0	3.7
							25–34	5.0	8.0	1.6
							35–44	6.0	8.2	1.4
							45–54	5.5	7.5	1.4
							55–64	3.0	7.0	2.3
							65+	1.0	2.0	2.0
80	Canadian Community Health Survey 1.2	Canada	15+	WMH-CIDI	12-month	36,984		2.9	5.0	1.72
81	Depres I & II	Belgium, France, Germany, the Netherlands, Spain, UK	16+	NR	6-month	80,342 (wave I & II)		7.6	14.9	2.0
82	Epidemiological Catchment Area Survey (ECA)	Christchurch, New Zealand	18–64	DIS/DSM III	6-month		Total	3.4	7.1	2.1
							18–24	3.5	6.5	1.86
							25–44	2.5	8.5	3.40
							45–64	2.5	7.6	3.04

Table 12.1 (*continued*)

Reference	Survey	Location	Age range	Definition	Time period	Sample size	Subgroup	Men (%)	Women (%)	Ratio W: M
4	European Study of the Epidemiology of Mental Disorders (ESEMED)	Belgium, France, Germany, Italy, the Netherlands, Spain	18+	NR	12-month	21,425		7.1	12.0	1.69
85	(*Example of a second generation PSE study; see text*)	Camberwell (London), UK	18–64	PSE (two-stage method) – any psychiatric disorder	Current	800; 210 interviewed	Total 18–24 25–34 35–44 45–54 55–64	6.1 1.5 5.5 11.1 7.5 6.9	14.9 4.2 23.6 12.5 26.7 7.4	2.4 2.8 4.3 1.1 3.6 1.1
86	Mexican National Comorbidity Survey	Mexico	18–65	WHO-CIDI	12-month	5,826		NR	NR	OR = 1.6
87	National Comorbidity Replication	USA	18+	WHO-CIDI	12-month	9,282		NR	NR	OR = 1.4
88	National Comorbidity Survey	USA	15–54	DSM-IIIR	12-month	8,098	15–24 25–34 35–44 45–54	9.5 7.9 8.1 4.0	16.3 11.6 12.7 11.0	1.7 1.5 1.6 2.8

Table 12.1 (continued)

Reference	Survey	Location	Age range	Definition	Time period	Sample size	Subgroup	Men (%)	Women (%)	Ratio W: M
89	National Population Health Survey	Canada	15–55+	CIDI-SFMD	12-month	16,650	15–54 55+	4.2 1.9	9.0 3.9	2.2 2.1
80	Canadian Community Health Survey 1.2	Canada	15+	WMH-CIDI	12-month	36,984		2.9	5.0	1.7
23	National Survey of Psychiatric Morbidity (UK)	UK	16–64	CIS-R		9,792	16–54 55–64	1.7 2.0	2.7 1.1	2.1 0.8
90	Netherlands Mental Health Survey and Incidence Study (NEMESIS)	Netherlands	18–64	DSM-IIIR	12-month Lifetime	7,076		5.7 10.9	9.7 20.1	1.8 1.8
19	World Health Organization (WHO) Multicentre Primary care study	Multi-centre	18–65	ICD-10	Current	25,900	All centres Ankara Athens Bangalore Berlin Groningen Ibaden Mainz Manchester	7.1 9.8 6.5 4.8 3.7 13.0 5.5 9.9 13.9	12.5 12.5 6.4 13.3 7.7 17.9 3.8 12.5 18.4	1.9 1.3 1.0 2.8 2.2 1.5 0.7 1.3 1.4

Table 12.1 (*continued*)

Reference	Survey	Location	Age range	Definition	Time period	Sample size	Subgroup	Men (%)	Women (%)	Ratio W: M
							Nagasaki	2.3	2.8	1.2
							Paris	9.3	18.8	2.2
							Rio de Janeiro	5.9	19.7	3.3
							Santiago	11.2	37.5	3.3
							Seattle	6.0	6.6	1.1
							Shanghai	3.3	4.5	1.3
							Verona	3.5	6.4	1.7
92		Germany	18–65	CIDI DSM IV	12-month	4,181		7.5	14.0	1.9
93		Finland	15–75	UM-CIDI-SF	12-month	5,993	Total	7.2	11.0	1.5
							15–24	6.2	8.1	1.3
							25–45	6.0	13.4	2.2
							35–44	9.1	11.3	1.3
							45–54	9.3	13.6	1.5
							55–64	6.4	8.6	1.3
							65–75	4.1	8.4	2.0

Table 12.2
Prevalence for depression in women, sub-populations

Reference	Survey	Age range	Definition	Time period	Sample size	Subgroup	Prevalence / OR	Note
1. Single motherhood								
94	NPHS 94–95	15–54	UM-CIDI-SF	12-month	2,968	Single Married	15.4 6.8	
95	NPHS 96–97	20–65	UM-CIDI-SF	12-month	13,225	Single Married	12.6 6.1	
96	NPHS 94–95	15–54	UM-CIDI-SF	12-month	3,061	Single Married	15 6.5	OR = 2.44 (1.81–3.27)
35	BNSPM	16–64	CIS-R		5,281	Single Supported	OR = 3.64 (reference = non-mothers) OR = 1.16 (ns; reference = non-mothers)	
34	NPHS 96–97	20–65	UM-CIDI-SF	12-month	13,225	Single Married	11.7 5.0	OR = 1.7 (95% CI = 1.2–2.6)
97	NPHS 98–99	24–45+	CIDI-SF	12-month	2,184	Single	14	
98	NCS 92–93	15–55	UM-CIDI	12-month	1,346	Single Married Separated	11.7 11 20.7	

Table 12.2 (continued)

Reference	Survey	Age range	Definition	Time period	Sample size	Subgroup	Prevalence / OR	Note
2. Urban/Rural								
37	ODIN study	18–64	Beck Depression Inventory	12-month	8,764	Finland – rural	3.8	
						Finland – urban	6.6	
						Ireland – rural	5.9	
						Ireland – urban	15.2	
						Norway – rural	10	
						Norway – urban	9.4	
						Spain – rural	NR	
						Spain – urban	1.8	
40	NPHS 96–97	12–55+	CIDI-SFMD	12-month	9,220	Rural	3.8	OR = 0.80 (0.62–0.97)
						Urban	5	
3. Socioeconomic status								
44	Stirling County	18+	DPAX	Current	3,600	Low SES	12.7	
						High SES	4.6	
99	ANSMH	18+	CIDI (affective disorder)	12-month	10,641	Unemployed	14.6	
						Employed	7.5	
						Income from gov't benefits	13.6	
						Other income sources	7	

Table 12.2 (continued)

Reference	Survey	Age range	Definition	Time period	Sample size	Subgroup	Prevalence / OR	Note
4. Ethnicity								
55	SWAN 1995, 1997	40–55	CES-D >16	12-month	3,015	African American	OR = 0.98 (reference=white)	
						Hispanic	OR = 1.38 (reference=white)	
						Chinese	OR = 0.56 (reference=white)	
						Japanese	OR = 0.67 (reference=white)	
102	NGHS (Wave II)	21–23	SCID-IV	Lifetime	378	White	34	p<0.05
						Black	18	
	NCS	15–54	DSM-III-R	Lifetime	3,749	White	22	p<0.05
						Black	15	
59	ECA	20–74	DSM-III	12-month	14,699	White	12.1	
						Black	5.5	
						Hispanic	7.1	
5. Lesbian, gay, bisexual, trans-gendered (LGBT)								
49	NCS	15–54	CIDI	Lifetime psychiatric disorder	8,098	Same-sex partners	34.5	OR = 1.9 (1.0–3.3)
						Opposite-sex partners	12.9	
101	NEMESIS	18–64	CIDI	12-month	7,076	Homosexual	11.6	OR = 1.03 (0.38–2.80)
						Heterosexual	7.3	
				Lifetime		Homosexual	44.2	OR = 2.44 (1.26–4.72)
						Heterosexual	20	
48	MIDUS	25–74	CIDI-SF	12-month	2,917	Lesbian or bisexual	33.5	OR = 1.88 (0.71–4.98)
						Heterosexual	16.8	

(see chapters 1 and 3).[6–10] The findings from this early phase of the rural Stirling County study complemented the urban data being generated about the same time from the Midtown Manhattan study of 1,664 White adults aged 20 to 59 years, 858 of whom were followed-up 20 years later in 1974.[11] The Manhattan study, however, did not show a gender difference and this is best explained by the coarse assessment methods used. Respondents in this project had their overall mental health graded into six symptom severity categories – well, mild, moderate (= unimpaired); marked, severe, incapacitated (= impaired). This approach would, in today's terms, include mood disorders as well as substance abuse disorders, in which men predominate. The third and fourth projects from this phase, both Scandinavian, found a female predominance in psychiatric morbidity. One in Iceland was based on the clinical notes from one practising psychiatrist, supplemented by diverse sources of additional data and gave a female:male rate of 2:1;[12,13] the other in Sweden used a community sample and generated a female:male ratio of 15:12 evolving to 15:8 at follow-up.[14]

In summary, despite very different assessment methods, a robust trend of greater female psychiatric morbidity was shown in three of four of these early studies. The fourth can be explained easily by considering the measurement approach taken.

In the next phase, eight surveys used the present state examination (PSE) as the case-finding instrument and were conducted in England, Australia, Spain, the Netherlands, Finland, and Africa. One typical example only, from London, England, is included in table 12.1.[15] Six of the eight projects showed a clear female preponderance of psychiatric disorder; the short version of the PSE, which they used, gives rates for combined depression-anxiety omitting substance abuse. Two of the eight studies, however, produced male:female rates which did not differ statistically. The report on one study, conducted in Uganda, commented that there may have been some confusion in the terminology used when translated into the local language.[16] Also, the annual prevalence rates were very high: 23.5% for men and 27.0% for women. The other, in the Netherlands, linked psychiatric disorder to employment rather than gender.[17] The rates, with the exception of the African data, were similar ranging for women from 7.5%–22.6% and men 6.1%–8.8% per annum.[7]

Overall, as with the earlier studies discussed, these later studies showed a remarkable consistency for the female excess in depression and related conditions.

Recent Whole Population Studies

Over the last two decades, the governments of a number of first world countries, specifically those with developed economies, have committed substantial resources to undertaking major nation-wide studies of the prevalence of mental disorders. The awareness of the importance of doing so was highlighted by the Global Burden of Disease Study.[18] This redirected attention from mortality to morbidity, the years lived with disability, and this has reshaped dramatically our earlier concepts of the relative importance of different illnesses. By doing so, the heavy burden generated by psychiatric disorders, which typically start early and last many years, became evident. These chronic disabling conditions are those which tax health and welfare budgets and which can result in immense personal suffering and economic impact. Many nations have conducted only one major study, where as Statistics Canada produces annual surveys and has a tradition of making these data sets available to independent researchers.

Table 12.1 summarizes the methods and results from all of these various national studies.

Overall Comment

This brief overview of fifty years of research endeavour reveals a very consistent picture of greater female depression. The methods used in these studies ensure that the gender findings are not an artifact of either help-seeking or regional variations in prevalence rates. The female to male ratio for 12-month prevalence of depression of the studies shown in table 12.1 ranges from 0.8 to 4.6 (omitting the WHO primary care study of Maier and colleagues).[19] Most fall in the 1.5 to 3.0 range, and low ratios are found in older groups. This profile is found despite significant variations in the total population rate by country and era. Such a consistent set of findings immediately stimulates the need to generate a testable, explanatory theory and many writers have begun addressing themselves to this challenge.

Current Areas of Uncertainty and Disagreement

In case we should be lulled into thinking that the state of psychiatric epidemiology is in total harmonious agreement, there are two key areas which are currently being hotly disputed, and both have gender relevance. These are age of maximal prevalence and course of illness.

The prevalence of depression at different ages based on some studies is given in table 12.1. Mainstream thinking about the interplay of psychiatric disorder, gender, and age has reversed dramatically during our review period. Forty years ago, studies suggested that elderly people had poorest mental health. Twenty years ago, Jorm published a pair of reviews summarizing the gender ratios for depressive disorder and depressive symptoms and showed that the highest rates of disorder for women and the greatest female:male discrepancy in rates occurred in middle adulthood, ages 25 to 40.[20,21] While a biological explanation implicating reproductive psychoendoimmunology could be advanced, Jorm considered that social roles were a more likely explanatory contender. Women bear the brunt of child and elder care, without financial and social status rewards, during these years. Social isolation may also have played a part.

Since then, a number of studies have suggested that young people, those aged 15 through 25, are burdened with the highest prevalence rates; these included many of the studies reviewed in this chapter and indeed testing for this concept was one of the rationales for the National Comorbidity study. A number of recent studies have reported low prevalence rates for depression in late adulthood and early old age. In the Australian study, depression was lowest in the over 65 years age group for both men and women;[22] in the UK NSPM study, depression for women was lowest in the over 55 years age group but not for men,[23] and in Canada, a steady decline was found over the age of 55 years.[24]

A number of authors have reported that the frequency of depressive disorders has increased in the last 20 years.[25,26] The interpretation of these findings are tricky as it needs to separate out statistically the effects of age, period, and cohort.[27,28] We await with great interest the forthcoming analyses of the National Comorbidity Replication study which has been designed to address so-called time trends in common psychiatric disorders.[29]

The Course of Illness in Each Gender

A prevalence excess may arise because more people in one group develop the condition; or because once started, the episode may last longer in one group; or both may occur. There is currently no consensus about the course of depression in each gender. Some projects have attempted to examine which explanation better applies, but most of these have used clinic samples, which do not generalize to the whole population. The Baltimore ECA follow-up study found an essentially similar course of unipolar depression for men and women,[30] suggesting that the reported differences in prevalence between men and women seem to be due to the differences in incidence, not chronicity. Similarly, Patten and Lee[31] have examined several Canadian data sets using Markov models and reported that gender differences in prevalence of major depression are due primarily to differences in incidence rather than episode length. A number of studies using non-population samples have found a higher relapse rate or non-remission rate for women but these cannot generate a community wide picture. This, then, is another aspect of the debate, which awaits more research before it can be resolved clearly.

Subgroup Studies

Several authors have examined the prevalence of depression among various subpopulations of women considered to be at potentially increased risk. An examination of populations of women who are at increased risk for depression may further our understanding of the mechanisms for the gender difference in depression prevalence: these data enable us to highlight that which may also differ between the genders. Table 12.2 provides a summary of relevant studies.

Lone Mothers

Studies from Canada, Australia, and the United Kingdom have all reported increased rates of depression among lone mothers relative to partnered mothers. An approximately 2.3-fold increase in risk of 12-month depression has been consistently reported.[32–35] In an analysis of the British National Survey of Psychiatric Morbidity, Targosz and colleagues[35] compared single mothers to a reference group of women not caring for children under 16, and found a 3.64-fold increase in risk of 12-month depression among the single mothers. Notably, risk of depression among supported mothers did not differ significantly from risk among the non-parenting sample (OR = 1.16, 95% CI 0.75–1.79).

Several variables that could potentially mediate the relationship between lone parenthood and depression among women have been examined. For example, Butterworth and colleagues[33] found that in their Australian sample, exposure to violence (specifically, sexual molestation and physical attack) explained 30% of the difference in prevalence of affective disorders between single and partnered mothers. Consistent with other studies, sociodemographic variables, particularly low levels of education, were also significant, explaining 26% of the difference in depression rates.[36] Finally, using multivariate modelling of 1994–1995 National Population Health Survey data, Cairney and colleagues[32] found that the interaction between lack of social support and stressful life events accounted for nearly 40% of the relationship between depression and lone parent status.

Rural vs. Urban Samples

We identified three published reports from population-based studies comparing prevalence of depression among rural and urban women. These studies, including data from Canada, the United Kingdom, Finland, Norway, and Spain, report lower rates of depression among rural women relative to their urban counterparts. Table 12.1 shows the results from two studies.[37,38] The third did not provide results in a form suitable for our table.[39] A fourth, by the first author and colleagues, found a lower risk of depression amongst rural dwellers, which was associated with a stronger sense of community belonging. The reasons for this decreased rate of depression among rural women remains unclear. Potential contributors include adverse living environments in urban areas,[39] lack of access to mental health services and therefore lower detection rates in rural areas,[40] and finally, systematic differences in sociodemographic characteristics (e.g., age) between urban and rural samples.[39] Social support has also been suggested as a potential mediating variable between risk for depression and rural residence. Some researchers have suggested that people in rural communities may be more likely than their urban counterparts to have immediate family close by, and to be willing to use family and friends for help and support.[41,42] Indeed, when community belonging was assessed in the Canadian Community Health Survey (CCHS) cycle 3.1, those living in rural communities reported significantly higher levels of belonging than did those living in urban areas.[43]

The definition of 'rural' used in these comparisons may also be particularly important. For example, in the 2004 Canadian study by Wang,[40] any respondent living outside a major urban centre was classified as rural. It is conceivable that rates of depression may differ substantially between those living in geographically isolated rural communities and those living within commuting distance of an urban centre.

Low Socioeconomic Status

Reports have examined risk for depression among women of low socioeconomic status, with all indicating an increase in prevalence rates.[44] The magnitude of this increase in risk appears to be approximately 2.0-fold–2.8-fold, and is consistent across variable definitions of socioeconomic status.

These findings support early conclusions from the Stirling County study in Atlantic Canada that the stress of poverty may be causally related to both the onset and persistence of depression.[44] However, it has also been noted that the functional impairment associated with depression can lead to a drop in socioeconomic status over time.[44] The relationship between poverty and depression may be particularly salient for women, considering the disproportionate number of women living in poverty, the contribution of women's unpaid labour to the global economy, and the continuing gender disparity in employment wages worldwide.[45] The implications of these results for provision of not only mental health, but also social and economic services, to those with and at risk for depression have been noted.[46]

Lesbian and Bisexual Women

Three population-based studies, originating from the United States and the Netherlands, have reported risk for psychiatric disorders among lesbian/bisexual women relative to heterosexual women.[47–49] All found increased rates of major depression and mood disorders in lesbian/bisexual women relative to heterosexual women, though the differences tended to be statistically significant only for lifetime, and not 12-month, prevalence.

The increased risk for depression in lesbian and bisexual women noted in these population-based studies is consistent with reports using other, non-representative samples,[50,51] and has been clearly linked to the experience of minority stress; that is, the experience of being denied access to equal rights and the consequential lack of access to resources and opportunities.[52,53] However, there are methodological limitations of epidemiological survey data for examining rates of depression among lesbian and bisexual women – a small and potentially invisible population. First, while the total populations sampled in each study were large, the numbers of women identified as lesbian/bisexual in each survey were relatively small, ranging from 37 to 96. These small sample sizes result in imprecise prevalence estimates and, possibly, insufficient power to show statistically significant differences. As such, the increased risk among lesbian and bisexual women may be more significant than the available data would suggest. Further, all of the epidemiological data reported here grouped lesbian and bisexual women together. The limited available data that examine bisexual people separately indicate that the risk for psychiatric disorders among bisexuals may be elevated relative to those individuals who identify themselves as gay or lesbian.[54] Finally, the data reported here assume truthful disclosure of sexual orientation, which may not occur in all cases. Indeed, the low rates of non-heterosexual orientation reported in epidemiological surveys such as CCHS 1.2 (0.7% of women identifying as homosexual and 0.9% of women identifying as bisexual) are suggestive of under-reporting.

Ethnic Minority Women

Several studies have reported rates of depression among various groups of ethnic minority women in the United States. The data indicate either no significant difference in prevalence of depression in ethnic minority women relative to non-Hispanic White women[55] or significantly lower rates of depression among ethnic minority women, particularly Black/African-American women.[56–58]

Oquendo and colleagues[59] examined the female-male ratios for depression prevalence among non-Hispanic White and ethnic minority women in the ECA and Hispanic Health and Nutrition Epidemiologic (HHNES) Surveys. Their results revealed wide confidence intervals, and as a result, significant overlap in ratios between ethnic groups. However, the reported ratios were highest among Mexican American (3.4, 95% CI = 2.1–5.5) and Black (3.1, 95% CI = 1.9–5.0) participants, and lowest among White (2.1, 95% CI = 1.6–2.6) and Hispanic (1.8, 95% CI = 1.0–3.5) participants. It should be noted that the ratio reported for Hispanic participants in the ECA survey is lower than the ratio obtained for any of the individual Hispanic ethnic groups examined in the HHNES (including Mexican American, Cuban American, and Puerto Rican).

The finding of no increased risk for depression among ethnic minority populations is puzzling when considered from the perspective of social determinants of health framework.[60] This framework would suggest that the relative levels of socioeconomic deprivation, discrimination, and other social disadvantages faced by ethnic minority individuals would be causally associated with depression. However, although the data suggest that prevalence rates of depression are no higher in ethnic minority women than in White women, Breslau and colleagues[61] found that ethnic minority individuals had an increased risk for persistent disorders, relative to White individuals. The authors propose that this may be due to a lack of economic resources and disadvantages in access to mental health services through the labour market; i.e., that ethnicity does not determine likelihood of developing depression, but that ethnic minorities may be less likely to have access to resources to facilitate recovery from the disorder. Others, however, have suggested that there may be an as yet unidentified genetic or culturally specific factor that protects from depression among the ethnic groups studied.[59] A final possibility that requires consideration relates to methodological issues such as language barriers, recall bias, and general cultural appropriateness of the diagnostic instruments used in these studies.[58]

It is important to note that all of the available data relating to ethnicity and depression in women come from epidemiological studies conducted in the United States. Canadian research is urgently needed in this area, since there may be many important contextual differences between ethnic minority status in the United States versus Canada, including the particular composition of the ethnic minority community, number of generations in the host country, and relevant social policies (e.g., universal health insurance). Data from other countries will also contribute to our understanding.

Discussion

We are in a strong position now to understand whether women have a greater prevalence of depression than men. Recent studies addressing the question have been undertaken in a range of countries using exemplary methods and large samples, and have generated a very consistent result. These nation-wide studies add to the results from previous generations of research and confirm that women are more at risk of depression. It should be noted that our current understanding of the nature of depression, with the precise diagnostic criteria, is itself very recent and continues to evolve with new and better studies.[62] Considering this, the consistency of the gender findings seems even more remarkable.

Although not addressed here, gender rates of psychiatric morbidity become similar if substance abuse disorders, in which men predominate, are included. Should the greater prevalence of depression in women be dismissed as insignificant if this is considered? If we want to stop portraying women as the weaker gender, frail and needing protection from the rigours of adult life outside the home, this may be a valid position to take. However, it is not sensible if we want to develop a robust framework for understanding the vulnerability and disease maintenance factors so that prevention strategies can be developed and the overall burden of these disorders minimized to the benefits of both individuals and societies. Those aims will be accomplished by having finely grained pictures of depression rates across countries and decades, dissected by key demographic variables. This review has shown that major advances have been made so far. There are significant gaps, still, in the form of populations missing from our bank of data. These include subpopulations of indigenous people, aboriginals, the disabled, sub-literate, deaf, those in institutions and the armed forces, ethnic minorities, and immigrants. Most of these understudied groups will need focused and creative recruitment strategies. As we worked through the construction of the tables, a number of papers were not included because of our rigorous criteria noted in the methods. Further, the lack of studies from developing nations is of great concern, as the patterns of illness may be quite different, as hinted at by the Ugandan second generation study already mentioned.[16]

A wide range of explanations has been advanced to explain the female prevalence of depression but none so far has been comprehensive or genuinely satisfying. We have only some pieces of a complex jigsaw puzzle. In major measure, this arises from the available methodologies. Cross sectional studies give very valuable snapshots but usually have a limited focus. Risk factors identified by surveys may not be the real causal ones, although they can be useful in identifying who needs assessment and treatment. These risk factors also may need to be categorized as vulnerability, precipitating, or maintaining factors and studied separately. Although it has long been known that prevention techniques can be developed and shown to be effective without the causal mechanisms of the disorder being fully understood, there would seem to be a need for new epidemiological theory to explain the current data and to guide new studies. Krieger[63] has suggested that there are two frameworks for understanding disease patterns: (1) diseases can be prenatal, or due to poverty or affluence; this is the framework from McKeown,[64] which is commonly understood as either genetic or due to lifestyle; and (2) the more traditional, multi-causal social factor approach, which uses a traditional public health approach of examining social groups rather than individuals.

Most writers seem to adopt the second approach when discussing their findings and few classify identified risk factors into conceptually useful groupings, such as necessary or sufficient causes, or distal versus proximal, or precipitating versus maintaining factors. Most of the studies have focused on a few variables, which may differ in their impact at different stages of the life cycle.

A number of authors have called for longitudinal data collection so that approaches can begin to address causality in ways which cross-sectional data cannot.[65–67] Longitudinal study designs, however, do bring some unique problems of their own: attrition (which may not be random but essentially linked to the nature of the disorders being studied); the ethical mandate to intervene when disorders are detected, which may result in a sample which is atypically healthy; and, of course, the sophisticated statistics which are necessary if the data are to reveal their secrets fully.

There is one recurring theme in many of these studies and it is one which may allow an explanation of at least some of the reported findings. This concerns social networks and how they differ for women and men. Our review of special subpopulations suggests the importance of social support and connectedness for women. The interaction between psychiatric disorder and social isolation is complex and may be bidirectional. Evidence from other studies not reviewed here attests to the importance of poor social networks preceding and possibly being causal for later depression and that this effect is greater for women than men.[68–70] Women have larger social networks than men and are more emotionally involved in those they do have. The theorists from the 'growth in relation' school of developmental psychology have emphasized the importance of relationships for adolescent girls and young women as part of identity development in a way that does not apply for men.[71,72] These differences may have a biological basis.[73]

A detailed understanding of social support for women has the potential to explain the traditional findings related to marital status and employment. It will need to address how women use their time – their employment and non-paid work patterns and conditions.[74,75]

Social networks themselves can be further understood as located in the wider community, which brings an evaluation of social capital – a characteristic of a community – into relevance. The quality of a social network a woman creates for herself is in part determined by her internal psychological resources but can be enhanced or diminished by the wider social environment. The increasing interest in social capital is likely to bring new insights into the ways in which gender and social support determine poor mental health.[76–78]

Despite the progress made in recent years, we have to agree with the opinion of one senior epidemiologist that the sex difference in incidence and prevalence of depressive disorders is a major and unsolved problem in psychiatric epidemiology.[23] The explanations remain elusive and need more work.

REFERENCES

1   Instel TR, Fenton WS. Psychiatric epidemiology: It's not just about counting anymore. *Arch Gen Psychiatry* 2005;62:590–2.

2   Morris J. *Uses of Epidemiology*, Baltimore: Williams and Wilkins, 1964.

3   Maier W, Falki IP. The epidemiology of comorbidity between depression, anxiety disorders and somatic diseases. *Int Clin Psychopharmacol* 1999;14(suppl 2):s1–6.

4   Alonso J, Angermeyer MC, Bernert S, et al. 12-Month comorbidity patterns and associated factors in Europe: Results from the European Study of the Epidemiology of Mental Disorders (ESEMeD) project. *Acta Psychiatr Scand Suppl* 2004:28–37.

5   Andrade L, Caraveo-Anduaga JJ, Berglund P, et al. The epidemiology of major depressive episodes: Results from the International Consortium of Psychiatric Epidemiology (ICPE) Surveys. *Int J Methods Psychiatr Res*, 2003;12:3–21.

6   Henderson A. The present state of psychiatric epidemiology. *Aust N Z J Psychiatry* 1996;30:9–19.

7   Romans SE. Gender differences in psychiatric disorder: In: Romans SE, eds.) *Folding Back the Shadows: A Perspective on Women's Mental Health.* Dunedin: University of Otago Press, 1998:43–61.

8   Leighton DC, Harding JS, Macklin D, et al. Psychiatric findings of the Stirling County Study. *Am J Psychiatry* 1963;119:1021–26.

9   Leighton DC, Harding JS, Macklin et al. *The Character of Danger. The Stirling County Study of Psychiatric Disorder and the Sociocultural Environment.* New York: Basic Books, 1963.

10 Murphy JM, Laird NM, Monson RR, et al. A 40-year perspective on the prevalence of depression: The Stirling County Study. *Arch Gen Psychiatry* 2000;57:209–15.

11 Srole L, Fischer AK. The Midtown Manhattan Longitudinal Study vs 'the Mental Paradise Lost' doctrine. A controversy joined. *Arch Gen Psychiatry* 1980;37:209–21.

12 Helgason TC. Epidemiology of mental disorder in Iceland. *Acta Psychiatrica Scandinavica* 1964;60:355–74.

13 Helgason TC. Prevalence and incidence in mental disorder estimated by health questionnaire and a psychiatric case register. *Acta Psychiatr Scand* 1964;58:256–66.

14 Essen-Moller E, Hagnell O. The frequency and risk of depression within a rural population group in Scania. *Acta Psychiatr Scand Suppl* 1961;37:28–32.

15 Bebbington P. Misery and beyond: The pursuit of disease theories of depression. *Int J Soc Psychiatry* 1987;33:13–20.

16 Orley J, Wing J. Psychiatric disorders in two African villages. *Arch Gen Psychiatry* 1979;36:513–20.

17 Hodiamont P, Peer N, Sybern N. Epidemiological aspects of psychiatric disorder in a Dutch health area. *Psychol Med* 1987;17:495–505.

18 Murray CJL, Lopez AD (Eds). *The Global Burden of Disease: A Comprehensive Assessment of the Mortality and Disability from Diseases, Injuries and Risk Factors in 1990 and Projected to 2020.* Boston: Harvard School of Public Health on behalf of the World Health Organization and the World Bank, 1996.

19 Maier W, Gansicke M, Gater R, et al. Gender differences in the prevalence of depression: A survey in primary care. *J Affect Disord* 1999;53:241–52.

20 Jorm AF. Sex and age differences in depression: A quantitative synthesis of published research. *Aust N Z J Psychiatry* 1987;21:46–53.

21 Jorm AF. Sex differences in neuroticism: A quantitative synthesis of published research. *Aust N Z J Psychiatry* 1987;21:501–6.

22 Wilhelm K, Mitchell P, Slade T, et al. Prevalence and correlates of DSM-IV major depression in an Australian national survey. *J Affect Disord* 2003;75:155–62.

23 Bebbington PE, Dunn G, Jenkins, R, et al. The influence of age and sex on

the prevalence of depressive conditions: Report from the National Survey of Psychiatric Morbidity. *Psychol Med*1998;28:9–19. [Erratum in *Psychol Med* 1998;28:1253]

24 Streiner DL, Cairney J, Veldhuizen S. The epidemiology of psychological problems in the elderly. *Can J Psychiatry,* 2006;51:185–91.

25 Wickramaratne PJ, Weissman MM, Leaf PJ, et al. Age, period and cohort effects on the risk of major depression: Results from five United States communities. *J Clin Epidemiol* 1989;42:333–43.

26 Klerman GL, Weissman MM. Increasing rates of depression. *JAMA* 1989;261:2229–35.

27 Murphy JM. Trends in depression and anxiety – men and women. *Acta Psychiatr Scand* 1986;73:113–27.

28 Murphy JM, Horton NJ, Laird NM, et al. Anxiety and depression: A 40-year perspective on relationships regarding prevalence, distribution, and comorbidity. *Acta Psychiatr Scand* 2004;109:355–75.

29 Kessler RC, Berglund P, Chiu WT, et al. The US National Comorbidity Survey Replication (NCS-R): Design and field procedures. *Int J Methods Psychiatr Res* 2004;13:69–92.

30 Eaton WW, Anthony JC, Gallo J, et al. Natural history of Diagnostic Interview Schedule/DSM-IV major depression. The Baltimore Epidemiologic Catchment Area follow-up. *Arch Gen Psychiatry* 1997;54:993–9.

31 Patten SB, Lee RC. Epidemiological theory, decision theory and mental health services research. *Soc Psychiatry Psychiatr Epidemiol* 2004;39:893–8.

32 Cairney J, Boyle M, Offord DR, et al. Stress, social support and depression in single and married mothers. *Soc Psychiatry Psychiatr Epidemiol* 2003;38:442–9.

33 Butterworth P. Lone mothers' experience of physical and sexual violence: Association with psychiatric disorders. *Br J Psychiatry* 2004;184:21–7.

34 Wang JL. The difference between single and married mothers in the 12-month prevalence of major depressive syndrome, associated factors and mental health service utilization. *Soc Psychiatry Psychiatr Epidemiol* 2004;39:26–32.

35 Targosz S, Bebbington P, Lewis G, et al. Lone mothers, social exclusion and depression. *Psychol Med* 2003;33:715–22.

36 Lipman EL, Offord DR, Boyle MH. Single mothers in Ontario: Sociodemographic, physical and mental health characteristics. *Can Med Assoc J* 1997;156:639–45.

37 Ayuso-Mateos JL, Vazquez-Barquero JL, et al. Depressive disorders in Europe: Prevalence figures from the ODIN study. *Br J Psychiatry* 2001;179:308–16.

38 Lehtinen V, Michalak E, Wilkinson C, et al. Urban-rural differences in the occurrence of female depressive disorder in Europe – evidence from the ODIN study. *Soc Psychiatry Psychiatr Epidemiol* 2003;38: 283–9.

39 Paykel ES, Abbott R, Jenkins R, et al. Urban-rural mental health differences in Great Britain: Findings from the national morbidity survey. *Psychol Med* 2000;30:269–80.

40 Wang JL. Rural-urban differences in the prevalence of major depression and associated impairment. *Soc Psychiatry Psychiatr Epidemiol* 2004;39:19–25.

41 Romans-Clarkson SE, Walton VA, Herbison GP, et al. Social networks and psychiatric morbidity. *Aust N Z J Psychiatry* 1992;26:485–92.

42 Amato, P. Urban-rural differences in helping friends and family members. *Soc Psychol Quart* 1993;56:249–62.

43 Statistics Canada. *Community Belonging and Self-perceived Health: Early CCHS Findings*. Ottawa: Minister of Industry, 2005.

44 Murphy JM, Olivier DC, Monson RR, et al. Depression and anxiety in relation to social status: A prospective epidemiologic study. *Arch Gen Psychiatry* 1991;48:223–9.

45 Arber S, Khlat M. Introduction to 'social and economic patterning of women's health in a changing world.' *Soc Sci Med* 2002;54:643–7.

46 Taylor R, Page A, Morrell S, et al. Mental health and socio-economic variations in Australian suicide. *Soc Sci Med* 2005;61:1551–9.

47 Cochran SD, Mays VM. Relation between psychiatric syndromes and behaviorally defined sexual orientation in a sample of the US population. *Am J Epidemiol* 2000;151:516–23.

48 Cochran SD, Mays VM, Sullivan JG. Prevalence of mental disorders, psychological distress, and mental health services use among lesbian, gay, and bisexual adults in the United States. *J Consult Clin Psychol* 2003;71: 53–61.

49 Gilman SE, Cochran SD, Mays VM, et al. Risk of psychiatric disorders among individuals reporting same-sex sexual partners in the National Comorbidity Survey. *Am J Public Health* 2001;91:933–9.

50 Matthews AK, Hughes TL, Johnson T, et al. Prediction of depressive distress in a community sample of women: The role of sexual orientation. *Am J Public Health* 2002;92:1131–9.

51 King M, McKeown E, Warner J, et al. Mental health and quality of life of gay men and lesbians in England and Wales: Controlled, cross-sectional study. *Br J Psychiatry* 2003;183:552–8.

52 Mays VM, Cochran SD. Mental health correlates of perceived discrimina-

tion among lesbian, gay, and bisexual adults in the United States. *Am J Public Health* 2001;91:1869–76.

53 Meyer IH. Prejudice, social stress, and mental health in lesbian, gay, and bisexual populations: Conceptual issues and research evidence. *Psychol Bull* 2003;129:674–97.

54 Jorm AF, Korten AE, Rodgers B, et al. Sexual orientation and mental health: Results from a community survey of young and middle-aged adults. *Br J Psychiatry* 2002;180:423–7.

55 Bromberger JT, Harlow S, Avis N, et al. Racial/ethnic differences in the prevalence of depressive symptoms among middle-aged women: The Study of Women's Health Across the Nation (SWAN). *Am J Public Health* 2004;94:1378–85.

56 Franko DL, Striegel-Moore RH, Bean J, et al. Self-reported symptoms of depression in late adolescence to early adulthood: A comparison of African-American and Caucasian females. *J Adolesc Health* 2005;37:526–9.

57 Franko DL, Thompson D, Russell R, et al. Correlates of persistent thinness in black and white young women. *Obes Res* 2005;13:2006–13.

58 Riolo SA, Nguyen TA, Greden JF, et al. Prevalence of depression by race/ethnicity: Findings from the National Health and Nutrition Examination Survey III. *Am J Public Health* 2005;95:998–1000.

59 Oquendo, MA, Ellis SP, Greenwald S, et al. Ethnic and sex differences in suicide rates relative to major depression in the United States. *Am J Psychiatry* 2001;158:1652–8.

60 Raphael D. Social determinants of health: Present status, unanswered questions, and future directions. *Int J Health Serv* 2006;36:651–77.

61 Breslau J, Aguilar-Gaxiola S, Kendler KS, et al. Specifying race-ethnic differences in risk for psychiatric disorder in a USA national sample. *Psychol Med* 2006;36:57–68.

62 Hirshbein LD. Science, gender, and the emergence of depression in American psychiatry, 1952–1980. *J Hist Med Allied Sci* 2006;61:187–216.

63 Krieger N. Epidemiology and the web of causation: Has anyone seen the spider? *Soc Sci Med* 1994;39:887–903.

64 McKeown T. *The Origins of Human Disease.* Oxford: Oxford University Press, 1988.

65 Gater R, Tansella M, Korten A, et al. Sex differences in the prevalence and detection of depressive and anxiety disorders in general health care settings: Report from the World Health Organization Collaborative Study on Psychological Problems in General Health Care. *Arch Gen Psychiatry* 1998;55:405–13.

66 De Graaf R, Bijl RV, Ravelli A., et al. Predictors of first incidence of DSM-

III-R psychiatric disorders in the general population: Findings from the Netherlands Mental Health Survey and Incidence Study. *Acta Psychiatr Scand* 2002;106:303–13.

67 Bebbington P, Dunn G, Jenkins R, et al. The influence of age and sex on the prevalence of depressive conditions: Report from the National Survey of Psychiatric Morbidity. *Int Rev Psychiatry* 2003;15:74–83.

68 Henderson AS. Social support and depression. In: Veiel H, Baumann R, eds. *The Meaning and Measurement of Social Support.* New York: Hemisphere Publication, 1992:85–92.

69 Kendler KS, Myers J, Prescott CA. Sex differences in the relationship between social support and risk for major depression: A longitudinal study of opposite-sex twin pairs. *Am J Psychiatry* 2005;162:250–6.

70 Huurre T, Eerola M, Rahkonen O, et al. Does social support affect the relationship between socioeconomic status and depression? A longitudinal study from adolescence to adulthood. *J Affect Disord* 2007;100, 55–64.

71 Jordan JV, Kaplan AG, Miller JB, et al. *Women's Growth in Connection.* New York: Guilford Press, 1991.

72 Miller JB. *Toward A New Psychology of Women.* Boston: Beacon Press, 1986.

73 Pedersen CA. Biological aspects of social bonding and the roots of human violence. *Ann N Y Acad Sci* 2004;1036:106–27.

74 Lennon MC. Work conditions as explanations for the relation between socioeconomic status, gender, and psychological disorders. *Epidemiol Rev* 1995;17:120–7.

75 Lennon MC, Rosenfield S. Women and mental health: The interaction of job and family conditions. *J Health Soc Behav* 1992;33:316–27.

76 Kawachi I, Berkman LF. Social ties and mental health. *J Urban Health* 2001;78:458–67.

77 McKenzie K, Whitley R, Weich S. Social capital and mental health. *Br J Psychiatr,* 2002;181:280–3.

78 Helliwell JF, Putnam RD. The social context of well-being. *Philos Trans R Soc LondB Biol Sci* 2004;359:1435–46.

79 Henderson S, Andrews G, Hall W. Australia's mental health: An overview of the general population survey. *Aust N Z J Psychiatr,* 2000;34:197–205.

80 Patten SB, Wang JL, Williams JV, et al. Descriptive epidemiology of major depression in Canada. *Can J Psychiatry* 2006;51:84–90.

81 Angst J, Gamma A, Gastpar M, et al. Gender differences in depression. Epidemiological findings from the European DEPRES I and II studies. *Eur Arch Psychiatry Clin Neurosci* 2002;252:201–9.

82 Oakley-Browne MA, Joyce PR, Wells JE, et al. Christchurch Psychiatric

Epidemiology Study, Part II: Six month and other period prevalences of specific psychiatric disorders. *Aust N Z J Psychiatry* 1989;23:327–40.

83 Weissman MM, Bland R, Joyce PR, et al. Sex differences in rates of depression: cross-national perspectives. *J Affect Disord* 1993;29:77–84.

84 De Girolamo G, Polidori G, Morosini P, et al. Prevalence of common mental disorders in Italy, risk factors, health status and use of health services: The ESEMeD-WMH (European Study of the Epidemiology of Mental Disorders-World Mental Health) project. *Epidemiol Psichiatr Soc* 2005;14:1–100.

85 Bebbington P, Hurry J, Tennant C, et al. Epidemiology of mental disorders in Camberwell. *Psychol Med* 1981;11:561–79.

86 Medina-Mora ME, Borges G, Lara C, et al. Prevalence, service use, and demographic correlates of 12-month DSM-IV psychiatric disorders in Mexico: Results from the Mexican National Comorbidity Survey. *Psychol Med* 2005;35:1773–83.

87 Kessler RC, Berglund P, Demler O, et al. The epidemiology of major depressive disorder: Results from the National Comorbidity Survey Replication (NCS-R). *JAMA* 2003;289:3095–105.

88 Kessler RC, McGonagle KA, Swartz M, et al. Sex and depression in the National Comorbidity Survey. I: Lifetime prevalence, chronicity and recurrence. *J Affect Disord* 1993;29:85–96.

89 Cairney J, Wade TJ. The influence of age on gender differences in depression: Further population-based evidence on the relationship between menopause and the sex difference in depression. *Soc Psychiatry Psychiatr Epidemiol* 2002;37:401–8.

90 Bijl RV, Ravelli A, Van Zessen, G. Prevalence of psychiatric disorder in the general population: Results of The Netherlands Mental Health Survey and Incidence Study (NEMESIS). *Soc Psychiatry Psychiatr Epidemiol* 1998;33:587–95.

91 Kruijshaar ME, Barendregt J, Vos T, et al. Lifetime prevalence estimates of major depression: An indirect estimation method and a quantification of recall bias. *Eur J Epidemiol* 2005;20:103–11.

92 Jacobi F, Wittchen H-U, Holting C, et al. Prevalence, co-morbidity and correlates of mental disorders in the general population: Results from the German Health Interview and Examination Survey (GHS). *Psychol Med* 2004;34:597–611.

93 Lindeman S, Hamalainen J, Isometsa E, et al. The 12-month prevalence and risk factors for major depressive episode in Finland: Representative sample of 5993 adults. *Acta Psychiatr Scand* 2000;102:178–84.

94 Cairney J, Thorpe C, Rietschlin J, et al. 12-month prevalence of depression among single and married mothers in the 1994 National Population Health Survey. *Can J Public Health* 1999;90:320–4.

95 Wade TJ, Cairney J. Major depressive disorder and marital transition among mothers: Results from a national panel study. *J Nerv Ment Dis* 2000;188:741–50.

96 Cairney J, Wade TJ. Single parent mothers and mental health care service use. *Soc Psychiatry Psychiatr Epidemiol* 2002;37:236–42.

97 Young LE, James AD, Cunningham SL. Lone motherhood and risk for cardiovascular disease: The National Population Health Survey (NPHS), 1998–99. *Can J Public Health* 2004;95:329–35.

98 Cairney J, Pevalin DJ, Wade TJ, et al. Twelve-month psychiatric disorder among single and married mothers: The role of marital history. *Can J Psychiatry* 2006;51:671–6.

99 Taylor R, Page A, Morrell S, et al. Socio-economic differentials in mental disorders and suicide attempts in Australia. *Br J Psychiatry* 2004;185:486–93.

100 Matheson FI, Moineddin R, Dunn JR, et al. Urban neighborhoods, chronic stress, gender and depression. *Soc Sci Med* 2006;63:2604–16.

101 Sandfort TG, De Graaf R, Bijl RV, et al. Same-sex sexual behavior and psychiatric disorders: Findings from the Netherlands Mental Health Survey and Incidence Study (NEMESIS). *Arch Gen Psychiatry* 2001;58:85–91.

102 Franko DL, Thompson D, Barton BA, et al. Prevalence and comorbidity of major depressive disorder in young black and white women. *J Psychiatr Res* 2005;39:275–83.

13 Migrants and Epidemiology of Psychiatric Disorders in Canada

DOUGLAS W. MACPHERSON AND BRIAN D. GUSHULAK

> Both physical bodies and political bodies are ever in the process of trans-
> formation, analogous one to the other. Hence it is possible to formulate
> laws descriptive of processes in each area.
>
> Machiavelli, *The Prince*

Introduction

The population characteristics of Canada and the perceived and documented health outcomes of Canadians are in a dynamic interaction
with a complex array of factors. Shifting demographic and biometric
population characteristics, and the impact of those shifts on health
outcomes, are increasingly being influenced by factors originating
external to Canada. The consequences of the increasing pace of glob-
alization that has occurred over the past half century are reflected
both in the traditionally described determinants of health of Canadians and in the manner in which the determinants of health relate to
each other. The relative significance of each of those determinants –
socioeconomic, genetic-biologic, environmental, and behavioural
factors – and how they affect each other, are also increasingly influenced by global and international factors. International population
mobility and its underlying components are emerging as a process
that is affecting the appreciation, measurement, and interpretation of
the significance of several classical health determinants in nations,
such as Canada, that receive high numbers of migrants for permanent
and temporary residency or settlement. Depending upon time and
location, these mobile populations often introduce both diversity and

disparity across the determinants of health through the processes of international relocation.

This chapter will describe the relationships between international population mobility and health with a focus on mental health. These relationships include the population-based health characteristics of mobile communities, the processes influencing the volumes and typology of international mobility, and the impact of transferring inter-regional disparities in disease prevalence. Using the context of mental health characteristics of migrants in Canada, we will describe the existing differences in population health parameters and public health care services infrastructures as well as differences in the recognition and perception of risk in diverse and disparate mobile populations. Last, the significance of this discussion will be presented in terms of future research that will be required to support policy development and influence program design and implementation to better address mental health issues for internationally mobile populations.

I What Does the Rest of the World Have to Do with Mental Health in Canada?

A. Population-Based Health Characteristics. Between 2001 and 2006, Canada experienced the greatest proportional population growth of any G8 nation.[1] The 2006 census reported the Canadian population at 31,612,897 persons, a growth of 5.4% since 2001. Two-thirds of Canada's population growth in this period was attributable to net international migration (almost 1.2 million people) in comparison to the U.S. population growth which resulted mostly from natural increase. If children born to foreign-born mothers are included in this perspective, the potential impact of ethnic diversity and intra-regional disparity relevant to health outcomes emerges as an even more significant factor in health discussions. In addition, in a change from historical patterns of immigration to Canada, the vast majority of foreign-born arrivals during the past five decades have settled in large urban centres. Currently more than 95% of immigrants in Canada live in urban areas, compared to 64% of the total Canadian population who live in cities.[2] In particular, three major urban centres – Vancouver, Toronto, and Montreal – are home to nearly 75% of new immigrant arrivals to Canada.

Canada has experienced several waves of population-driven nation building based on immigration. From the mid-seventeenth century to the 1950s, the preponderance of these movements could be described as the 'Europeanization' of Canada. During this early time period, the source regions of immigration to Canada represented a relatively comparable 'profile' across the determinants of health. A major shift in the source countries for immigration to Canada occurred beginning in the middle of the last century. This shift was associated with a series of technological, social, and geo-political changes that affect the willingness, ability, and capacity of individuals to migrate. Those changes included greater accessibility and affordability of international transportation, primarily through the expansion of air travel. Additionally, regional political and civil security changes that occurred after the Second World War, coupled with the process of de-colonialization, both facilitated and supported international migration patterns that differed from earlier waves of immigration to North America.

At the same time, 'pull' factors, including a national policy of multiculturalism and humanitarianism, falling birth rates in Canadian-born women compared to foreign-born women,[3] and increasing labour market demands in Canada, attracted markedly different migrant populations to Canada than in the previous century. Facilitated by a modernizing national immigration policy,[4] these movements became geographically and culturally more diverse and often included refugee resettlement or humanitarian components. They were subsequently modified by external international forces and legislative and regulatory procedures that supported active family reunification. Demographically, they generated greater population-based cultural diversity in Canada with continued links and relationships to source nations that are supported by modern communications and transportation technologies. The net result of these events, working in combination, has been the regional outward pressure for the international movement of people with Canada being one of the preferred host destinations.[5] As a result, Canada has one of the highest growth rates of foreign-born citizens of any western nation.[6,7] In 2005, the population growth rate in Canada was 10 per 1,000 persons of which 7.8 persons per 1,000 arrived via immigration compared to a natural growth rate (births in excess of deaths) of 2.2 per 1,000. Approximately 20% of all people living in Canada in 2005 were born elsewhere.[8,9] See table 13.1 and figure 13.1.

B. *The Processes Influencing International Mobility.* There are several cultural, medical, epidemiological, and methodological factors associated with international variations in reported rates of psychiatric diseases

Table 13.1
Immigration admissions of new permanent residents in 2002

	Total	Male	Female
Economic class			
Skilled workers	123,357	66,764	56,593
Business immigrants	11,041	5,764	5,277
Provincial/territorial nominees	2,127	1,111	1,016
Live-in caregivers	1,981	348	1,633
Total economic class (including dependants)	138,506	73,987	64,519
Family class			
Spouses, partners, and children	42,775	15,856	26,917
Parents and grandparents	22,502	9,615	12,887
Total family class	65,277	25,471	39,804
Protected persons			
Government-assisted refugees	7,504	3,953	3,551
Privately sponsored refugees	3,044	1,518	1,526
Protected persons landed in Canada	10,544	6,059	4,485
Dependants abroad of protected persons			
landed in Canada	4,019	1,712	2,307
Total protected persons	25,111	13,242	11,869
Other	197	111	86
Total permanent residents	229,091	112,811	116,278

Source: Citizenship and Immigration Canada. Facts and Figures 2006 Immigration Overview: Permanent Residents. http://www.cic.gc.ca/english/resources/statistics/facts2006/permanent/12.asp.

(see table 13.2). If these factors are not considered in national assessments of mental health status, particularly as applied to migrants, similar challenges to the interpretation of studies in Canada can be made.

In addition to these thematic factors, international migration introduces process-related factors that affect the comparability of disease prevalence rates in source country and resettled populations in Canada. For example, seriously ill individuals, unless they are joining family under a family reunification application, may be unlikely to initiate or complete the onerous processes associated with an application for permanent resettlement. This may result in different prevalence levels between origin and destination for those with psychological and psychiatric problems, particularly those that are inadequately

Figure 13.1 Canada – Permanent residents by category and source area, 2006

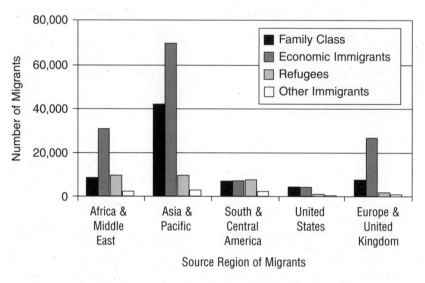

Adapted from Citizenship and Immigration Canada, Facts and Figures[9]

managed, due to the level of social dysfunction associated with unmanaged mental health disorders.

In addition, Canada is one of the major immigrant receiving nations that requires a pre-acceptance and pre-arrival immigration medical examination for all permanent and some temporary residency applicants.[10] Through this process, an individual's health status can be a factor used to determine immigration acceptance or admissibility. In Canada, medical inadmissibility for immigration purposes reflects the individual's danger to public health, danger to public safety, and risk of generating excessive demands on medical and social services. The latter two criteria are particularly relevant in the context of psychosocial health. They can provide grounds to exclude persons who have a history of violent or criminal behaviour, and those who are projected to be an excess cost burden or to increase wait times for medical and social services in Canada.

In reality, however, few permanent or temporary residency applicants are deemed medically inadmissible to Canada (approximately

Table 13.2
Disease burden of selected major psychiatric disorders by World Bank region.

	World Bank Region							
	Sub-Saharan Africa	Latin America and the Caribbean	Middle East and North Africa	Europe and Central Asia	South Asia	East Asia and the Pacific	High-income countries	World
Total [a]	688	528	310	477	1,388	1,851	9,29	6,159
Burden [b]	15,151	18,781	8,310	14,108	37,734	42,992	31,230	168,304
Percentage of neuro-psychiatric disease burden								
Schizophrenia	7.56	5.74	8.38	5.52	7.67	9.15	3.57	6.92
Bipolar disorder	7.95	4.70	6.82	4.74	5.93	7.25	3.38	5.78
Depression	21.82	27.79	24.39	30.26	38.64	32.69	26.92	30.80
Panic disorder	3.45	2.18	3.18	2.41	2.86	3.26	1.72	2.70

Adapted from table 1.1 in World Health Organization, Disease control priorities related to mental, neurological, developmental, and substance abuse disorders.
[a] Population in millions
[b] Total neuro-psychiatric disease burden (1000s DALYs)

400/450,000 applicants per year, or less than .001% of all applicants), and most of those exclusions are due to pre-existing chronic and progressive medical end-organ failures, malignancies, or developmental conditions associated with diminished mental capacity. Additionally, some categories of applicants for permanent residency in Canada are exempted from the excessive demand assessments, meaning that the presence of diseases or disorders that could deny admission to Canada in one group may not have the same outcome in others. Currently, the exemptions to admission that may occur in the case of high cost or service demand illnesses are extended to some family reunification applicants and migrants of the humanitarian group. The latter include refugees selected abroad for resettlement in Canada and refugee claimants (known in some locations as asylum seekers) who arrive in Canada by other means and make a subsequent claim for refugee status.

The differential application of medical admission criteria based on the administrative classification of migrant populations can, over time, be expected to influence the epidemiology of the involved diseases. This has particular relevance in the case of refugee populations, which are vulnerable groups known to be at increased risk of psychosocial and mental health disorders.

Finally, irregular arrivals in Canada, those who by-pass the system of immigration application (refugee claimants, persons who change their legal status while in Canada by over staying the conditions of an issued visa, and persons who are smuggled or trafficked into Canada) do not undergo an immigration medical examination outside of Canada. Only those who officially enter the immigration administrative system through their voluntary actions of making a refugee claim once arrived in Canada, or involuntarily enter the system by detection and detention by the civil authorities who require them to have an immigration medical examination in Canada, are assessed. As noted, those assessments for humanitarian applicants such as refugees and refugee claimants deal with inadmissibility only in terms of public health and public safety criteria. An important feature of the pre-arrival medical assessment for immigration exclusion purposes is that, being a one-time exercise conducted during the twelve months preceding the individual's arrival in Canada, it will not detect 'incubating' medical conditions. Factors that predispose a person to intrinsic or acquired mental illness expressed later on in the process are unlikely to be detected in the pre-arrival immigration medical screening examination.

Given the lack of specific screening tools in the immigration process that would detect sub-clinical or pre-clinical expression of psychiatric disorders in regular migrants, and in the absence of other self-selective, exclusive factors, the mental health of migrants could be expected to reflect the rate of mental health disorder in their source country. As will be discussed, the observed outcomes may not consistently match the expected outcomes in various migrant populations.

While existing individual or geographic factors affecting the development of mental disorder may pre-date the immigration application process, there are also factors associated with the transit and post-arrival phases of relocation[11,12] that may also contribute to the occurrence of mental health outcomes in migrants. It is important to note that these health outcome influences associated with migration are not always deleterious. While some influences that may be associated with the process of international relocation generate negative health outcomes, other migration-associated health factors may have no effect on mental health, while some may even support positive or improved outcomes.

It is also important to note that the modern post-arrival phase of migration now frequently includes the potential for return travel to source, ancestral, or other higher prevalence disease destinations. Acute illness outcomes associated with what has become to be known as immigrant 'visiting friends and relatives' travel (VFR), are an emerging area of research interest but have yet to focus on mental health outcomes.[13,14]

Temporary resident movements to Canada, such as business travel, tourism, and stays for under six months from non-visa source countries, generally have no pre-departure medical assessment requirements for Canada. Many migrant workers, including most farm worker programs which can be for durations of under six months, do have a requirement for an immigration medical examination. Irregular international movements (asylum seekers/refugee claimants, trafficking and smuggling of persons, and over-staying visa requirements) fall outside of the process of immigration and medical assessment.[15,16] These populations differ significantly from each other and also differ in demographic and biometric indicators from permanent residency applicants. Post-traumatic stress disorders and studies on victims of torture, rape, and other abuses on these vulnerable migrant populations are beyond the scope of this chapter.[17–19]

C. Inter-regional Disparities in Disease Prevalence. Comparisons of health outcome characteristics between international regions may show similar, greater, or lesser prevalence of mental health indictors than those observed and reported during the general assessment of the health of people in Canada. As a consequence, depending upon migrant origin, migrant selection factors, and other location-specific issues, these inter-regional differences may be reflected in or influence emerging rates of specific health outcomes in communities when measured in Canada.

The global estimates of neuro-psychiatric disease burdens are shown in table 13.2 by regional population census, disability life years (DALY's) by population-region, and selected major psychiatric disorders.[20,21] In all categories of disorders, except for depression rates which are more evenly distributed globally, the major psychiatric disorders represented by schizophrenia, bipolar, and panic disorders are less commonly reported in high-income countries.

In a recent review paper examining the 'healthy immigrant effect,'[22] several emerging considerations not examined during earlier considerations of this effect[23] were noted. In particular, the use of self-reported assessments of health and provincial health services billing data may not reflect true health status of diverse ethnic and recently arrived populations. It was also observed that rates of chronic diseases in ethnic migrant populations may evolve over time for several reasons, including acculturalization factors related to the process of migration, migration status, and post-arrival factors such as social and socioeconomic integration in Canada.[24] The complexity of evaluating the mental health characteristics of ethnically diverse migrants in Canada was noted to be an issue requiring more research.

Several studies reporting on mental health in immigrants in Canada have been published.[25-38] A selection of these studies is presented in table 13.3 describing the population studied, the mental health indicator of interest, and the outcome.

The challenge in interpreting these studies is in addressing the diversity of the population of migrants across outcome dependent criteria that are difficult to measure. Those criteria include population-based mental health determinants in the source country, the impact of the migration process itself that can differ between classes of migrants (e.g., refugees vs. other immigrants), economic and linguistic capacities, and the post-arrival consequences of residency in Canada.

An appreciation and knowledge of migrant-based factors in mental health services utilization are emerging. Whitley and colleagues[39] identified three issues that Canadian immigrants identified as sources of reluctance to use mental health services: the perception of both an over-willingness of doctors to prescribe medications as interventions, as well as a dismissive attitude and lack of time from physicians encounters in previous health services, and the belief in the curative power of non-medical interventions, most notably God and, to a lesser extent, traditional folk medicine.

Changing patterns of clinical research and methodology in this area may itself be exerting influence on how essential information is being gathered, analysed, and interpreted with a consequence of emerging gaps in knowledge for an increasingly important sector of the Canadian population.[40-42] Few Canadian studies have considered the consequences of changing social policy on the health of immigrants or refugees.[43] No identified studies have examined the combined influences of population health/disorder prevalence, social policy, and the migration processes, including the administrative status of the migrant, and how these factors can impact on health or mental health disorders in foreign-born persons in Canada. Table 13.3 shows some of the varied mental health outcomes in immigrant populations.

Each of these studies has taken a different perspective on the analysis of mental health observations. These perspectives and the factors taken into account in the study can create challenges in interpreting and generalizing the outcomes. As well, 'immigrants' as a single label for analysis and interpretation does not reflect their complexity and non-homogeneity, for example: the prevalence of the disorder of interest in the source country compared to Canadians or a non-migrating source country population; the use of culturally and linguistically validated measurement tools; stratification of the migrant population by status on arriving in Canada; duration in Canada and the means of transiting between source country, intermediary countries, and Canada, and the shifting impact of health determinants over time and place, and other characteristics specific to migrants post-arrival. In the context of the migrant health paradigm[44] summarized in table 13.4, the assessment variables for migrants' health outcomes are generally much more complex than available in the cited studies.

Addressing these issues will require improved understanding of both the nature and processes of migration and population mobility. The interest in migration and mental health is global and increasing.

Table 13.3
Selected mental health studies on immigrants to Canada

Population studied	Syndrome	Outcome
Southeast Asian 'boat people' – refugees	Depression	High levels of depression post-arrival; lack of social integration associated with persistence of depression at 2 years. 10 year follow up: importance of pre-arrival mental status, post arrival social programs, language training, and personal coping skills.[a,b]
Foreign born children	Emotional and behaviour problems	Poverty impact less than on Canadian born children; transient component of the resettlement process.[c]
Southeast Asia refugees – men and women employment status	Depression	Depression on arrival predicted depression at 10 years; language attainment and employability negatively correlated on employability (women > men).[d]
Immigrant adolescents	Suicide	Lower rate compared to Canadian adolescent; associated lower drug use at time of crisis.[e]
Multi-ethnic university undergraduates	Suicide – ideation, planning, attempts	No differences across post-generations or by ethnic group; close cultural heritage identification associated with suicidal thoughts only.[f]
Ethnic Chinese students	Measures of suicide, hostile and aggressive behaviour	Higher levels of suicide and hostile thoughts, but lower levels of self or outward aggression. The latter interpreted as related to Chinese ethnic cultural constraints.[g]
Canadian Vital Statistics Data Base and the World Health Statistics Annual of the World Health Organization	Suicide rates in immigrant and Canadian born.	Suicide rates in immigrants from the top 10 source countries were half the Canadian rate, although suicide in immigrants tended to be by older males: female rates similar.[h]
Cross-sectional study of race/ethnicity and mental health using data from the 1996–97 National Population Health Survey	General mental health	East and Southeast Asian, Chinese, South Asian, and black Canadians have better mental health than English Canadians. Jewish Canadians have poorer mental health than English Canadians. All other racial/ethnic groupings have similar mental health as English Canadians. Socioeconomic, social resource, and interaction effects were identified but they did not fully explain racial/ethnic mental health variation.[i]
Kosovars humanitarian evacuees and Czech Roma refugees	General socio-economic and health self-assessments	Posttraumatic stress was higher in the Kosovars potentially related to differences in pre-migration status, migration process, and post-migration factors; including duration in Canada.[j]

Table 13.3 (*continued*)

Population studied	Syndrome	Outcome
European immigrants (Britain, continental Europe) to British Columbia, Canada; study period: 1902–1913	Schizophrenia and other undefined psychosis syndromes	Increased rate compared to Canadian born (1.54 x) that increased over time associated with socioeconomic stress.[k]
Communal Hutterite colonies in Manitoba	Psychosis and neurosis	Lower prevalence of psychosis in communal vs. non-communal and general population, although neurosis rates were elevated in communal and comparison group of Hutterites.[l]
General population-based mental health survey	Bipolar disorder	Male gender, lower educational attainment, and immigrant status were predictors of not accessing treatment services.[m]
General population-based mental health survey	Any psychiatric, mood, and anxiety disorders	Of persons who immigrated to Canada after the age of 18 years, those aged 55 to 64 years had lifetime and 1-year prevalence rates for these disorders that were roughly one-half those for people who were born in Canada.[n]

[a] Beiser M[25]
[b] Beiser M[26]
[c] Beiser M, How F, Hyman I, et al.[27]
[d] Beiser M, Hou F[28]
[e] Greenfield B, Rousseau C, Slatkoff J, et al.[29]
[f] Kennedy MA, Parhar KK, Samra J, et al.[30]
[g] Aubert P, Daigle MS, Daigle JG[31]
[h] Malenfant EC[32]
[i] Wu Z, Noh S, Kaspar V, et al.[33]
[j] Redwood-Campbell L, Fowler N, Kaczorowski J, et al.[34]
[k] Smith GN, Boydell J, Murray RM, et al.[35]
[l] Nimgaonkar VL, Fujiwara TM, Dutta M, et al.[36]
[m] Schaffer A, Cairney J, Cheung AH, et al.[37]
[n] Streiner DL, Cairney J, Veldhuizen S[38]

This increased interest is reflected in the growth of medical literature and investigations in the field. However, the diversity in migrant communities and populations extends to the national level, and, while investigators commonly use similar terms to describe foreign born populations, the demographics of migrants can differ markedly between nations. Terms such as refugee, asylum seeker, immigrant and migrant worker, depending on the location, may actually refer to

Table 13.4
Epidemiological issues in assessing health of mobile populations

Factor	Source country	Receiving country	Issues
Prevalence of outcomes of interest	Changing local factors in health measurements, interventions, and outcomes. Cultural and linguistically appropriate health measurement tools. Differential health priorities and programs.	Lack of comparable baseline health measurements in newly arrived persons, absence of homogeneity in population characteristics	Differential demographics and bio-metrics in highly mobile and repetitively internationally mobile populations.
Population characteristics	Determinants of health: social economics, genetics-biology, environmental, behavioural	Relative importance and impact of determinants on pre-departure, transit, post-arrival factors on acculturalization; next generation; vulnerable populations; duration of settlement or resettlement factors	Shifting importance of traditional determinants of health over time, place, and population and significance of the rate of change in globalization (telecommunications, transportation, technology, trade)
Processes in administration of migration: transportation, classification, selection	Administrative classification of the migrant: regular versus irregular; means of transportation; duration of transition through which countries	Social policy in access to status determination, inclusion/exclusion, stratified identification of population by process	Means of arrival, classification of process or arrival, duration of stay, role and responsibilities in source or host country, selective pressures of admission determination or selection process
Phases of Migration	Pre-departure: health and social services infrastructure, access, availability, affordability	Post-arrival: linguistic and cultural components of health and health services utilization; ethnic, traditional, and alternative health care services.	Transition country factors
Perceptions of Threat and Risk to Personal and Public Health	Health programs and policy priorities; funding infra-structures	Existing barriers to health services: administrative, willingness, access, availability, affordability.	Training and education health care providers, shifting health and disease priorities, cultural and linguistically appropriate services. Regulation of health care providers.

different populations with different characteristics, histories, health backgrounds, and access to services. Women, for example, can be under-represented in asylum seekers depending on the nature of the journey.[45]

Additionally, access to certain migrant populations or communities can be inequitable, meaning that the amount of data available for a particular migrant population, such as refugees, may reflect the ability to undertake the investigation rather than need or disease prevalence. As migration plays an ever greater role in Canadian demography, providers and researchers alike will require improved understanding and awareness of the nature of the relationships between population mobility and health.

As a footnote to the process of international mobility and mental health in Canada, Canadian born citizens can themselves be migrants to foreign lands for the purpose of tourism, business, study, permanent or temporary residency, or as part of the foreign diplomatic or military commitments abroad,. Very little is known about the mental health outcomes in these populations. Two studies have reported on cause of death in Canadians abroad.[46,47] The consular services specifically records cause of death as natural, accidental, murder, or suicide in Canadian civilians abroad. In these studies, suicide was less frequent than suicide in non-travelling Canadians but followed the national pattern of higher frequency in males than in females.

II Population and Public Health Services, Perception of Risk, and the Future of Migrant Mental Health in Canada

In a rapidly globalizing world, variations in population health determinants and differences in the use and capacities in public health services that exist between regions can rapidly be bridged by mobile populations. An international health policy approach encompassing this new dynamic of global pressures[48] has been described. It includes and addresses issues related to chronic disease and mental health but given current global attention to the risks of infectious diseases and security, this approach is struggling to find a balance with other programs on the international stage.

Diversity and disparity provide the new basic parameters of health determination in fields where migrants are an important component of clinical practice. The emergence of international population mobility is creating increasingly complex paradigms that frequently challenge current research approaches. The ability to account for the diversity in factors that previously were relatively homogeneously distributed in study populations is becoming more important as the populations diversify as a consequence of migration. Balancing those differences will require greater effort in study design, improved validation of study tools for cultural and linguistic appropriateness, and a consideration that the very process of international migration brings with it multiple dimensions of research opportunity.

In a security conscious world tending at times to xenophobia, risk associated with immigrants and health concerns may be interpreted in one narrow way. In the context of mental and psychosocial health however, the perceptions of risk and migration can themselves provide an opportunity for greater understanding of population mobility and mental health. This understanding generates the potential for demographically appropriate study and interventions that go beyond the simple traditional basics of gender, age, education, and marital status to include an appreciation of the importance of the global community in the process of health determination. This may lead to the formulation of laws that describe the interaction between physical and political bodies and their synergistic impact on mental health.

REFERENCES

1 Statistics Canada. *Population and Dwelling Count Highlight Tables, 2006 Census. Data tables.* http://www12.statcan.ca/english/census06/data/popdwell/Tables.cfm. Accessed August 12, 2007.
2 Statistics Canada. *Canada's Ethnocultural Portrait: The Changing Mosaic.* 2003. http://www12.statcan.ca/english/census01/products/analytic/companion/ etoimm/contents.cfm. Accessed August 22, 2007.
3 Statistics Canada. *Report on the Demographic Situation in Canada.* 2002. http://www.statcan.ca/english/freepub/91-209-XIE/91-209-XIE2002 000.pdf. Accessed August 19, 2007.
4 Department of Manpower and Immigration. *White Paper on Immigration: Canadian Immigration Policy, 1966.* Ottawa: Queen's Printer, 1966.
5 Vembar D. *Canada – Preferred Destination of International Migrants.* Chennaionline. April 1, 2002. http://www.chennaionline.com/columns/variety/variety45.asp. Accessed August 22, 2007.
6 Statistics Canada. *Annual Demographic Estimates: Canada, Provinces and Territories.* 2005–2006. http://www.statcan.ca/english/freepub/91-215-XIE/91-215-XIE2006000.pdf. Accessed August 19, 2007.

7 Statistics Canada. *Report on the Demographic Situation in Canada. 2003 and 2004*. http://www.statcan.ca/english/freepub/91-209-XIE/91-209-XIE2003000.pdf. Accessed August 19, 2007.

8 Citizenship and Immigration Canada. *Annual Report to Parliament on Immigration 2006*. http://www.cic.gc.ca/english/pdf/pub/immigration2006_e.pdf. Accessed August 12, 2007.

9 Citizenship and Immigration Canada. *Facts and Figures 2006 Immigration Overview: Permanent Residents*. http://www.cic.gc.ca/english/resources/statistics/ facts2006/permanent/12.asp. Accessed August 12, 2007.

10 Justice Canada. *Immigrant and Refugee Protection Act. 2001*. http://laws.justice.gc.ca/en/showdoc/cs/I-2.5//20070819/en?command=searchadvanced &caller=AD&fragment= immigration%20refugee&search_type=bool&day=19&month=8 &year=2007&search_domain=cs&showall=L&statuteyear=all&length-annual=50&length =50. Accessed August 19, 2007.

11 MacPherson DW, Gushulak BD. Human mobility and population health. New approaches in a globalizing world. *Perspect Biol Med* 2001;44: 390–401.

12 MacPherson DW Gushulak BD. The basic principles of migration health. Population mobility across prevalence gaps and disparity. *Emerging Themes in Epidemiology* 2006;3:3 doi:10.1186/1742-7622-3-3.

13 Leder K, Tong S, Weld L, et al. Illness in travelers visiting friends and relatives: A review of the GeoSentinel Surveillance Network. *Clin Infect Dis* 2006;43:1185–93.

14 Behrens RJ. Hatz CH, Gushulak BD, et al. Illness in travelers visiting friends and relatives: What can be concluded? *Clin Infect Dis* 2007;44:761–2.

15 Gushulak BD, MacPherson DW. Health issues associated with the smuggling and trafficking of migrants. *J Immigrant Health* 2000;2:67–78.

16 MacPherson DW, Gushulak BD. *Irregular migration and health. For the Global Commission on International Migration*. Research paper series – No. 7. (October 2004). http://www.gcim.org/ir_gmp.htm.

17 Office of the United Nations High Commissioner for Human Rights. *Special rapporteur on torture and other cruel, inhuman or degrading treatment or punishment*. http://www.ohchr.org/english/issues/torture/rapporteur/ Accessed September 1, 2007.

18 Office of the United Nations High Commissioner for Human Rights. Committee against Torture. *Monitoring the prevention of torture and other cruel, inhuman or degrading treatment or punishment*.http://www.ohchr.org/english/bodies/ cat/ Accessed September 1, 2007.

19 Canadian Centre for Victims of Torture. http://130.227.3.66/usr/irct/home.nsf/unid/JREW-5MSCRN. Accessed September 1, 2007.

20 World Health Organization. *Global burden of disease estimates.* http://www.who.int/healthinfo/bodestimates/en/ Accessed August 12, 2007.

21 World Health Organization. *Disease control priorities related to mental, neurological, developmental and substance abuse disorders.* http://whqlibdoc.who.int/ publications/2006/924156332X_eng.pdf. Accessed August 12, 2007.

22 Joint Centre of Excellence for Research on Immigration and Settlement – Toronto. *Working paper series: Immigration and health: Reviewing evidence of the healthy immigrant effect in Canada.* Ilene Hyman. CERIS working paper 55. April 2007. http://ceris.metropolis.net/Virtual%20Library/WKPP%20List/ WKPP2007/CWP55.pdf. Accessed August 19, 2007.

23 Health Canada. Health Policy Working Paper Series. *Immigration and Health. Hyman I. Working paper 01-05.* September 2001. http://www.hc-sc.gc.ca/sr-sr/alt_formats/iacb-dgiac/pdf/pubs/hpr-rps/wp-dt/2001-0105-immigration/2001-0105-immigration_e.pdf. Accessed August 19, 2007.

24 Beiser M. The health of immigrants and refugees in Canada. *Can J Pub Health* 2005;96(suppl 2):s30–44.

25 Beiser M. Longitudinal research to promote effective refugee resettlement. *Transcult Psychiatry* 2006;43:56–71.

26 Beiser M. Influences of time, ethnicity, and attachment on depression in Southeast Asian refugees. *Am J Psychiatry* 1998;145:46–51.

27 Beiser M, How F, Hyman I, et al. Poverty, family process, and the mental health of immigrant children in Canada. *Am J Public Health* 2002;92:220–7.

28 Beiser M, Hou F. Language acquisition, unemployment and depressive disorder among Southeast Asian refugees: A 10-year study. *Soc Sci Med* 2001;53:1321–34.

29 Greenfield B, Rousseau C, Slatkoff J, et al. Profile of a metropolitan North American immigrant suicidal adolescent population. *Can J Psychiatry* 2006;51:155–9.

30 Kennedy MA, Parhar KK, Samra J, et al. Suicide ideation in different generations of immigrants. *Can J Psychiatry* 2005;50:353–6.

31 Aubert P, Daigle MS, Daigle JG. Cultural traits and immigration: Hostility and suicidality in Chinese Canadian students. *Transcult Psychiatry* 2004;41:514–32.

32 Malenfant EC. Suicide in Canada's immigrant population. *Health Report* 2004;15:9–17.

33 Wu Z, Noh S, Kaspar V, et al. Race, ethnicity, and depression in Canadian society. *J Health Sco Behav* 2003;44:426–41.

34 Redwood-Campbell L, Fowler N, Kaczorowski J, et al. How are new refugees doing in Canada? Comparison of the health and settlement of the Kosovars and Czech Roma. *Can J Public Health* 2003;94:381–5.

35 Smith GN, Boydell J, Murray RM, et al. The incidence of schizophrenia in European immigrants to Canada. *Schizophr Res* 2006;87:205–11.

36 Nimgaonkar VL, Fujiwara TM, Dutta M, et al. Low prevalence of psychoses among the Hutterites, an isolated religious community. *Am J Psychiatry* 2000;157:1065–70.

37 Schaffer A, Cairney J, Cheung AH, et al. Use of treatment services and pharmacotherapy for bipolar disorder in a general population-based mental health survey. *J Clin Psychiatry* 2006;67:386–93.

38 Streiner DL, Cairney J, Veldhuizen S. The epidemiology of psychological problems in the elderly. *Can J Psychiatry* 2006;52:185–91.

39 Whitley R, Kirmayer LJ, Groleau D. Understanding immigrants' reluctance to use mental health services: A qualitative study from Montreal. *Can J Psychiatry* 2006;51:205–9.

40 Bland RC, Orn H. Schizophrenia: Sociocultural factors. *Can J Psychiatry* 1981;26:186–8.

41 Jarvis GE. The social causes of psychosis in North American psychiatry: A review of a disappearing literature. *Can J Psychiatry* 2007;52:287–94.

42 Trovato F. Violent and accidental mortality among four immigrant groups in Canada, 1970–1972. *Soc Biol* 1992;39:82–101.

43 Steele LS, Lemieux-Charles L, Clark JP, Glazier RH. The impact of policy changes on the health of recent immigrants and refugees in the inner city. A qualitative study of service providers' perspectives. *Can J Public Health* 2002;93:118–22.

44 Gushulak BD, MacPherson DW. *Migration medicine and health: Principles and practice.* Toronto: BC Decker, 2006.

45 Boyd M. Gender, refugee status and permanent settlement. *Gender Issues* 1999;17:5–25.

46 MacPherson DW, Guérillot F, Streiner DL, et al. Death and dying abroad – The Canadian experience. *J Travel Medicine* 2000;7:227–33.

47 MacPherson DW, Gushulak BD, Sandhu J. Death and international travel – The Canadian experience: 1996 to 2004. *J Travel Med* 2007;14:77–84.

48 MacPherson DW, Gushulak BD, Macdonald L. Health and foreign policy: Influences of migration and population mobility. *Bull World Health Organ* 2007;85:200–6.

14 Mental Disorders and Social Stigma: Three Moments in Canadian History

HEATHER STUART

An epidemiology of stigma, either in the sense of having a coherent picture of the distribution and determinants of stigma at the population level, or in the sense of having a unified body of researchers who share the same disciplinary roots, does not yet exist. Significant contributions to the field have been made by sociologists, social psychologists, geographers, psychiatrists, and, only recently, epidemiologists. What has unified the field, and perhaps conferred an epidemiologic flavour, has been the underlying goal of reducing the burden of disability caused by mental illness by acting on the social factors that determine its occurrence, severity, and duration.[1] Thus, if we can't speak of an epidemiology of stigma per se, we can certainly trace the historical path of public mental health efforts aimed at eradicating it.

Public mental health doctrine builds on three basic principles: (1) a significant portion of mental morbidity is preventable through community action designed to reduce social pathogens such as psychosocial stress or early childhood deprivation; (2) the burden of mental illness can be alleviated through secondary prevention designed to reduce symptoms through early intervention and effective treatment; and (3) social disability can be reduced through tertiary prevention designed to reduce functional impairments and promote social inclusion.[2]

Stigma has been variously defined depending on whether the focus is on knowledge (mental health literacy and incorrect attributions), attitudes (stereotypes and prejudices), or behaviours (discrimination and inequity). From a public health perspective, however, it is useful to conceptualize 'stigma' as a complex social process involving interactions between individual-level factors (such as cognitions, attributions, stereotypes, and behaviours) with social structural elements (such as laws, policies, institutional practices, power imbalances, and norms) that create and maintain social inequities that are based on an individual's psychiatric status.[3]

The early history of stigma reduction in Canada – the first moment – predated sociological theories that defined the nature and effects of psychiatric stigma. The second moment coincided with deinstitution-alization and the community mental health movement. If the first moment defined itself in relation to the stigmatizing and iatrogenic effects of institutionalization, then the second moment crystallized around the stigmatizing after-effects of community living. Finally, the third moment is characterized by a growing international recognition of the disabling effects of stigma for recovery. Each of these eras is marked in Canada by a first – the first documented attempt to change public attitudes, the first ever replication study to examine secular trends in attitude change, and the first contribution to a global program to fight stigma and discrimination because of schizophrenia. This chapter will consider Canadians' contributions to stigma reduc-tion from 1950 onward, not only to celebrate these accomplishments, but to garner insight along the way into principles and practices that may guide future made-in-Canada solutions.

The First Moment – 1950 to 1970:
Closed Ranks – Stigma in a Prairie Town

The first Canadian contribution to stigma research, *Closed Ranks*, was published in 1957. Canada's Stirling County Study, initiated in 1948,[4] deserves special attention for its early contributions to social epidemi-ology, and the Cummings' *Closed Ranks*[5] deserves equal attention for its landmark contributions to understanding the epidemiology of psy-chiatric stigma. It is of interest to note that both studies were rooted in a public health model that recognized the social determinants of mental health and illness, and both contributed to a strong presence of social psychiatry in Canada. As the first published account of public perceptions of mental illness, *Closed Ranks* achieved both national and international importance. It is all the more remarkable because public health principles were at odds with the mental health treatment system during the asylum era, when mental illness was considered to be chronic and largely untreatable. At that time, there were few theo-ries about the causes of mental illness and no epidemiologic base of information about the incidence, prevalence, or modifiable determinants on which to base prevention efforts.[6]

The beginnings of a public mental health philosophy in Canada, and the initial impetus for stigma reduction programs, began in the middle of the twentieth century when several factors coalesced: the epidemiologic transition denoting a shift from infectious to chronic diseases as the main sources of morbidity and mortality; the corresponding rise of chronic disease epidemiology; the creation of disease classification systems for mental disorders; the completion of the first large scale community psychiatric epidemiologic studies – the Stirling County Study in Canada and the Midtown Manhattan Study in the United States – documenting the high prevalence of mental illness in the community and highlighting the role of potentially modifiable social determinants of mental disability; the discovery of chlorpromazine, which became available in the early 1950s, changing conceptions about the treatability of mental illness and making it possible to release many mentally ill into community settings; the rise of a community mental health philosophy which emphasized the iatrogenic characteristics of institutionalization and community treatment alternatives; changes to legislation emphasizing civil liberties and least restrictive alternatives; and deinstitutionalization policies that shifted the locus of care from the institutional system to the community.[6,7]

At the time of this study (1951), Canada's asylum system was still in a period of vigorous growth, reaching a bed capacity of approximately 66,000 in 1960, having doubled over the preceding thirty years. Most of the buildings were obsolete, dating from the Victorian era (1840 to 1880), with a patchwork of new construction to increase bed spaces and ease overcrowding. In 1932, asylums were running at 30% over capacity, but by 1960, overcrowding had fallen below 10%.[8] General hospital psychiatric units were just beginning to be developed. In 1952, for example, only 11 general hospitals – all in urban centres – had psychiatric facilities.[9] There were no community treatment services or supports, and patients' vocational and social rehabilitation needs received virtually no attention.[8] Thus, patients who returned to their communities often experienced considerable hardship.

Public funding for psychiatric hospitalization (or any hospitalization) did not yet exist and private insurance carriers often discriminated against the mentally ill. Although there had been a number of attempts to ensure that the emerging medicare system would include funding for psychiatric hospitalization,[9] public sentiment was such that the final legislation excluded psychiatric services provided in a provincial psychiatric hospital.[10] However, general hospitals were federally reimbursed for psychiatric services provided no more than 10% of their beds were assigned to psychiatric care.[11] This gave significant impetus to the development of general hospital-based treatment systems, but negatively affected the development of psychiatric services in the provincial facilities, effectively creating a two-tiered system of psychiatric care,[10] ultimately compounding problems of stigma for ex-mental patients.

The report of the Royal Commission on Psychiatric Services (published in 1964) indicates that Canadians considered mental illness a deep disgrace, which evoked strong feelings of shame and hopelessness. Admission to a mental hospital (although often a last resort) was usually obtained painfully, using legal means and often with the cooperation of the police. Once admitted, patients 'disappeared' and family members often lost contact with them. Although conditions were deplorable, members of the general public were generally comfortable segregating the mentally ill in large overcrowded and geographically isolated institutions (housing up to 5000 patients).[8] The rural communities, where the mental hospitals were located, valued them as a source of employment.[11]

Closed Ranks provides a view of Canadians' perceptions of mental illness at the close of the asylum era in a small prairie town. Although conditions in prairie mental hospitals were deplorable, as they were in the rest of Canada, Blackfoot residents expressed considerable confidence in the ability of psychiatric hospitals to treat the mentally ill. When asked directly whether the mentally ill should hospitalized, almost half of the survey sample indicated that they ought to because mental hospitals have *the finest treatment available* and skilled staff who are trained to handle the mentally ill. In fact, they thought it was *downright unfair* to deprive the mentally ill of such facilities. The Cummings attributed the population's unshakable belief in the efficacy of mental hospitals to a patterned response that involved social and physical isolation of the mentally ill (when denial of deviance was no longer possible), followed by a secondary denial that the 'solution' was also a serious problem. Indeed, the ordinary Blackfoot citizen, like most Canadians of the day, felt little social responsibility for the plight of the mentally ill and remained happily uninformed about the nature of mental illness and its treatments.

The central goals of the Cummings' six-month educational experiment was to reduce feelings of social distance toward the mentally ill and to improve citizens' sense of social responsibility for the management of mental illness. They had no formal sponsor in the community, so worked with a variety of voluntary groups with mandates relevant to mental health (such as the Parent-Teacher Association, the Civil Servants' Association, or the local branch of the Canadian Legion). The program was fluid, taking advantage of community events that could be platforms for stigma reduction. They considered that relatively immovable ideas would not be particularly receptive to the usual didactic methods or mass media interventions, so, whenever possible, they relied on small group interactions and personal communication. Sponsored events, such as an essay contest and mental health film festival, were also used. Direct discussions of social distance toward the mentally ill and social responsibility regarding mental illness were left to later stages in the program, once the attitudinal groundwork had been laid. Through a variety of means, they repeated three main educational messages: (1) behaviour was understandable and subject to change, (2) there was a continuum between normality and abnormality, and (3) there was a wider variety of normal behaviour than people generally realized. A post survey showed that 56% of the community residents had some direct contact with the educational program and were aware of its content, indicating that the program had reached a large share of its target audience.

Initial community reactions were cordial and friendly, although people were somewhat puzzled as to the researchers' motivations. As program momentum and intensity grew, so did community reactions. One month into the program, several rumours circulated, one indicating that the program was a clerical plot. By three months, the townspeople began to withdraw, conveying the message that things had probably *run their course* and should *wind down*. People who had been supportive, now distanced themselves from the program and displayed mounting concern about the researchers' continued presence in the town. When the interview team arrived to conduct the post-survey, they were surprised to be met with open hostility. The mayor indicated that the town had *had too much of this sort of thing, were not interested*, and encouraged the researchers to leave. The ranks had closed and the study team had been ousted from the community.

Analysis of the pre/post survey data showed that community members were no more willing to get closer to someone with a mental illness, or willing to take more responsibility for the problem after the program, than before the program began. In the Cummings' own words:

> Generally, we conclude that the six-month educational program, in its all-out attempt to improve the attitudes toward mental illness, produced virtually no change in the general orientation of the population either toward the social problem of mental illness or toward the mentally ill themselves.[5(p88)]

Subsequent critical appraisal of the assumptions on which the program was based revealed that they had badly missed the mark. Thematic analysis of interview data showed that the townspeople accepted a much wider spectrum of 'normal' behaviour than did the mental health educators who were trying to teach them to be more tolerant of abnormality. For most people, mental illness was narrowly conceived and synonymous with psychiatric hospitalization. Among those who had never been hospitalized, a wide range of serious psychopathological symptoms were tolerated. A second false assumption was that the lay population was ignorant of the social and biological causes of abnormal behaviour and needed professional advice in this regard. Once they realized that the mentally ill suffered from illnesses with causes that could be understood, they would feel more sympathetic toward the mentally ill. In fact, the population was already quite knowledgeable about the causes of mental illness. Finally, their third message, that there was an arbitrary and artificial line between normality and abnormality, turned out to be entirely unacceptable. Residents saw a sharp distinction between the mentally ill and the mentally well centering on the unpredictability of mentally disordered behaviour. The message that these behaviours existed on a continuum was anxiety provoking for a population that had fixed and non-continuous ideas about the nature of mental illness – anxiety that was not appreciated by the educational team and not adequately addressed.

Although the Cummings had appreciated the scope of the task before them, they had significantly underestimated the intensity of public prejudices and the immutability of stigmatizing views. Most important, they failed to empirically validate their theory of change and their educational messages *before* the program began. In their closing statement they summarized their main mistake with reference to Kurt Lewin's [12](p346) now-famous epigram, *'there is nothing so practical as a good theory'*.

The Cummings received international acclaim for their careful analysis and their intellectual candor. Thus, *Closed Ranks* remains one of the most thoughtful treatises on public mental health and stigma yet achieved. The disappointing results reverberated throughout the public mental health community in Canada (and elsewhere). Another large-scale public mental health attempt to reduce stigma was not repeated in Canada for almost forty years.

The Second Moment – 1970 to 1990: Blackfoot Revisited

The next 15 years brought a revolution in thinking about mental illness that had far reaching social and structural consequences. In the early 1960s, Erving Goffman published two seminal volumes analysing the social experiences of the mentally ill, both of which emphasized the exclusionary nature of society's response to mental illness and the negative impact this had for the mentally ill. In *Asylums: Essays on the Social Situation of Mental Patients and Other Inmates*,[13] Goffman followed the moral career of mental patients throughout the process of hospitalization, noting that they started out with rights and relationships, but ended up with little of either. In *Stigma: Notes on the Management of Spoiled Identity*[14] Goffman described a process of self-mortification experienced by the mentally ill in response to stigma and discrimination. For Goffman, mental illness was a mark of disgrace that engendered shame, guilt, and a wish for concealment. In 1966, Scheff published his sociological theory on the effects of labelling.[15] Building on Goffman's work, labelling theory maintained that the label of mental illness, created through contact with the mental health system, and the resulting stigma were the main etiological factors in creating and maintaining mental disability. This sparked a heated debate. Proponents of labelling theory challenged the traditional psychiatric model arguing that the consequences of being diagnosed or treated were more malevolent that the disease itself. Critics contended that appropriate diagnosis and treatment were ultimately benign and minimized their stigmatizing effects.[16] These now classic texts not only reflect the genesis of scholarly interest in stigma, but continue to form the basis for modern conceptions of stigma and its psychosocial effects.[3]

Other influential publications appeared during this same time, such as Laing's *The Divided Self*,[17] Rosenhan's *Being Sane in Insane Places*,[18] Foucault's *Madness and Civilization*,[19] and Szasz's *The Myth of Mental Illness*,[20] and *Psychiatric Slavery*.[21] These provided a significant counterpoint to the medical model, raised questions about the therapeutic qualities of psychiatric treatment, and laid the theoretical underpinnings for the anti-psychiatry and community mental health movements. The vilification of psychiatric hospitals was echoed in popular novels such as Kesey's *One Flew over the Cuckoo's Nest*, published in 1962,[22] which was made into an Academy Award winning movie in 1975. Other movies, such as *The Snake Pit* (1948) and *Pressure Point* (1962), had vividly documented the inhumane treatment of patients in mental institutions.[23] In a relatively short span of time, mental hospitals had become the object of public derision and the focus of structural reforms, the effects of which continue to be felt today.

By the mid to late 1960s, Canada's asylum system had reached its zenith, with a rated bed capacity of almost 70,000. By 1975, this had decreased to 54,000 and by 1980, to 20,000, reflecting an overall decline of approximately 70%. Provincial governments were increasingly investing in general hospital psychiatric units and, in the wake of rising inpatient costs, community-based services. Saskatchewan had been the first province to begin deinstitutionalizing psychiatric hospitals and by 1976, its bed capacity had decreased by 80%.[24] The asylum era was coming to a close.

By 1960, research had established that public recognition of psychiatric syndromes was improving. More than a dozen studies showed that the public was better able to recognize the symptoms of serious mental disorders such as schizophrenia than in previous decades. Whether increasing public knowledge of mental illness was also associated with more tolerant attitudes and more socially accepting behaviours was the topic of considerable debate. Incomparability across surveys of attitude conducted at different times limited any conclusions that could be made.[25] A large population study in Toronto conducted by a team of geographers demonstrated that the majority of their sample was favourably disposed to community mental health care. A third of the sample thought they would do nothing if a community mental health program were located in their neighbourhood, suggesting that community opposition to mental health facilities was probably limited to a small vociferous minority. However, a clear distance-decay pattern emerged. Whereas 25% of those living within 7–12 blocks of a hypothetical facility would take action to oppose it (ranging from signing a petition to moving), 53% of residents in a 2–6 block radius, and 58% of those in a 1 block radius would take such action. Indeed, 22% of those in a one block radius would consider moving. Residents worried about reduced property values, violence and unpredictability of patients, and reduced satisfaction with neighbourhood ambiance.[26]

To determine whether public perceptions of the mentally ill had improved since the 1950s, D'Arcy and colleagues revisited the Blackfoot community originally studied by the Cummings to determine whether the ranks had opened in the intervening years.[25,27] They used the identical study design and survey instruments originally used by the Cummings, making this the first study to eliminate methodological confounds and directly assess the extent to which stigmatizing attitudes had improved over time.

Blackfoot had changed little in the ensuing years. It remained a stable, prosperous community. Census data showed that it continued to have a larger than provincial average proportion of older residents and slightly more females than males. The predominant ethnic group continued to be British, and three quarters of the townsfolk were Protestant. The educational level had increased between 1951 and 1971, as it had in most of Canada. Table 14.1 summarizes the results from this research showing the percentage improvement in the 12 social distance items used. The table has been reconstructed from that originally published to highlight the proportion of respondents providing stigmatizing responses. Rows are organized by the magnitude of reduction in stigma noted over the 23 years.

The 1974 re-survey showed slight reductions in stigma, but these patterns were not consistent across all items. Only the first two items show reductions greater than 10%. Similarly, an analysis of descriptive vignettes showed that residents' recognition of the signs and symptoms of mental illness had not changed substantially in 23 years; D'Arcy concluded that *public attitudes towards the mentally ill and recognition of psychiatric symptoms have changed little in the last quarter-century.*[26(p289)] These results are noteworthy given the substantial mental health reforms that were ongoing during this time. Blackfoot residents continued to adopt a narrow view of mental illness that corresponded with only the most aberrant behaviours – behaviours that fell beyond the spectrum of acceptability. For the wide range of behaviours that were considered indicative of 'something wrong,' but not necessarily of mental illness, Blackfoot residents appeared to be quite

Table 14.1
Percentage improvement in social distance, 1951 to 1974, Blackfoot community

Social distance item	1951 Baseline (%)	% Change
Wouldn't marry a member of a family in which there was mental illness	58	−24
We should strongly discourage our children from marrying someone who has been mentally ill	73	−18
Would hesitate to rent an apartment to a former mental hospital patient	40	−9
Could not imagine falling in love with a person who had been mentally ill	68	−8
Wouldn't work for someone who had been mentally ill	29	−6
Would be unwilling to trust someone with financial matters who had been mentally ill	50	−5
Wouldn't lend money to a person who had been mentally ill	29	−4
Wouldn't trust someone to look after my children, even for a short period, who had been mentally ill	45	−2
Would be willing to sell an empty lot beside my house to a former mental hospital patient	29	−1
Would hesitate to share an office at work with someone who had been mentally ill	71	1
Would be unwilling to sponsor a person who had been mentally ill for membership in a favourite club or society	22	1
Would be unwilling to room with a former mental hospital patient	44	8

Note: Table was constructed from tabular data reported by D'Arcy[27]

open, leading D'Arcy to wonder to what extent the ranks were really closed to the mentally ill in the first place.

Uninformed or Misinformed?

By 1989, the community mental health movement in Canada was in full swing and by 1990, there were almost as many days of psychiatric care provided in general hospital psychiatric units (201 per 1,000 population) as there were in psychiatric hospitals (255 per 1,000). Although funding for community-based services was increasing,[24] it remained wholly inadequate to support the large numbers of deinstitutionalized mentally ill, thereby creating a problem that would preoccupy provincial governments during the last decade of the century.[28]

Canadian researchers were echoing findings from their U.S. counterparts that documented poor social and treatment outcomes for deinstitutionalized patients.[29–31] The first Canadian epidemiologic study to use modern diagnostic methods was conducted in Edmonton. Not only did it confirm the high prevalence of mental illness in community samples, [32,33] it linked mental illness to a wide range of social problems such as family violence,[34] suicide attempts,[35] unemployment,[36] and child abuse.[37]

U.S. research began to paint a more optimistic picture of public conceptions of mental illness. People recognized a much wider array of difficulties as 'psychiatric,' they were more comfortable seeking care for psychiatric problems, and were using more psychiatric services.[38] Optimistic news was also emanating from the United Kingdom. In 1985, a Team for the Assessment of Psychiatric Services (TAPS) was established to study the clinical and social outcomes of patients who were relocated from large psychiatric institutions to local community facilities.[39] Attitude surveys conducted prior to resettlement showed that the majority of neighbourhood residents viewed the opening of community mental health facilities in their neighbourhood positively. A focused educational campaign that was implemented in a single neighbourhood had also shown positive results. Residents in the neighbourhood that received the educational campaign were more understanding and less fearful of the mentally ill than before the intervention. The ex-patients living in the targeted neighbourhood had more social contacts with neighbours and larger social networks than those in a control community. Not only did the public appear to be more accepting of the mentally ill, these results suggested that localized educational campaigns could improve the social integration of deinstitutionalized patients and reduce neighbourhood opposition to the placement of residential and treatment facilities.

Between 1978 and 1989, a second set of replication studies were conducted in Canada to assess changing public perceptions, making this the only country examining secular trends in public attitudes over four decades. The first survey of the pair was conducted in 1976 by Trute and Lowen.[40] It questioned whether the Canadian public was simply lacking facts about mental illness or holding false and prejudicial beliefs – in short, whether Canadians were uninformed or misinformed. If the former were true, then attempts to alter public opinion should focus on education and literacy. If the latter were true, then educational approaches would need to be reconsidered in light of the difficulty of changing prejudicial beliefs and discriminatory behaviours. The main study hypothesis was that members of the general public having had direct experience with people who were mentally ill would have more positive and less socially rejecting attitudes. Such a relationship, if borne out, might have important implications for public mental health strategies.

A random sample of ex-patients living in sheltered care facilities in Winnipeg was drawn. Two households were then randomly selected on the same city block and one adult aged 18 to 65 was selected from each household by chance, thereby anchoring the sample in neighbourhoods where sheltered housing already existed. Sixty-two randomly selected neighbours formed the study sample. The survey questionnaire contained social distance items as well as an experience scale to determine the extent to which community neighbours had previously interacted with the mentally ill. One third of the sample had no previous experience. Another third had some previous contact, and the final third had more extensive contact, yielding groups with high, moderate, and low experience. The higher the level of direct experience with the mentally ill, the less rejecting were a person's attitudes. These findings suggested that anti-stigma programs should incorporate direct exposure to a wider cross-section of those identified as mentally ill. Previously, knowledge had been considered the most central modifiable characteristic of stigma. To improve community tolerance, these findings suggested that anti-stigma programs would have to go beyond improving mental health literacy, to the more difficult task of correcting misperceptions and dispelling prejudices. Further, they suggested that contact-based approaches might be effective.

The replication survey was published in 1989 by Trute, Teft, and Segal, employing the same methods and measures as a decade earlier.[41] The two community samples, one surveyed in 1976 and the other in 1986, were comparable with respect to demographic characteristics such as gender and age distribution. Using the identical social rejection scale, the researchers determined that social distance toward the mentally ill had remained unchanged. The general improvement in public awareness of human rights issues that had occurred in Canada had not liberalized views toward the mentally ill. Further, there appeared to be important differences between public views of social relationships with the mentally ill versus broader feelings of social responsibility for appropriate treatment and management of mental illness, but neither dimension of stigma had improved.

The differentiation of situations involving personal interactions from those involving social responsibility was thought to have implications for public education. Acceptance of social relationships was associated with close personal experiences with the mentally ill, whereas feelings of social responsibility were not. Improved feelings of social responsibility were associated with indirect exposure to mental illness through educational materials, formal education, and mass media. Thus, if the goal were to increase public feelings of social responsibility, more educational campaigns, including use of the mass media, made sense. If, on the other hand, the goal was to improve social integration of the mentally ill, then programs that fostered direct contact with people who were living with a mental illness would be more effective. Consistent with past research, this study also showed that rejecting public attitudes were associated with older age, lower education, and perceptions of the mentally ill being dangerous and unpredictable. With this research, the groundwork was now laid for more effective anti-stigma programming.

The Third Moment – 1990 to 2006: Stigma and the Global Village

By 1990, a two-tiered system of inpatient psychiatric care was well established in Canada. Psychiatric units in general hospitals provided acute care amounting to approximately 44% of the total days of inpatient psychiatric care (accounting for 201 days of care per 1,000 population and an average length of stay of 33 days), and psychiatric institutions provided long-term care (accounting for approximately 255 days of care per 1,000 population with an average length of stay of 223 days). General hospital psychiatric units now accounted for approximately 60% of institutional expenditures for the treatment of mental disorders and expenditures on psychiatric institutions was decreasing. Between the late 1980s and the late 1990s expenditures on psychiatric institutions and general hospital psychiatric units decreased by about 60%, and expenditures on community-based services increased by over 1200%, signalling a trend toward dehospitalization. Between 1985 and 1998, the combined days of care in psychiatric hospitals and general hospital psychiatric units decreased by almost 40% from 464 per 1,000 population to 286 per 1,000 population.[24] Despite their physical presence in the community and the therapeutic and social supports they received, clients of community-based treatment programs continued to feel rejected by their local communities.[42]

In support of deinstitutionalization, legal criteria for involuntary admission had narrowed the focus of inpatient care to individuals who were dangerous to themselves or others. Thus, over time, there had been a progressive convergence of mental illness and violence in day to day clinical practice, and mental health practitioners were now expected to be proficient in predicting and managing violent behaviours. Indeed, a growing number of risk assessment tools were designed for this purpose.[43] An important replication study conducted by U.S. researchers, comparing public conceptions of mental illness between 1950 and 1996, showed that definitions of mental illness had indeed broadened, but at the same time, had become increasingly associated with notions of social deviance, violence, and other frightening characteristics. Whereas Americans in the 1950s defined mental illness in narrow and extreme terms, with associated attitudes that were fearful and rejecting, in the 1990s they were much more eclectic in their definition of mental illness. At the same time, the stereotype of the violent psychotic person had become more entrenched.[38] The American public was also becoming more discerning in its application of stereotypes, linking violence and unpredictability to substance abuse and psychotic disorders. People were also more likely to support legal and coercive measures when dangerousness was at issue.[44] Previous attitudinal research had tended to be generic, asking respondents about people with a 'mental illness.' Given the link between social intolerance and attributions of violence, these findings highlighted the need for greater diagnostic specificity, both in attitude surveys and in anti-stigma programming.

Two Canadian surveys, one conducted in Quebec[45] and the other in Alberta,[46] examined public perceptions of people with schizophrenia. Both confirmed that Canadians were quite knowledgeable about the biological basis of schizophrenia and the need for medical treatment, but varied in their view of dangerousness. Among Quebec respondents, 54% considered that people with schizophrenia were violent and dangerous, and 40% disagreed with the strategy of integrating people with schizophrenia into the community. Among Alberta respondents, 18% considered that people with schizophrenia were dangerous. They were as likely to believe that people with schizophrenia were a public nuisance due to panhandling, poor hygiene, or odd behaviour. Seventy per cent thought that people with schizophrenia could be successfully treated outside of hospital in the community. Attributions of violence were now fairly well accepted as a major determinant of stigma. If there was any lingering doubt, a remarkable series of replication surveys conducted in Germany before and after violent attacks on public figures by people suffering from psychiatric disorders convincingly demonstrated the extent to which stigmatizing public views were influenced by incidents of violence.[47]

Prompted by public perceptions, the relationship of mental illness to violence became a topic of increasing policy and scientific debate. Scientists who had once been comfortable unequivocally stating that the mentally ill were no more, and probably less violent than the average citizen, were now recanting, suggesting that mental illness conferred some (albeit small) risk. However, unresolved methodological and sampling limitations made these results difficult to interpret.[48] In a reanalysis of the Edmonton epidemiologic survey data, Canadian researchers reconfirmed the association of mental illness to a wider range of social problems than had previously been considered – alcohol abuse, drug abuse, divorce, unemployment, suicide attempts, felony convictions, spousal abuse, and child abuse – and further highlighted a possible relationship between mental illness, social dysfunction, violence, and criminality.[49] To consider the question of public risk, data from a large epidemiologic study of mental illness in a jail population were reanalysed to estimate that 3% of violent crimes in Alberta (and probably Canada) could be attributed to inmates with a primary mental disorder that was not substance related. An additional 7% of violent crimes were attributed to inmates with a primary substance abuse disorder.[48]

The decade of the 1990s also brought international recognition of the burden caused by mental disorders and their associated stigma. The Global Burden of Disease Study estimated that in 1990, 5 of the top 10 leading causes of disability were attributable to mental disorders, accounting for 22% of the total years lived with a disability worldwide.[50] Despite the high burden associated with mental disorders, the World Health Organization determined that the majority of the world's population still had little or no access to even basic mental health treatments. A third of the countries reporting data to the World Mental Health's Atlas Project in 2005 had no specific budget for mental health programming and one in five spent less than 1% of their total budget on mental health. Two-thirds of the world's population had access to fewer than one psychiatric bed per 10,000 population and more than half of these were in large custodial institutions known to have poor psychosocial and clinical outcomes and a propensity toward human rights violations.[51] Epidemiologic data from the World Health Organization's Mental Health Consortium Surveys further revealed that in developed countries, 35% to 50% of people with serious mental disorders living in the community had not received treatment in the year prior to the survey. In developing countries, unmet need was as high as 85%. Stigma and discrimination were widely considered as to account for these treatment gaps.[52]

To raise awareness of these emerging global issues, the World Health Organization devoted the 2001 World Health Report to mental disorders, declaring that stigma was 'the single most important barrier to overcome in the community.'[51(p98)] They followed up with a global advocacy campaign to raise awareness of the burden associated with mental disorders and the hidden burden associated with psychiatric stigma[53,54] and a call for action to World Health Ministers at the 54th World Health Assembly,[55] including the necessity of fighting stigma and associated human rights violations.[56] In 2004, a consortium of international agencies (the World Association for Social Psychiatry, World Psychiatric Association, World Association for Psychosocial Rehabilitation, World Federation for Mental Health, and the Japanese Society for Social Psychiatry) issued a joint statement urging the United Nations to recognize the burden of mental disability and promote activities and programs designed to improve acceptance of people with mental disorders.[57] There were also a number of official declarations, mental health system reviews, and action plans highlighting the disabling effects of stigma on recovery across much of Europe,[58] the United States,[59,60] and Canada.[61,62] It is of interest to note that the national review of mental health and addiction treatment systems undertaken by the Canada's Standing Senatorial Committee on Social Affairs, Science, and Technology was the first parliamentary interest shown in mental health in almost half a century, since the 1964 Royal Commission.[10] In addition to system reviews, several nationally coordinated population-based anti-stigma campaigns emerged, such as in Australia,[63] New Zealand,[64] the United Kingdom,[65] and Japan.[66]

In 1996, the World Psychiatric Association launched a global program to fight stigma and discrimination because of schizophrenia. Based on input from experts from more than 20 countries, the program was founded on the following three principles: (1) the experiences of individuals living with the illness should guide the program's activities and, wherever possible, these individuals should be directly involved; (2) the program should encourage participation from a broad range of stakeholders throughout the community; and (3) the program should be a long-term effort rather than a brief or time-limited campaign. The Open the Doors global anti-stigma program is now active in over 20 countries with over 200 different interventions.[67,68]

Canada, specifically Alberta, was the pilot site for the Open the Doors global anti-stigma program. The aim of the pilot program was to evaluate a range of approaches to stigma reduction in order to provide guidance as to possible best practices. The pilot program had a compressed time frame in which to complete its activities (approximately 18 months, the amount of time normally devoted to start-up). A Local Action Committee composed of a broad base of stakeholders (mental health professionals, people with schizophrenia, family members, advocates, decision makers, and researchers) developed and evaluated a number of smaller scale interventions targeted toward specific population groups such as the media, members of the general public, hospital decision makers, and high school students.[67,69]

The media have been widely criticized by mental health professionals for producing a vast store of negative imagery containing some of the most malignant depictions of mental illness, mental health professionals, and psychiatric treatments.[70] It is not surprising, therefore, that anti-stigma advocates often find media professionals an irresistible target for their activities; and the Canadian Local Action Team was no different. In an effort to determine whether it was possible to influence media messages and create positive news, the Canadian Pilot Project targeted a local newspaper. Previous literature had suggested that the public depended on print media generally, and on newspapers specifically, as a source of information about health-related matters (more so than the broadcast media). There was also evidence that Canadian newspapers portrayed the mentally ill and mental illness in a generally negative light.[71] The objectives were to increase the number of positive news stories and their word length by at least 10% over the 18-month intervention period. Committee members worked to increase positive communication between members of the Local Action Committee and local reporters by helping to develop new story ideas, providing background information for breaking news, holding press events, and inviting local reporters to all conferences and program activities. A senior editor joined the Local Action Committee.

A content analysis of stories in the targeted newspaper was conducted to evaluate the success of this component of the program. Positive stories about mental health increased by 33% in the post intervention period and their word length increased by 25%. Positive stories about schizophrenia also increased by 33% but their word count declined by 10%. Concomitantly, negative stories about mental illness increased by 25% and their word count increased by 100%. Negative stories about schizophrenia also increased by 46% and their word count increased by over 200%. Global events (dubbed the 'CNN effect') easily overshadowed the local efforts. The most damaging stories appeared to be those that presented facts in a balanced way as this made negative stereotypes appear to be more credible. Thus, while it was possible to improve opportunities for positive news, increases in negative news items meant that the overall effort probably lost ground. While results were positive, they were meager, showing that local efforts can have, at best, only limited effect on media portrayals of mental illness.[72]

The speed and penetration of negative news in Canadian newspapers was illustrated by Webster, who traced the path of two violent incidents perpetrated by people with a mental illness.[73] Within one month of one of the incidents, over 100 articles had been published in 35 different papers – 11 of which had a print circulation exceeding 1.4 million copies – making the story available to Canadians from coast to coast. All of the articles noted that the shooter had a mental illness and most focused on this aspect of the case almost exclusively, limiting information about the victim to a line or two. Few articles reflected on the double nature of the tragedy – that not only the victim died, but the perpetrator had also been shot and killed by police. In a country that is not known for its yellow press, this is a sobering reminder that violence and mental illness is often a winning news combination.

The willingness of the Canadian news press to promulgate negative and stereotypical stories of the mentally ill is puzzling in light of data that showed that Canadian reporters were not negatively predisposed to the mentally ill. Matas and colleagues administered an attitudinal questionnaire to a systematic sample of 20 reporters, 20 psychiatrists, 20 medical outpatients with no previous psychiatric history, and 40 psychiatric inpatients.[74] In spite of the negative news they produced, media reporters were not negatively predisposed to the mentally ill, suggesting that the oft-times controversial and negative role played by media could not be explained by attitudinal differences. These authors considered that media coverage was negative in spite of the fact that reporters were not found to be unaccepting of mental illness. A number of possible explanations for this disparity were considered: (1) sensationalism sells, (2) cost and time pressures preclude many reporters from undertaking in-depth analyses of positive 'non-news' stories dealing with the mentally ill, (3) reporters' knowledge of mental illness may be as limited as that of the general pubic, and (4) the reporter has no control over what is edited by superiors, suggesting that negativity is layered onto a story by more senior editorial staff in the fight for audience appeal.

The second component of the pilot project assessed the effectiveness of a public education campaign, even though past research had demonstrated problems with this approach. The Local Action Committee tested a radio-based campaign to convey the message that schizophrenia was treatable, incorporating a component of direct contact in an effort to improve on previous fact-based approaches. Contact was established through a story narrated by a person with schizophrenia and a local psychiatrist. More than 500 radio messages were aired at different times during the day for several months.

The evaluation used a pre-test/post-test survey design to assess changes in knowledge, attitudes, and expressions of social distance. Both surveys were conducted using random digit dialing with a 70% response. The pre-test survey showed that Albertans were relatively knowledgeable about schizophrenia and had largely adopted a community mental health attitude. However, direct interpersonal contact with someone who had schizophrenia was not associated with greater tolerance, even among people who reported working in mental health agencies[46] or advocacy groups.[75] Pre- and post-public opinion surveys were conducted to assess changes in knowledge, attitudes, and socially distancing behaviours. About a third of the samples remembered seeing a news items referring to schizophrenia and this did not change from pre- to post-test. However, those who remembered hearing something on the radio rose significantly from 2% to 27%, suggesting that the radio intervention was successful in connecting with its intended target audience. Despite this, there were no improvements in knowledge, attitudes, or socially distancing behaviours. As in previous research, higher social distance was associated with increased age.[69]

A third component of the pilot program targeted grade 9 and 11 high school students. In addition to upgrading the educational materials contained in teacher manuals dealing with schizophrenia (the material was outdated by almost half a century), a poetry and art contest was held. The main focus of the high school intervention was a 1 to 2 hour contact-based educational session offered by people living with schizophrenia. A pre-test/post-test evaluation design was used to measure changes in students' knowledge and attitudes. Significant improvements in knowledge and social distance were noted immediately following the intervention – findings that were replicated in a similar classroom-based active-learning program offered in the United Kingdom.[76] It is noteworthy that the UK high school program demonstrated significant improvements even after six months, suggesting that direct contact with people who have a mental illness in the context of active learning can bring about lasting improvements in high school students' conceptions of the mentally ill.[77] A subsequent evaluation of a school-based intervention in eight Canadian schools that used video depictions of people with schizophrenia combined with a teacher resource to support active learning demonstrated comparable effects. Students were four times more likely to get a high knowledge score (defined as 80% or more correct) following the program and twice as likely to get a correct social distance score following the program.[78] This finding is noteworthy as it opens up the possibility of using indirect contact through video depictions of mental illness to mount more extensive and standardized educational efforts in Canadian schools.

Other components of the programs were not so extensively evaluated. They included a review of local emergency room policies and procedures with five key recommendations: (1) that the examination and interview process and space be adequate for the safety, security, and privacy of patients and staff (none of the hospitals reviewed had private interview space in the emergency department for psychiatric patients), (2) that there be enough interview rooms available to ensure privacy, (3) that interview rooms be located with easy access to hospital security personnel, (4) that security staff be available on a timely basis, but as needed, (so that security personnel do not have to be routinely involved in psychiatric assessments), and (5) a policy be implemented governing the use of restraints. In addition to reviewing these recommendations with local hospitals, they were sent to the Canadian Council on Health Services Accreditation where they were integrated into the country's national hospital accreditation process. By focusing

effects. Interventions that have targeted broad policy changes have also been effective. No large-scale population-based study of stigma experienced by people with mental illness has yet been conducted in Canada, and instruments that could be used for this purpose are only now becoming available.[80] This makes it difficult to assess whether anti-stigma activities are improving the lives of those who bear the greatest burden of stigma. Perhaps as we move into our fourth moment in history, research will focus less on what the general public thinks and more on what people who live with mental illnesses (both consumers and family members) feel.

REFERENCES

1 Wagenfeld MO, Lemkau PV, Justice B. *Public Mental Health: Perspectives and Prospects*. Beverly Hills: Sage Publications, 1982.

2 Jablensky A. Public health aspects of social psychiatry. In: Goldberg D, Tantam D, eds. *The Public Health Impact of Mental Disorder*. Toronto: Hogrefe & Huber, 1990:5–13.

3 Link B, Phelan JC. Conceptualizing stigma. *Annu Rev Sociol* 2001;27:363–85.

4 Leighton DC, Harding JS, Macklin DB, et al. *The Character of Danger*. New York: Basic Books, 1963.

5 Cumming E, Cumming J. *Closed ranks: An Experiment in Mental Health Education*. Cambridge, Massachusetts: Harvard University Press, 1957.

6 Pickett G, Hanlon JJ. *Public Health Administration and Practice* (9th ed). Toronto: Times Mirror/Mosby College, 1990.

7 Holland W, Fitzsimons B. Public health concerns: How can social psychiatry help? In: Goldberg D, Tantam D, eds. *The Public Health Impact of Mental Disorder*. Toronto: Hogrefe & Huber, 1990:14–19.

8 Richman A. *Royal Commission on Health Services. Psychiatric Care in Canada: Extent and Results*. Ottawa: Queen's Printer, 1964.

9 Greenland C, Griffin JD, Hoffman BF. Psychiatry in Canada from 1951 to 2001. In: Rae-Grant Q, ed. *Psychiatry in Canada: 50 Years*. Ottawa: Canadian Psychiatric Association, 2001:1–16.

10 Pankratz WJ. The history of the Canadian Psychiatric Association, 1951 to 2001. In: Rae-Grant Q, ed. *Psychiatry in Canada: 50 Years*. Ottawa: Canadian Psychiatric Association, 2001:29–48.

11 Hartford K, Schrecker T, Wiktorowicz M, et al. Four decades of mental health policy in Ontario, Canada. *Adm Policy Ment Health* 2003;31:65–73.

12 Lewin K. *Field Theory in Social Science: Selected Theoretical Papers*, London: Tavistock, 1952.
13 Goffman E. *Asylums: Essays on the Social Situation of Mental Patients and Other Inmates*. New York: Anchor Books, 1961.
14 Goffman E. *Stigma: Notes on the Management of Spoiled Identity*. New York: Simon and Schuster, 1963.
15 Scheff T. *Being Mentally Ill: A Sociological Theory*. Chicago, IL: Aldine, 1966.
16 Weinstein RM. Labelling theory and attitudes of mental patients. *J Health Soc Behav* 1983;24:70–84.
17 Laing RD. *The Divided Self: An Existential Study in Sanity and Madness*. Baltimore: Penguin Books, 1965.
18 Rosenhan DL. On being sane in insane places. *Clin Soc Work J* 1974;2:237–56.
19 Foucault M. *Madness and Civilization*. London: Tavistock, 1975.
20 Szasz TS. *The Myth of Mental Illness: Foundations of a Theory of Personal Conduct*. Rev ed. New York: Harper Row, 1974.
21 Szasz TS. *Psychiatric Slavery: When Confinement and Coercion Masquerade as Cure*. New York: Free Press, 1977.
22 Kesey K. *One Flew over the Cuckoo's Nest*. Toronto: Penguin Books, 1962.
23 Wedding D, Boyd MA, Niemiec RM. *Movies and Mental Illness*. 2nd rev. Cambridge, MA: Hogrefe & Huber, 2005.
24 Sealy P, Whitehead PC. Forty years of deinstitutionalization of psychiatric services in Canada: An empirical assessment. *Can J Psychiatry* 2004;49:249–57.
25 D'Arcy C, Brockman J. Changing public recognition of psychiatric symptoms? Blackfoot revisited. *J Health Soc Behav* 1976;17:302–10.
26 Dear MS, Taylor M, Hall GB. External effects of mental health facilities. *Ann Assoc Am Geogr* 1980;70:342–52.
27 D'Arcy C. Opened ranks? Blackfoot revisited. In: Coburn D, D'Arcy C, Torrance GM, Newman P, eds. *Health and Canadian Society: Sociological Perspectives*. 2nd ed. Richmond Hill, Ontario: Fitzhenry & Whiteside, 1987:280–94.
28 Wasylenki D. The paradigm shift from institution to community. In: Rae-Grant Q, ed. *Psychiatry in Canada: 50 Years*. Ottawa: Canadian Psychiatric Association, 2001:95–110.
29 Wasylenki DA, Goering PN, Lancee W, et al. Psychiatric aftercare in a metropolitan setting. *Can J Psychiatry* 1985;30:329–35.
30 Holley HL, Arboleda-Flórez J. Criminalization of the mentally ill: Part I. Police perceptions. *Can J Psychiatry* 1988;33:81–6.

31 Arboleda-Flórez J, Holley HL. Criminalization of the mentally ill: Part II. Initial detention. *Can J Psychiatry* 1988;33:87–95.

32 Bland R, Orn H, Newman SC. Lifetime prevalence of psychiatric disorders in Edmonton. *Acta Psychiatr Scand Suppl* 1988;338:24–32.

33 Bland R, Newman SC, Orn H. Period prevalence of psychiatric disorders in Edmonton. *Acta Psychiatr Scand Suppl* 1988;338:33–42.

34 Bland R, Orn H. Family violence and psychiatric disorder. *Can J Psychiatry* 1986;31:129–37.

35 Dyck RJ, Bland RC, Newman SC, et al. Suicide attempts and psychiatric disorders in Edmonton. *Acta Psychiatr Scand Suppl* 1988;338:64–71.

36 Bland RC, Stebelsky G, Newman SC, et al. Psychiatric disorders and unemployment in Edmonton. *Acta Psychiatr Scand Suppl* 1988;338:72–80.

37 Bland RC, Orn H. Psychiatric disorders, spouse abuse, and child abuse. *Acta Psychiatr Belg* 1986;86:444–9.

38 Phelan JC, Link BG, Stueve A, et al. Public conceptions of mental illness in 1950 and 1996: What is mental illness and is it to be feared? *J Health Soc Behav* 2000;41:188–207.

39 Leff J, Trieman N, Knapp M, et al. The TAPS Project: A report on 13 years of research, 1985–1998. *Psychiatr Bull* 2000;24:165–8.

40 Trute B, Loewen A. Public attitude toward the mentally ill as a function of prior personal experience. *Soc Psychiatry* 1978;13:79–84.

41 Trute B, Teft B, Segall A. Social rejection of the mentally ill: A replication study of public attitude. *Soc Psychiatry Psychiatr Epidemiol* 1989;24:69–76.

42 Prince PN, Prince CR. Perceived stigma and community integration among clients of assertive community treatment. *Psychiatr Rehabil J* 2002;25:323–31.

43 Stuart H. Violence and mental illness: An overview. *World Psychiatry* 2003;2:121–4.

44 Pescosolido BA, Monahan J, Link BG, et al. The public's view of the competence, dangerousness, and need for legal coercion of persons with mental health problems. *Am J Public Health* 1999;89:1339–45.

45 Stip E, Caron J, Lane CJ. Schizophrenia: People's perceptions in Quebec. *Can Med Assoc J* 2001;164:1299–300.

46 Stuart HL, Arboleda-Flórez J. Community attitudes toward people with schizophrenia. *Can J Psychiatry* 2001;46:245–52.

47 Angermeyer MC, Matschinger H. Violent attacks on public figures by persons suffering from psychiatric disorders. Their effect on the social distance toward the mentally ill. *Eur Arch Psychiatry Clin Neurosci* 1995;245:159–64.

48 Stuart H, Arboleda-Flórez J. A public health perspective on violent offences among persons with mental illness. *Psychiatr Serv* 2001;52:654–9.

49 Thompson AH, Bland RC. Social dysfunction and mental illness in a community sample. *Can J Psychiatry* 1995;40:15–20.

50 Murray CJL, Lopez AD. Global mortality, disability, and the contribution of risk factors: Global burden of disease study. *Lancet* 1997;349:1436–42.

51 World Health Organization. *The World Health Report 2001. Mental Health: New Understanding, New Hope.* Geneva: World Health Organization, 2001.

52 The WHO World Mental Health Survey Consortium. Prevalence, severity, and unmet need for treatment of mental disorders in the World Health Organization World Mental Health Surveys. *JAMA* 2005;291:2581–90.

53 World Health Organization. *Results of a Global Advocacy Campaign.* Geneva: World Health Organization, 2001.

54 World Health Organization. *Investing in Mental Health.* Geneva: World Health Organization, 2003.

55 World Health Organization. *Mental Health: A Call for Action by World Health Ministers.* Geneva: World Health Organization, 2001.

56 Arboleda-Flórez J. Stigma and human rights violations. In World Health Organization. *Mental Health: A Call for Action by World Health Ministers.* Geneva: World Health Organization, 2001:57–70.

57 Kobe Declaration. *World Association of Social Psychiatry,* 2004. http://www.wpanet.org/bulletin/wpaeb2103.html. Accessed February 28, 2005.

58 *Science and Care.* 2004;4(October–December):12.

59 U.S. Department of Health and Human Services. *Mental health: A Report of the Surgeon General – Executive Summary.* Rockville, MD: U.S. Department of Health and Human Services, Substance Abuse and Mental Health Services Administration, Center for Mental Health Services, National Institutes of Health, National Institute of Mental Health, 1999.

60 Druss BG, Goldman HH. Introduction to the special section on the President's New Freedom Commission report. *Psychiatr Serv* 2003;54:1465–66.

61 The Standing Senate Committee on Social Affairs, Science, and Technology. *Mental Health, Mental Illness, and Addiction. Issues and Options for Canada.* Ottawa: Interim Report of the Standing Committee on Social Affairs, Science, and Technology, 2004.

62 The Standing Committee on Social Affairs, Science and Technology. *Out of the Shadows at Last: Transforming Mental Health, Mental Illness, and Addiction Services in Canada.* Ottawa: Parliament of Canada, 2006. www.parl.gc.ca.

63 Rosen A, Walter G, Casey D, et al. Combating psychiatric stigma: An overview of contemporary initiatives. *Australas Psychiatry* 2000;8:19–26.

64 Vaughan G, Hansen C. 'Like minds, like mine': A New Zealand project to counter the stigma and discrimination associated with mental illness. *Australas Psychiatry* 2004;12:113–7.

65 Crisp AH, ed. *Every Family in the Land*. Rev. ed. London: Royal Society of Medicine, 2004.

66 Desapriya EBR, Nobutada I. Stigma of mental illness in Japan. *Lancet* 2002;359:1866.

67 Sartorius N. The World Psychiatric Association global programme against stigma and discrimination because of stigma. In: Crisp AH, ed. *Every Family in the Land*. Rev. ed. London: Royal Society of Medicine Press, 2004:373–5.

68 Sartorius N, Schulze H. *Reducing Stigma of Mental Illness: A Report from the Global Program of the World Psychiatric Association*. Cambridge: Cambridge University Press, 2005.

69 Stuart H. Stigmatisation. Leçons tirées des programmes de réduction. *Santé Ment Québec*, 2003;28:37–53.

70 Stuart H. Media portrayals of mental illness and its treatments. What effect does it have on people with mental illness. *CNS Drugs* 2006;20:99–106.

71 Day DM, Page S. Portrayal of mental illness in Canadian newspapers. *Can J Psychiatry* 1986;31:813–7.

72 Stuart H. Stigma and the daily news: Evaluation of a newspaper intervention. *Can J Psychiatry* 2003;48:651–6.

73 Webster CL. News media critique: 'Crazies in the streets'. *Int J Ment Health Addiction* 2005;3:64–8.

74 Matas M, el-Guebaly N, Peterkin A, et al. Mental illness and the media: An assessment of attitudes and communication. *Can J Psychiatry* 1985;30:12–7.

75 Thompson AH, Stuart H, Bland RC, et al. Attitudes about schizophrenia from the pilot site of the WPA worldwide campaign against the stigma of schizophrenia. *Soc Psychiatry Psychiatr Epidemiol* 2002;37:475–82.

76 Pinfold V, Stuart H, Thornicroft G, et al. Working with young people: The impact of mental health awareness programs in schools in the UK and Canada. *World Psychiatry* 2005;4(S1):50–4.

77 Pinfold V, Toulmin H, Thornicroft G, et al. Reducing psychiatric stigma and discrimination: Evaluation of educational interventions in UK secondary schools. *Br J Psychiatry* 2003;182:142–6.

78 Stuart H. Reaching out to high school youth: The effectiveness of a video-based anti-stigma program. *Can J Psychiatry* 2006;51:17–23.

79 Schulze B, Angermeyer M.C. Subjective experiences of stigma. A focus group study of schizophrenic patients, their relatives and mental health professionals. *Soc Sci Med* 2003;56:299–312.

80 Stuart H, Milev R, Koller M. The Inventory of Stigma Experiences. Its development and reliability. *World Psychiatry* 2005;4(S1):35–9.

15 Epidemiology of Mental Illness among Offenders

JULIO ARBOLEDA-FLÓREZ

Introduction

The large number of mental patients in prisons and jails, and the challenges that they pose for provision of services by these institutions, have become a practically intractable problem. With public concern about the violence perpetrated by the mentally ill adding further to the problem, more research is required into coordination of services among branches of government, inter-institutional arrangements, and better community best practices on diversion programs for the mentally ill and to the prevention of reincarceration.

When serious and bizarre crimes come to the attention of the public and the courts, it is not unusual that mental illness is suspected as one of the reasons for the crime. Knowledge of the characteristics of the crime could help increase our understanding of potential associations between mental illness and criminality, or act as a 'marker' to indicate the presence of a mental condition. People suffering from any kind of illness commit crimes. Mental illness, however, is expressed through behavioural manifestations and it affects the cognitive, emotional, and volitional aspects and functions of the personality. These are the very functions that the law considers essential to assess to assign guilt, label the accused a criminal, and proffer a sentence.[1]

This chapter will deal first with general aspects of the relationship between systems and between mental illness and criminality. Secondly, it will review the prevalence of mental disorders at the different levels of the correctional system, with special emphasis on a study by the author on the prevalence of mental illness in a remand centre in Canada. Finally, it will deal with possible reasons for the seemingly large migration of mental patients into the correctional system, while also identifying potential risk factors for the development of mental disorders in prison. This will be achieved by reviewing issues related to research and ethics in corrections, with an emphasis on the contributions of correctional research on offender populations in Canada.

Parameters of a Relationship

The justice system covers all the state apparatus to keep peace internally in a nation-state, either by apprehending, processing, and sentencing wrongdoers (criminal law), or by mediating in disputes among citizens (civil law). While the label is all-encompassing, the justice system proper is that in between policing (apprehension) and prisons and that includes exclusively the mechanics of court work, court appearances, trial, and sentencing. In criminal law, once the person is found guilty, a set of variables, including mental condition, are considered before sentencing. Sentences may entail community supervision (probation) or time in prison, and are managed by the Department of Corrections. Corrections, as a general term, is applied to the branch of the criminal justice system that involves 'all agencies of social control which attempt to rehabilitate and neutralize deviant behaviour of adult criminals and juvenile delinquents for the protection of society.'[2(p444)] The study of how the mentally abnormal offender is handled within correctional settings is the purview of 'correctional psychiatry,' which in the strictest sense, refers to psychiatric practice in the corrections system.[3] More specifically, correctional psychiatry could be defined as the branch of forensic psychiatry that studies the incidence, prevalence, determinants, and management of mental disorders in prisons, the response of correctional systems to the mentally ill offender, and the relationship between criminality and mental illness.

Relationship between Mental Health System and Correctional System

The mentally ill, and by extension, mental health professionals, interact with legal systems at practically every junction of the different components of the system, be it law enforcement, administration of justice, or correctional systems. The close relationship between the two systems is dictated by the intrinsic needs of the population served by both psychiatry and corrections. In some communities, the transfer of patients back and forth between the two systems makes the correctional system, especially the jails, part and parcel of the mental health system.

Detention and Triage

In many jurisdictions, as a result of minor infractions by an individual or when public behaviour is obviously aberrant, police forces have the option to convey mentally abnormal individuals to a mental hospital or to a psychiatric emergency department for an examination as an alternative to laying criminal charges. Provincial mental health acts in Canada contain specific sections that give special powers to a police officer to bring the person for an examination to the emergency department of a local hospital, if the person was acting in a public place in such a manner that, in the opinion of the officer, the person's behaviour was abnormal. The basis for this type of legislation is the recognition that police officers have or can be taught skills to be able to recognize mental conditions among arrestees.[4,5]

Powers vested in police officers under these circumstances allow them to circumvent the justice system and to divert the person directly to the mental health system. Police officers become, *de facto*, 'extensions' of the mental health system. Studies have indicated that, given their familiarity with individuals who display abnormal behaviour, police officers can be relied upon to make this type of judgment.[6-9]

The failure of deinstitutionalization policies in the face of inadequate community resources makes it necessary for the mental health system to utilize other community agencies, such as the police force, to help the mentally ill person in the community. Allowing police officers to be part of the mental health system helps prevent further criminalization of the mentally ill and is one of the ways of dealing in the community with the mentally ill offender. The role of the police officer, however, is limited to bringing the person to a hospital; it is the role of clinicians at the hospital to make decisions on further management. The clinical team at the hospital, for example, could return the person to the care of the police or make arrangements for outpatient follow-up, level of community supervision, or admission to hospital, either voluntarily, or by invoking the commitment powers vested in clinicians within the provincial mental health act or similar legislation.

Community Disposition

To prevent the revolving door phenomenon and, at the same time, maximize treatment opportunities and provide a modicum of protection to the community, several jurisdictions have implemented outpatient commitment legislation.[10] Under this type of legislation, the court places the accused on probation on condition of treatment, or a physician discharges the patient to the community on a certificate that obligates the patient to continue receiving treatment and the medication for a specified period of time, usually one to two years. Two treatment modalities are used extensively in association with out-patient commitment: case-management and assertive community treatment. These are considered essential components of outpatient commitment as strategies aimed to maximize the impact of mental health care in the community and the effectiveness of other treatment alternatives. In case management, a mental health specialist follows a few assigned cases in the community and brokers their social and treatment needs; whereas in assertive community treatment (ACT), a specialized cadre of clinicians follows the patient and practically takes over community functioning with the intent to make sure that patients live within specified conditions and that they comply with all treatment recommendation for community tenure. Patients are reported back to the court or brought back to the hospital if they fail to comply. These strategies have been found highly effective in preventing relapses, rehospitalizations, and reincarcerations.[11–13] Outpatient commitment is based on the premise that seriously mentally ill persons, because of delusions and other symptoms, may not have the ability to make decisions regarding their need for treatment and, consequently, fail to avail themselves of treatment opportunities. Failure to take advantage of treatment opportunities because of the illness may constitute a denial of the patient's right to be treated. Although there may be concerns about possible threats to civil liberties, outpatient commitment is promoted as an alternative to imprisonment and as a preventative step to avoid relapses or criminalization. It is considered to be an enlightened alternative to rehospitalizations and reincarcerations,[14] especially if accompanied by provisions for community management, exemplified in Brian's Law in Ontario.[15]

Sentencing

Working arrangements between the police and local hospitals are difficult to implement, as they require administrative mechanisms and previously organized payment systems.[16] Thus, more frequently, and especially if the charge is of a serious nature, police follow the justice route and bring mental patients to local police lockups, jails, or remand centres. Some of these patients may be found not fit to stand trial and be sent for assessment and treatment to specialized institutions from where they are supposed to return to court once their mental conditions stabilize. Later on, during their trial, some of these patients may be found not criminally responsible because of mental disorder and sent, according to local legislation, for indeterminate periods of time to mental hospitals, special hospitals, or to special wings in a penitentiary. On the other hand, despite the presence of a mental condition, a mental patient may still be found guilty and sentenced to a prison term. These mentally ill offenders tend to suffer from chronic mental problems and are usually found in remand centres or local jails, either because they are detained while awaiting their legal disposition, or because they are sentenced to short periods of incarceration. Medium and maximum security prisons usually house inmates who have been sentenced to long terms for offences somewhat related to abnormal behaviours (antisocial, psychopathic), sexual deviations, or to addictions that, inevitably, bring them into conflict with the law.

Relationship between Mental Illness and Criminality

When a mental condition is suspected in relation to a crime, the unstated assumption is that the condition *preceded* the crime, and hence, may have actually *caused* the crime. However, the clinician and the epidemiologist assessing the association between mental illness and crime and conducting prevalence studies have to keep in mind that, often, mental illness may develop after a crime has been committed.

It may be that the number of mentally ill persons in prisons is a function of a putative relationship between mental illness and crime (defined as unlawful acts, by commission or omission, leading to an arrest). The study of such relationship, however, is difficult[17] and much work remains to be done before clear patterns emerge. However, there are some patterns and data from which we can begin to better understand the complex associations between mental illness and crime.

Many factors have been described as being associated with criminality, including mental conditions. Alcoholism and substance dependence, for example, carry a high risk of law-breaking.[18] Swanson et al.[19] found higher rates of depression, suicide attempts, and aggressive tendencies among a group of alcoholics compared to non-alcoholics. Hare and Hart[20] suggested that psychopathy is strongly associated with a high risk for criminal and violent behaviour. Yarvis found,[21] in a series of 100 murderers, that 29% had a diagnosis of 'psychosis,' 21% schizophrenia, and 8% affective disorders. Other factors that seem to mediate the association between mental illness and crime include gender,[22] age,[23] socioeconomic status,[24] previous criminality,[25] and previous forensic psychiatric involvement.[26]

A proper study on the relationship between criminology and psychopathology, however, would have to start by questioning whether a relationship exists at all, and if so, whether it is one of causality or of correlation. A causal relationship could be based on nosographic parallelism because psychopathology and criminology share mutual grounds so that symptoms are equal to crimes and vice-versa; or on epidemiological decisions that some mental states cause criminality. On the other hand, a relationship of correlation would have to specify the factors through which the association holds. Although interest in the association can be traced back to Aristotle,[27] the large number of mental patients in prisons and the publicity generated by major crimes in which a mental patient has been involved has increased the interest in recent years. In addition, depictions of criminals with twisted minds in movies and television spread the opinion that crime and mental illness are closely related. Unfortunately, with some regularity, the media provide realistic portrayals of violence by mentally ill persons along with social neglect, homelessness, and social disenfranchisement, which contribute to reasons why some mental patients are arrested.

Behavioural Manifestations and Criminality

In general, mental conditions are related to crime, but the problem is not that the two could converge, but the degree of relatedness between the two and whether a causal connection could be established.

For example, there are mental disorders whose very behavioural manifestations become, *ipso facto*, a criminal offence. The 'patient,' by virtue of having the disorder, is a criminal as seldom can the symptoms be controlled and the very symptoms of the disorder are by themselves criminal acts. Such is the case of most of the paraphilias (exhibitionism, voyeurism, frotteurism, pedophilia, necrophilia, etc.), pyromania, kleptomania, and others. In these cases, it could be determined that the relationship between mental disorder and criminality is one-to-one; it is absolute.

Other disorders, such as antisocial personality, borderline personality, pathological gambling, and impulse control disorders connote a criminological element, but the degree of relatedness is not one-to-one in that symptoms could be expressed without necessarily breaking the law. For example, while not all alcoholics end up breaking the law, alcoholism carries a high risk of law-breaking in the form of victimization at the time of intoxication.[18] Dependency on other substances is known to lead to income-generating crimes in order to finance the habit if the addicted person does not have the financial means to support it and psychopathy is strongly associated with a high risk for criminal and violent offences.[20]

The relationship becomes less and less straightforward when other mental conditions are considered. There is, for example, a clinically frequent association between delinquency and psychotic, schizophrenia-like disorders[28] and it is also known that individuals suffering from schizophrenia may get involved either in minor law-breaking or in serious, unexplainable violent crime.[29] Persons suffering from major depression may display violent behaviour against self or others.[30,31] In fact, dangerousness, or the potentiality to cause grievous bodily harm to self or others, is the main criterion for civil commitment in many jurisdictions.[32] Still, seldom is the relationship between these conditions and criminal offences a one-to-one. Furthermore, many mentally ill persons never commit a criminal offence in spite of the relatively high prevalence of mental disorders in the general population.

Mental Illness and Violence

The literature seems to provide support for the proposition that there is more than a correlation between mental illness and criminality, whether by itself or in association with other factors.[33] In a 30-year follow-up of a birth cohort in Sweden, a relationship between crime and mental disorder and between crime and intellectual deficiency was identified, with men who had a mental disorder being 2.5 times more likely to have been registered for a criminal offence and 4 times more likely to have been registered for a violent offence, compared to men not mentally ill or intellectually handicapped.[34]

A review of computerized records in a prison showed that 13.8% of inmates without a psychiatric history or history of substance abuse had a history of recent or remote violence, compared with 17% of inmates with history of either. Percentages for the same two groups for remote violence were 30.9 and 51.1 respectively, and 5.8% of those with a history of both mental illness and violence committed unmotivated violent acts, compared to only 1.2% among inmates without either history.[35] Another study showed similar findings; in a series of 100 murderers, 29% had a diagnosis of 'psychosis' (schizophrenia 21% and affective disorders 8%), and 35% had a diagnosis of substance abuse.[21] Thus, these and many other studies point toward clusters of complex, but yet distinct diagnoses that emerge associated with other variables.

In 1993, Monahan,[36] a major commentator and researcher, proposed that factors such as socioeconomic status and institutionalization should be considered integral parts of mental disorders as opposed to simple statistical noise in need of control. This reassessment about the central-ity of some symptoms to the understanding of mental disorders and epi-demiological findings pointing to a major association between mental illness and violence lead some authors to suggest that a strong associa-tion existed amounting to proof of a causal link between the two.[37]

Although it is known that persons suffering from mental conditions comorbid with alcohol and substance dependence, or with psychopa-thy, are at a higher risk for violent offending, studies that have linked mental illness to violence, however, have been criticized on multiple methodological grounds, especially because of selection biases or lack of proper controls for confounding factors. For example, in a thorough review of the literature on mental illness and violence, Arboleda-Flórez, Holley, and Crisanti concluded that 'as yet, there is no consis-tent evidence to support the hypothesis that mental illness, uncompli-cated by substance abuse, is a significant risk factor for violence or criminality, once past history of violence is controlled'.[38(p45)]

More importantly, from a public health perspective, the measure to be concerned about is not the relative risk (the ratio of the risk of vio-lence among the exposed mentally ill to the risk among the unexposed, those not mentally ill) as such, but the attributable risk (the rate of vio-lence among mentally ill that can be attributed to their exposure to mental illness). Despite a high relative risk, violence due to mental illness is not that frequent once all other causes of violence in society are taken into account. Stuart and Arboleda-Flórez[38] have measured such risk and concluded that if all causes of violence are taken care of, the contribution of mental illness would only be about 3%, jumping to about 10% if substance abuse and alcoholism are included. A similar finding has been reported by Swanson et al.[39] who estimated that the attributable risk among those with major mental disorder would be only 4.3% and it might be as low as 1%.[40]

Criminality and mental illness, however, may be related only at the level of availability of systems. For example, in the absence of adequate hospital services, and when systems also fail in community alternatives, an increase of services in prisons would be expected. This has been known since 1939 when Penrose[41] outlined his balloon theory that for a sector of the population a decrease in hospital beds is made up by an increase in prison spaces and vice-versa. Violence committed by mentally ill persons[42–47] creates the impression that the mental health system is in disarray when, in fact, what could be needed would be better risk-management strategies[48] and more enlightened community-corrections partnerships to prevent further criminal offending and reincarcerations.[49–52] These programs rely heavily on case management practices,[53] and ACT programs. An evidence-based best practice on these alternatives, however, may still be missing, as results of reviews by the Cochrane Library indicate that case management has no clear effect on imprisonment,[54] and that ACT is no better than standard community care on imprisonment, arrests, or police contacts.[55]

Work on risk management and on the relationship of mental illness and violence takes into consideration issues relating to the management of the mentally ill prisoner and the use of preventative and diversion measures[56] as well as violence committed against mentally ill persons in the community and in prisons. In the community, mental patients living in poor tenements and neighbourhoods tend to become the subject of abuse and violence, so their crimes are many times reactive and contextual.[43] In prisons, apart from inadequate psychiatric services, clinical staff usually work in isolation and receive little support from management, thus increasing the vulnerabilities and disadvantaged status of mentally ill prisoners.[57]

In summary, contemporary public policy, based on historically legal doctrine, is premised on the assumption that there is a specific population on whom mental disorder and criminal behaviour converge. This convergence, however, is predicated more on statistical correlations than on proof of a causality link – that mental illness *causes* violence. The consequences for the management of mentally ill persons in the community will be major, were this link ever to be proven. Apart from increasing the stigma against mentally ill persons in the community, proof of such link will lead to longer periods of incarceration and hospitalization and increased social control on the mentally ill.

Prevalence of Mental Illness in Corrections

Prisons have been the repositories of the mentally ill ever since their invention over 200 years ago, and ever since the mix of regular prisoners and mentally ill individuals has been considered an anomaly in need of rectification and demanding of solutions. Yet, despite multiple government commissions and voluminous parliamentary reports in many countries, and the introduction of several alternatives to care, the problem of incarceration of the mentally ill in the prison system persists and appears to be getting worse. In many cities, the large number of mental patients in local jails has made this setting a practical extension of the general mental health services. The trans-institutionalization of mentally ill persons from hospitals to prisons has been documented in a plethora of studies that have also estimated their numbers at different points of the justice-correctional system.[58]

Research reports on the prevalence of mental illness in jails, also known as remand centres in Canada, date back many years[59-65] as do reports on longer term prisons.[66-70] Prevalence estimates of the mentally ill in correctional facilities, however, vary widely, from 7%[71] to 90%.[72] Many reasons have been given to explain these disparities (*vide infra*), including methodological problems, type of institutions where the studies have been carried out, kind and size of samples used, and how mental conditions/problems are defined.[73-74]

In a study by the Department of Health and the Office for National Statistics in Great Britain,[75] the authors found that 7% of sentenced males, 10% of men on remand, and 14% of women in both categories had been affected by a psychotic illness in the previous year. Among women on remand, 75% reported neurotic symptoms, and 20% of men and 40% of women had attempted at suicide at least once (25% of women in the previous year and 2% of women and men in the previous week).

A study in Texas[76] suggested that the rise of mental patients in prisons is primarily due to the influx of inmates incarcerated for drug-related offences, which, in turn, may be predictive of suicidal behaviour. Through the use of clinical interviews using the Structure Clinical Interview for *DSM-IV (SCID-IV)*, the authors determined that, among 400 consecutive admissions, lifetime substance abuse or dependence disorders were present among 74% of inmates, and about 37% had abused or were dependent on alcohol or drugs in the previous 30 days.

Unfortunately, violence in prison also encompasses acts against the self that are committed more often than acts against others. To follow Durkheim's[77] characterization of suicide in relation to the organization patterns of society, prison environments could be described as hypernomic or overly regulated. Whether this social structure contributes to the high levels of suicide in jails and prisons is debatable, but the fact is that suicide in correctional environments is a major public health issue.[78,79] For example, an item posted in the Criminal Justice Internet System in Canada[80] reproduced a news release in the *Courant* of Hartford about inmate suicides in the Department of Corrections in Connecticut. According to the news item, the suicide of three inmates in a matter of a week had drawn attention to the larger problem of mentally ill prisoners. Reportedly, the number of inmates with a history of mental illness in the state prison population has surged from 24% in 1991 to 40% in the current year. A court officer attributed the surge to 'people with mental illness who don't function well in the community and are ending up in prison.' More people die by suicide in prison than from any other cause and, given that the majority of suicides occur within the first days of detention in jails or remand centres, special precautions and screening methods are highly recommended.[81]

In a review of the literature on the prevalence of mental illness in prisons, Lamb and Weinberger[74] searched for publications in Medline, *Psychological Abstracts*, and the *Index to Legal Periodicals and Books*. These authors found that the mentally ill are more frequently arrested compared to the population in general, and that up to 15% of inmates in city jails and in state prisons have severe mental illnesses, a majority of them having been homeless prior to incarceration.

Finally, a study of consecutive admissions to detect the prevalence of psychopathy in prisons using the Hare Psychopathy Checklist Revised (PCL-R) found that among 104 sentenced inmates arriving at a therapeutic prison in England, 26% had PCL-R scores of 30 or more and were, therefore, identified as psychopaths.[82]

Epidemiological Study in a Remand Centre

Mental illness in correctional facilities could develop in three different epidemiological populations: those who are mentally ill on entrance into the system; those who were well on entrance, but who have a history of mental illness and, eventually, relapse while in prison; and those who were well on entrance and have no previous history of mental illness, but who eventually succumb to the rigours of prison life and develop a mental disorder. While each one of these populations can give an idea of the extent of the mental pathology in prisons and the relationship between mental pathology and criminality, a way to study this relationship, including violent offences, is to assess the mental condition of a group of detainees (those individuals just arrested as being suspect of a crime). Obviously, the results of such a selected sample will not provide information on causality, given the cross-sectional nature of the design, but it can provide important clues on the prevalence of mental disorders in a newly remanded population and some clues on the relationship.[7] While it is possible to study the presence of mental illness at an earlier moment, such as the moment of arrest, the context of the situation makes it practically impossible to conduct a diagnostic interview at that time. Hence, the first point in time to do an in-depth epidemiological study is at detention in remand centres (jails); in fact, this point may be the best one to study the prevalence and the mental illness-crime relationship.[83,84]

This section reports on a descriptive, cross-sectional[85,86] study conducted by the author at the Calgary Remand Centre (local jail) in Alberta, Canada from mid-August to mid-December 1992.[87] The main purpose of the study was to obtain one-month and lifetime prevalence estimates of mental conditions.[88]

For the 1,200 interviewees, a principal diagnosis was made in 728 (60.7%) individuals. Of these, 664 (92.2%) were for Axis I conditions and 64 (8.8%) for Axis II. One-month prevalence estimates with 95% confidence intervals showed the prevalence of any disorder for females to be 49.5% (CI = 40.2–58.9) with alcohol dependency, 26.1% (CI = 18.0–34.3), being the most frequent condition. For males, the overall prevalence for any disorder was 56% (CI = 53–59), with alcohol dependency, 31.7% (CI = 29.0–34.5), being the most frequent, followed by cannabis dependency, 8.5% (CI = 6.8–10.1), polysubstance abuse dependence, 4.2% (CI = 3.0–5.4), and major depression, 3.3% (CI =

2.3–44.0). No case of schizophrenia was diagnosed among females; in males 1.2% (CI = 0.4–1.6) were so diagnosed. Schizophrenia and depression were more frequent among the two oldest groups, while drugs of any kind, except alcohol, appeared more frequently in the younger groups. In both males and females, over half the pathology was accounted for by alcohol and substance abuse.

The highest prevalence of mental illness, 77.9% (CI = 70.1–85.5), was found among the lowest-educated group (3 to 8 years of schooling), where the most common diagnoses were alcohol/substance abuse (61.9%) and personality disorder (8.8%). While the overall prevalence of mental disorders was highest among Aboriginals, (66.4%; CI = 60.5–72.3), alcohol/substance abuse was the most common problem (60.7%) and the prevalence of major mental disorders was the lowest among them (0.4%). Personality disorders were most frequent among Caucasians (6.7%), but no ethnic differences were noted for psychosis or affective disorders.

For both males and females, there was a paucity of hierarchical diagnoses on Axis II personality disorders, especially APD. There were only four females who received a diagnosis on Axis II, one each for dependent personality, histrionic personality, borderline personality, and personality disorder not specified. In contrast, 60 males (5.5%) received a diagnosis on Axis II, with the most frequent being personality disorder not specified (2.0%) and antisocial personality disorder (1.0%). The most common comorbid conditions were schizophrenia and substance abuse disorders (2.9%).

From the results presented in this study, it can only be concluded that remandees are more likely to be mentally ill if they have a low education, had a previous history of previous detentions (the larger the number, the more likely), and had a history of previous forensic assessments. This would indicate that there is a tendency to shuffle more regularly into prison those whom the mental health system had already failed once – *once a forensic case, always a forensic case.*

Issues Affecting Prevalence Studies in Corrections

Apart from the inherent methodological difficulties in any study of this nature, the restrictions of the system, the concerns about security, the bureaucratic red tape, and the ethical entanglements make studies in prisons difficult to mount and to perform. Although these may be reasons for the wide variability in estimates of prevalence, methodological deficiencies in the studies seem to be the real reason. It may be that the wide variation in the estimates point to design errors, poorly chosen samples, the use of unstandardized instruments or diagnostic techniques,[71] and problems in the definition of what constitutes a 'case.'[36] More specific reasons to explain these variations include:

1 Variety of diagnostic systems and different psychiatric classifications and versions of recognized nomenclature systems, such as the International Classification of Diseases or the DSM systems, which make it difficult to compare estimates obtained from different geographical regions or eras.

2 Comparison of estimates from results of studies that have been conducted in different kinds of institutions (jails, prison, penitentiaries, specialized hospitals, etc.), or sampling from different types of institutions, is hazardous given that different institutions accommodate different criminal populations according to the function of the institution. Clinical populations in institutions tend to vary according to the functions of the institution.

3 Jails and short-term prisons may hold a large number of acutely ill persons affected by drug reactions, psychoses, or serious depressions; while long-term penitentiaries may house a disproportionate number of persons with antisocial personality disorders. Specialized hospitals may have an over-representation of individuals suffering from mental deficiencies or sexual pathologies.

4 Finally, contrary to studies in jails, studies in long-stay institutions measure two kinds of pathology: the pathology pre-existing imprisonment and the pathology that has developed *de novo* following long years of incarceration.

5 Results of some studies may be affected by the types of samples chosen. For example, samples based on consecutive admissions[63,66] to jails may yield distorted estimates as arrest rates in a particular locality are prone to be influenced by historical events and, possibly, by seasonal variations.

6 Few studies have provided age- and sex-standardized estimates.[72] Generally, estimates provided in other studies tend to be crude prevalence estimates and do not make specific comparisons to the estimated prevalence in the population.[61,62]

7 Instruments used have varied and many have not been tested for reliability or validity. These instruments range from unstandardized clinical interviews whose reliability cannot be controlled,[69] to

retrospective review of records,[67] or computer record linkage[35] that depend on secondary data whose quality cannot be vouched for.

8 Even the use of standardized, structured clinical interviews, such as the Diagnostic Interview Schedule that was used in the Epidemiology Catchment Area studies[89] and in some prison studies, provide faulty estimates when applied to a criminal population, as some Axis I and Axis II diagnoses common among criminal populations are not included in the DIS and because the definition of antisocial personality disorder is based on *DSM-III*, which makes APD similar to plain criminality.

9 Studies have used multiple raters[90] without giving consideration to problems of inter-rater reliability.

10 Confounding may be caused by substance abuse and dependence.

Issues on the Definition of Antisocial Personality

The bulk of mental pathology in remanded populations is mostly associated with substance abuse and dependency, whereas the prevalence of serious mental disorders does not seem to be much higher than that of these disorders in the general population. Similarly, a more rigorous diagnosis of antisocial personality disorder (APD) that differentiates it from plain criminality brings down the frequency of this diagnosis in prisons. Thus, this study does not support the large presence of APD individuals that have been reported in other studies. The reason for this seems to be the tighter understanding of the concept through the use of the Hare PCL.

Population and Health Services Research

Research on the management and treatment of the mentally ill in prisons has a long tradition. For example, considerable research has been conducted in Germany since the 1850s on suicide, the prevalence of mental conditions among prisoners, and the influence of the prison environment as a risk factor to psychiatric illness. Ganser syndrome and the term *prison psychosis* originated from this research.[91] As the number of mental patients multiplies in prison settings, so too have the research efforts to study not only their characteristics, but also the cost and effectiveness of treatment, the issue of lodging, and a host of other factors. The following are select examples of research in this ever-expanding field.

A sample of 178 Danish prisoners was administered Hare's Psycho-pathic Checklist-Revised PCL-R, the Present State Examination, and semi-structured interviews in order to detect levels of psychiatric mor-bidity in each of the quartiles of the PCL-R.[92] High rates of psychiatric morbidity in all PCL-R quartile groups were found. The medium to high scorers represented the most vulnerable group with a high preva-lence of dependence disorders and a relatively high prevalence of neu-rotic and stress-related disorders. High scorers were more psychoso-cially maladjusted, had more often made previous suicidal attempts, and had a higher psychoticism score. Psychopathy was not as preva-lent in comparison to figures in similar studies elsewhere. More recently, further work with the use of the PCL-R has been undertaken in other countries with the intention of defining cut-off scores applica-ble to different cultures and populations.[93]

Psychopaths and inmates affected by severe antisocial personality disorder, however, present major challenges in prison environments. Their high crime rates and mental pathology continued in prison where boundaries between treatability and punishment are easily blurred.[94] A recent example, out of the many in the forensic literature, is the one that came to light in the Fallon Inquiry in England. This inquiry, on the situation at the high security unit of Ashworth, report-edly found that the place was 'a deeply flawed creation' in which the patients were running the hospital. Apparently, this inquiry recom-mended that services for personality disordered persons be delivered within small specialized units in both highly secure hospitals and prisons, with easy transfer between the two, and that nationally agreed assessment and treatment protocols be developed. The empha-sis on custody over treatment concerns may place further burdens on psychiatrists to protect public safety. This seems to be happening lately with the practice of 'gating,' whereby serious violent and sexual offenders who are expected to be released into the community at the end of their sentences are instead civilly committed to mental hospitals regardless of the patients' treatability, and at the expense of precious beds for the regularly mentally ill person in the community.

Further, much difficulty accrues when anti-sociality is comorbid with substance disorders that triggers increased antisocial behaviour.[95] In a study in Australia, 400 subjects were studied, half of whom were from a community methadone maintenance program, and half from prison inmates on methadone maintenance recruited from five metro-politan and rural prisons. Study findings showed that there were close associations between substance dependence and antisocial personality disorder (ASPD) as measured via *DSM-III-R*, and psychopathy via PCL-R. Seventy-seven per cent of the subjects, termed 'primary anti-socials,' had engaged in criminal behaviour prior to their first use of heroin, 'secondary antisocials' (20%) had initiated use after the beginning of their criminal activities, and only 3% reported no criminal behaviour before or after their dependence on heroin. 'Primary antisocials' were more likely to have an antisocial personality disorder (63%) than 'secondary antisocials' (39%), and were also more likely to be psychopathic (8% vs. 4%).

Behavioural difficulties often come associated with brain injuries that also abound in the prison population, but there is a paucity of research on this. Two authors,[96] however, have reported the incidence and outcomes of a history of traumatic brain injury (TBI) and substance abuse among prisoners in New Zealand, and on the neuropsychological outcomes of TBI and substance abuse among a sub-sample of 50 prisoners. Although methodological shortcomings limit conclusions to be drawn from this study, especially the oversight of not having reviewed the medical files and the unreliability of self-reports among samples of prisoners, the rates of sustained TBI at some time in the lives of the subjects merits further attention. Eighty-six per cent of subjects reported TBI, and 32% reported serious multiple events of TBI. The lower prevalence of alcohol use among the subjects, those who 'have ever used' alcohol (89%), compared to the general population (96%), may be an artifact produced by the sampling problems. This population reported higher use of illicit substances (cannabis, LSD, psilocybin, and amphetamines) than the general population. The subjects of the second study reported having been unconscious for 30 minutes or longer and had endorsed 10 or more problems on the symptom rating scale provided in the questionnaire used in the previous study. Findings of these studies suggest that TBI may be especially high in a prison population and is associated with difficulties in verbal memory and verbal abstract thinking which may have implications for inmates' functioning in prisons and on release afterward.

The function and management of special care units have become central to the forensic debate, especially in the U.K. Although secure units are, technically, not prisons, there are many similarities between them and prison environments in relation to administrative structures, the populations served, security issues,[97] and specialized pathologies such as paraphilias.[98] Although there are no accurate figures for the cost of looking after the mentally ill in prisons, the cost of caring for those transferred back to psychiatric services is staggering and has been calculated in the U.K. at £1.4 million per 100,000 population.[99]

Recidivism has become an area of research in the hope of finding common indicators or pathways that could be used to halt the double revolving door phenomenon of multiple hospitalizations and reincarcerations.[100–102]

More recently research efforts have been focused on research on the outcome of interventions[103,104] and their cost-effectiveness,[105] or at a larger level, the cost-effectiveness of diversion programs in the community.[106]

In the federal penitentiary system in Canada, apart from studies on the prevalence of mental illness among penitentiary prisoners, population-based research on prisoners and parolees has been conducted at two levels: studies on methodologies and instruments to measure risk and studies on recidivism. Based on internal studies, the Office of the Correctional Investigator Annual Report 2004/2005 stated that 'the proportion of federal offenders with significant, identified, mental health needs has more than doubled over the past decade.'[107] This statement echoes figures highlighted in research by the services in the same year[108] in which about 8% of inmates were considered to have a psychotic illness, about 21% were depressed, 44% suffered from anxiety, 41% from substance dependence, and 47% from alcoholism, aside from a host of other mental conditions.

Canada has had a leading role in the development of scales to measure risk. Apart from the Psychopathic Checklist (PCL-R) devised by Hare[109] and considered in many countries the gold standard to diagnose psychopathy, there is also the HCR-20, a very easy to use instrument to help clinicians mange risk[110] and, more in regard to classification of offenders, the SIR devised by Nuffield.[111] Similarly, significant research has also been done on recidivists through evaluation of treatment programs, identification of correctional outcomes, and development of methodologies for their measurement[112] in order to reduce the risk of re-offending following release.

Conclusions

Despite many efforts and initiatives to minimize the plight of the mentally ill in prison, and to prevent deterioration and imprisonment and especially to prevent reincarcerations, their numbers do not seem to cease climbing. The prevalence of mental conditions in prisons remains high, and more mental patients arrive at the local jails. Mental patients and the developmentally disabled are found in death row. Close cooperation among agencies and new service modalities may be required, including diversion programs and better treatment approaches, but concerns about violence among the mentally ill threaten to undo years of progress of readaptation and reintegration in the community, and set the clock back to a more pernicious form of institutionalization. Given that back in the early 1800s and afterwards in many countries, prisons were the usual place for mental patients in lieu of asylums, despite all that has been done, little seems to have changed and their plight remains the same. *Plus ça change, plus c'est la même chose.*

REFERENCES

1 Arboleda-Flórez J, Deynaka CJ. *Forensic Psychiatric Evidence.* Toronto: Butterworths, 1999.
2 Kruzich JM. Services for mentally ill offenders. In: Austin MJ, Hershey WE, eds. *Handbook on Mental Health Administration.* San Francisco: Jossey-Bass, 1982:436–55.
3 Travin S. History of correctional psychiatry. In: Rosner R, ed. *Principles and Practice of Forensic Psychiatry.* New York: Chapman & Hall, 1994:369–74.
4 Lamb HR, Weinberger LE, DeCuir WJ. The police and mental health. *Psychiatr Serv* 2002;53:1266–71.
5 Arboleda-Flórez J, Crisanti A, Holley H. *The Police Officer as a Primary Mental Health Resource.* Washington: The World Health Organization Centre for Research and Training in Mental Health (Pan American Health Organization), 1996.
6 Arboleda-Flórez J, Holley H. Criminalization of the mentally ill – Part I. *Can J Psychiatry* 1988;33:81–6.
7 Teplin LA. The criminalization of the mentally ill: Speculation in search of data. *Psychol Bull* 1983;94:54–67.
8 Price M. Commentary: The challenge of training police officers. *J Am Acad Psychiatry Law* 2005;33:50–4.
9 Keram EA. Commentary: A multidisciplinary approach to developing mental health training for law enforcement. *J Am Acad Psychiatry Law* 2005;33:47–9.

10 Hiday VA, Scheid-Cook TL. Outpatient commitment for 'revolving door' patients: Compliance and treatment. *J Nerv Mental Disease* 1991;179: 83–8.

11 Sheldon CT, Aubry TD, Arboleda-Flórez J, et al. Social disadvantage, mental illness and predictors of legal involvement. *Int J Law Psychiatry* 2006;29:249–56.

12 Lamberti JS, Weisman R, Faden DI. Forensic assertive community treatment: Preventing incarceration of adults with severe mental illness. *Psychiatr Serv* 2004;55:1285–93.

13 Lang MA, Davidson L, Bailey P, et al. Clinicians' and clients' perspectives on the impact of assertive community treatment. *Psychiatr Serv* 1999;50: 1331–40.

14 Petrilla J, Ridgely Ms, Borum R. Debating outpatient commitment: Controversy, trends, and empirical data. *Crime and Delinquency* 2003;49: 157–72.

15 Ontario Ministry of Health and Long-Term Care. *Public Information – Mental Health: Brian's Law (Mental Health Legislative Reform), 2000.* http://www.health.gov.on.ca/english/public/pub/ mental/brianslaw.html. Accessed August 30, 2006.

16 Arboleda-Flórez J. Holley H. Criminalization of the mentally ill – Part II. *Can J Psychiatry* 1988;33:87–95.

17 Joukamaa M. Mental health of Finnish prisoners. *J Forens Psychiatry* 1993;4:261–71.

18 Pihl RO, Peterson JB. Alcohol/drug and aggressive behavior. In: Hodgins S, ed. *Mental Disorder and Crime.* Newbury Park: Sage, 1993:263–83.

19 Swanson JW, Holzer III CE, Ganju VK, et al. Violence and psychiatric disorder in the community: Evidence from the Epidemiologic Catchment Area Surveys. *Hosp Comm Psychiatry* 1990;41:761–70.

20 Hare RD, Hart SD. Psychopathy, mental disorder and crime. In: Hodgins S, ed. *Mental Disorder and Crime.* Newbury Park: Sage, 1993:104–15.

21 Yarvis RM. Axis I and Axis II diagnostic parameters of homicide. *Bull Am Acad Psychiatry Law* 1990;18:249–69.

22 Mednick SA, Pollock V, Volavka J, et al. Biology and violence. In: Wolfgang ME, Weiner NA, eds. *Criminal Violence.* Newbury Park: Sage, 1982:21–80.

23 Nestor PG. Neuropsychological and clinical correlates of murder and other forms of extreme violence in a forensic psychiatric population. *J Nerv Ment Dis* 1992;4:418–23.

24 Hodgins S. Mental disorder, intellectual disability and crime: Evidence from a birth cohort. *Arch General Psychiatry* 1992;49:476–83.

25 Moore MH, Estrich SR, McGillis S, et al. *Dangerous Offenders: The Elusive Target of Justice*. Cambridge: Harvard University Press, 1984.

26 Menzies RJ. *Survival of the Sanest: Order and Disorder in a Pre-trial Psychiatric Clinic*. Toronto: University of Toronto Press, 1989.

27 Aristotle. *The Nichomachean Ethics*, Ross D, trans. Oxford: Oxford University Press, 1941.

28 Otnow-Lewis D. *Vulnerabilities to Delinquency*. New York: SP Medical & Scientific Books, 1981.

29 McKay RD, Wright RE. Schizophrenia and antisocial (criminal) behaviour: Some responses from sufferers and relatives. *Med Sci Law* 1984;24:192–8.

30 Goodwin FK, Jamison KR. *Manic-depressive Illness*. New York: Oxford University Press, 1990.

31 Taylor PJ. Schizophrenia and crime: Distinctive patters in association. In: Hodgins S, ed. *Mental Disorder and Crime*. Newbury Park: Sage, 1993:63–85.

32 Arboleda-Flórez J, Copithorne M. *Mental Health Law and Practice*. Toronto: Carswell, 1994.

33 McNeil DE, Binder RL. Psychiatric emergency service use and homelessness, mental disorder, and violence. *Psychiatr Serv* 2005;56:699–704.

34 Hodgins S. The criminality of mentally disordered persons. In: Hodgins S, ed. *Mental Disorder and Crime*. Newbury Park: Sage, 1993:3–21.

35 Toch H, Adams K. *The Disturbed Violent Offender*. New Haven: Yale University Press, 1989.

36 Monaham J, Steadman HJ. Crime and mental disorder: An epidemiological approach. In: Tonry M, Morris N, eds. *Crime and Justice*. An Annual Review of Research, Vol. 4. Chicago: The University of Chicago Press, 1983.

37 Link BG, Stueve A. Evidence bearing on mental illness as a possible cause of violent behavior. Epidemiol Rev 1995;17:1–10.

38 Swanson JW, Borum R, Swartz M, et al. Psychotic symptoms and disorders and the risk of violent behaviour in the community. *Crim Behav Ment Health* 1996;6:317–38.

39 Wesseley S, Castle D, Douglas A, et al. The criminal careers of incident cases of schizophrenia. *Psychol Med* 1994;24:483–502.

40 Stuart H, Arboleda-Flórez J. Mental illness and violence: Are the public at risk? *Psychiatr Serv* 2001;52:654–9.

41 Steuve A, Link BG. Gender differences in the relationship between mental illness and violence: Evidence from a community-based epidemiological study in Israel. *Soc Psychiatry Psychiatr Epidemiol* 1998;33:s61–s76.

42 Penrose LS. Mental disease and crime. Outline of a comparative study of European statistics. *Br Med Psychol* 1939;18:1–15.

43 Estroff SE, Swanson JW, Lachicotte WS, et al. Risk reconsidered: Targets of violence in the social networks of people with serious psychiatric disorders. *Soc Psychiatry Psychiatr Epidemiol* 1998;33:S95–S101.

44 Link BG, Steuve A, Phelan J. Psychotic symptoms and violent behaviours: Probing the components of 'threat/control override' symptoms. *Soc Psychiatry Psychiatr Epidemiol* 1998;33:s56–s60.

45 Eronen M, Angermeyer MC, Schulze B. The psychiatric epidemiology of violent behaviour. *Soc Psychiatry Psychiatr Epidemiol* 1998;33:s13–s23.

46 Mødestin J. Criminal and violent behaviour in schizophrenic patients: An overview. *Psychiatry Clin Neurosci* 1998;52:547–54.

47 Mitchell EW. Does psychiatric disorder affect the likelihood of violent offending? A critique of the major findings. *Med Sci Law* 1999;39:23–30.

48 Belfrage H. Implementing the HCR-20 scheme for risk assessment in a forensic psychiatric hospital: Integrating research and clinical practice. *J Forens Psychiatry* 1998;9:328–38.

49 Draine J, Solomon P. Describing and evaluating jail diversion services for persons with serious mental illness. *Psychiatr Serv* 1999;50:56–61.

50 Deane MW, Steadman HJ, Borum R, et al. Emerging partnerships between mental health and law enforcement. *Psychiatr Serv* 1999;50:99–101.

51 Chung MC, Cumella S, Wensley J, et al. A follow-up study of mentally disordered offenders after a court diversion scheme: Six-month and one-year comparison. *Med Sci Law* 1999;39:31–7.

52 Wolff N. Interactions between mental health and the law enforcement systems: Problems and prospects of cooperation. *J Health Politics Policy Law* 1998;23:133–74.

53 Ventura LA, Cassel CA, Jacoby JE, et al. Case-management and recidivism of mentally ill persons released from jail. *Psychiatr Serv* 1998;49:1330–7.

54 Marshall M, Gray A, Lockwood A, et al. Case-management for people with severe mental disorders. *The Cochrane Library* 1999;1:11–25.

55 Marshal M, Lockwood A. Assertive community treatment for people with severe mental disorders. *The Cochrane Library* 1999;1:1–11.

56 Lurigio AJ. Persons with serious mental illness in the criminal justice system: Background, prevalence, and principles of care. *Crim Jus Policy Rev* 2000;11:312–28.

57 Exworthy T. Institutions and services in forensic psychiatry. *J Forens Psychiatry* 1998;9:395–412.

58 Brink JH, Doherty D, Boer A. Mental disorder in federal offenders: A Canadian prevalence study. *Int J Law Psychiatry* 2001;4–5:339–56.

59 Petrich J. Rate of psychiatric morbidity in a metropolitan county jail population. *Am J Psychiatry* 1976;133:1439–44.

60 Allodi F, Kedward HB, Robertson M. Insane but guilty: Psychiatric patients in jail. *Can Ment Health* 1977;25(2):3–7.

61 Whitmer GE. From hospitals to jails: The fate of California's deinstitutionalized mentally ill. *Am J Orthopsychiatry* 1980;50:65–75.

62 Lamb HR, Grant RW. The mentally ill in an urban county jail. *Arch Gen Psychiatry* 1982;39:17–22.

63 Gingell CR. *The Criminalization of the Mentally Ill: An Examination of the Hypothesis*. Burnaby: Simon Fraser University, 1991.

64 Watt F, Thomison A, Torpy D. The prevalence of psychiatric disorder in a male remand population: A pilot study. *J Forens Psychiatry* 1993;4:75–83.

65 Abram KM. The effect of co-occurring disorder on criminal careers: Interaction of antisocial personality, alcoholism and drug disorders. *Int J Law Psychiatry* 1989;12:133–48.

66 Glueck B. A study of 608 admissions to Sing-Sing Prison. *Mental Hygiene* 1918;2:85–151.

67 Robinson CB, Patten JW, Kerr WS. A psychiatric assessment of criminal offenders. *Med Sci Law* 1965;5:140–6.

68 Faulk M. A psychiatric study of men serving a sentence in Winchester Prison. *Med Sci Law* 1976;16:244–51.

69 James JF, Gregory D, Jones RK, et al. Psychiatric morbidity in prisons. *Hosp Comm Psychiatry* 1980;31):674–7.

70 Cote G, Hodgins S. Co-occurring mental disorders among criminal offenders. *Bull Am Acad Psychiatry Law* 1990;18:271–81.

71 Coid JW. How many psychiatric patients in prisons? *Br J Psychiatry* 1984;145:78–86.

72 Bland RC, Newman SC, Dyck RJ, et al. Prevalence of psychiatric disorders and suicide attempts in a prison population. *Can J Psychiatry* 1990;35:407–13.

73 Arboleda-Flórez J. In review – Mental illness and violence: An epidemiological appraisal of the evidence. *Can J Psychiatry* 1998;43:989–96.

74 Lamb HR, Weinberger LE. The shift of psychiatric inpatient care from hospitals to jails and prisons. *J Am Acad Psychiatric Law* 2005;33:529–34.

75 Fryers T, Brugha Y, Grounds A, et al. Severe mental illness in prisoners (editorial). *Br Med J* 1998;317:1025–6.

76 Peters RH, Greenbaum PE, Edens JF, et al. Prevalence of DSM-IV sub-

stance abuse and dependence disorders among prison inmates. *Am J Drug Alcohol Abuse* 1998;24:573–87.

77   Durkheim E. *Suicide*. Paris: Alcan, 1897.

78   Arboleda-Flórez J, Holley H. Development of a suicide screening instrument for use in a remand centre setting. *Can J Psychiatry* 1988;33: 595–8.

79   Goss JR, Peterson K, Smith L, et al. Characteristics of suicide attempts in a large urban jail system with an established suicide prevention program. *Psychiatr Serv* 2002;53:574–9.

80   Stuart H. Suicide behind bars. *Curr Opin Psychiatry* 2003;16:559–64.

81   Hobson J, Shine J. Measurement of psychopathy in a UK prison population referred for long term psychotherapy. *Br J Criminol* 1998;38:504–15.

83   Teplin LA. Criminalizing mental disorder – The comparative arrest rate of the mentally ill. *Am Psychologist* 1984;34:794–803.

84   Teplin LA. The prevalence of severe mental disorder among male urban jail detainees: Comparison with the Epidemiological Catchment Area. *Am J Public Health* 1990;80:663–9.

85   Feinstein AR. *Clinical Epidemiology – The Architecture of Clinical Research.* Toronto: WB Saunders, 1985.

86   Rothman KJ. *Modern Epidemiology*. Toronto: Little Brown and Company, 1986.

87   Arboleda-Flórez J. *The Epidemiology of Mental Illness and Crime*. Calgary: University of Calgary, 1994.

88   Last JM. *A Dictionary of Epidemiology*. Toronto: Oxford University Press, 1988.

89   Eaton WW, Regier DA, Locke BZ, et al. The NIMH Epidemiologic Catchment Area Program. In: Weissman MM, Myers JK, Ross CE, eds. *Community Surveys of Psychiatric Disorders*. New Jersey: Rutgers University Press, 1986:209–19.

90   Krefft KM, Brittain TH. A Prisoner Assessment Survey: Screening of a municipal prison population. *Int J Law Psychiatry* 1983;6:113–24.

91   Ganser SJM. Über einen eigenartigen hysterischen Dämmerzustand. *Arch Psychiatr Nerven-kr* 1898;38:633–7.

92   Andersen HS, Sesstoft D, Lillebeck T, et al. Psychopathy and psychopathological profiles in prisoners in remand. *Acta Psychiatr Scand* 1999;99:33–9.

93   Morana H, Arboleda-Flórez J, Portela Câmara F. Identifying the cutoff score for the PCL-R (Psychopathic Checklist-Revised) in a Brazilian forensic population. *Forens Sci Int* 2005;147:1–8.

94 Eastman N. Who should take responsibility for antisocial personality disorder? *Br Med J* 1999;318:206–7.

95 Kaye S, Darke S, Finlay-Jones R. The onset of heroin use and criminal behaviour: Does order make a difference? *Drug Alcohol Depend* 1998;53:79–86.

96 Barnfield TV, Leathem JM. Neuropsychological outcomes of traumatic brain injury abuse in a New Zealand prison population. *Brain Injury* 1998;12:951–62.

97 Watson W. Designed to cure: The clinician-led development of England's regional secure units. *J Forens Psychiatry* 1998;9:519–31.

98 Sahota K, Chesterman P. Sexual offending in the context of mental illness. *J Forens Psychiatry* 1998;9:267–80.

99 James D, Cripps J, Gray N. What demands do those admitted from the criminal justice system make on psychiatric beds? Expanding local secure services as a development strategy. *J Forens Psychiatry* 1998;9:74–102.

100 Kushel MB, Hahn JA, Evans JL, et al. Revolving doors: Imprisonment among the homeless and marginally housed population. *Am J Public Health* 2005;95:1747–52.

101 Quanbeck CD, Stone DC, McDermott BE, et al. Relationship between criminal arrest and community treatment history among patients with bipolar disorder. *Psychiatr Serv* 2005;56:847–52.

102 Lovell D, Gagliardi GJ, Peterson PD. Recidivism and use of services among persons with mental illness after release from prison. *Psychiatr Serv* 2002;53:1290–6.

103 Hartwell S: Short-term outcomes for offenders with mental illness released from incarceration. *Int J Offender Ther Comp Criminol* 2003;47:145–58.

104 Ruddell R. Jail interventions for inmates with mental illnesses. *J Correctional Health Care* 2006;12:118–31.

105 Szykula SA, Jackson DF. Managed mental health care in large jails: Empirical outcomes on cost and quality. *J Correctional Health Care* 2005;11:223–40.

106 Cowell AJ, Broner N, Dupont R. The cost-effectiveness of criminal justice diversion programs for people with serious mental illness co-occurring with substance abuse. *J Contemporary Crim Jus* 2004;20:292–315.

107 Office of the Correctional Investigator of Canada. *Annual Report 2004–2005*. http: //www..oci.bec.gc.ca/reports/AR200405_download _e.asp. Accessed on November, 10, 2007.

108 Corrections Services of Canada. A health care needs assessment of Federal inmates in Canada. *Can J Public Health* 2004;95(suppl 1).

109 Hare, RD. The Hare PCL-R: Some issues concerning its use and misuse. *Legal and Criminological Psychology* 1998;3:99–119.

110 Webster CD, Douglas KS, Eaves D, et al. *HCR-20, Assessing Risk for Violence*. Version 2. Vancouver: Mental Health Law and Policy Institute, Simon Fraser University, 1997.

111 Nuffield J. The SIR Scale: Some reflections on its applications. *Forum on Corrections Research* 1989;1(2):19–22.

112 Motiuk LL. *Contributing to Safe Reintegration: Outcome Measurement*. Correctional Service of Canada. http: //www.csc-scc.gc.ca/text/rsrch/compendium/ 2000/chap_23.e.shtml. Accessed on November 10, 2007.

16 The Epidemiology of Suicide in Canada

ISAAC SAKINOFSKY AND GREG WEBSTER

Almost a decade ago, one of us (Isaac Sakinofsky) published a book chapter with the same title as this in *Suicide in Canada*.[1] At that time, it was the cumulative year by year increase in suicide rates, particularly in young persons, that clamoured for attention. Cohort studies were published during the 1980s showing that successive waves of birth cohorts were going forward into the future burdened by an increased potential for suicide, each incrementally larger than that in the preceding cohort.[2–7] Increasing incidences of depressive illness in young people were being blamed for this sorry state of affairs[8,9] as well as the surge in the prevalence rates in youth for the abuse of illicit substances.[10–13]

The problem was not uniformly distributed across the country and it varied greatly among Canada's provinces and territories. It was observed that as one travelled from east to west there was an increasing suicide trend but especially in Quebec, Alberta, and at that time British Columbia.[14] (Of note, Thompson has developed an index to measure regional social problems[15] and found that the index increased from east to west in Canada together with the prevalence of depression and mania.[16]) As regards Quebec, Boyer and colleagues[17] remarked that in the span of two decades the suicide rate in Quebec nearly doubled and, until 1970, suicide in Quebec primarily involved older men. However, a new trend had emerged, that of much greater frequency of suicide among young males. 'What sets Quebec apart more than all else from the other Canadian regions, however, is a marked uptrend in the incidence of overall male suicide.'[17(p68)]

Currently, we are fortunate to be experiencing a downturn in suicide rates in western countries, including Canada, and suicide prevalence in young people is also declining. However, sizeable problems persist.

Suicide among males has not diminished at nearly the same rate as among females, perhaps because males are still more reluctant to come forward for help on account of depressed mood, which they consider to be stigmatized as unmanly and demeaning.[18] They are also less likely to accept and adhere to treatment.[19,20] The high suicide rates in Nunavut, the Yukon and Northwest Territories, and among indigenous people in general are shocking, to say the least. In the more populous provinces, the higher than elsewhere suicide rates found in Quebec and Alberta remain disturbing to all Canadians.

During 2004, the most recent year for which mortality data are currently available, nearly one quarter of a million persons (exactly 226,584) died of all causes in Canada – an age-standardized mortality rate of 587 per 100,000. Suicide accounted for 2%, only a small proportion of these deaths, pale when compared with the larger proportions attributable to cardiovascular causes (32%) or cancer (30%). But the cold statistics understate the reality that in 2004, approximately 4,000 Canadian residents (actually 3,613) of both genders intentionally took their lives, and their deaths might, at least in theory, have been preventable. Their deaths and the manner of their dying must have caused a great deal of sorrow and agonizing to their relatives and friends, not to mention the economic consequences to their families and society, and the suicide victims would have endured a great deal of anguish and suffering before taking the final decision to end their lives.

The total number of Canadians who lost their lives during 2000–2004 was 18,326, with a male:female ratio of 3.4:1. Although this gender ratio is lower than that found in Canada in previous years (for example, between 1988–1992 it was 3.7:1),[21] in 2000–2004 male suicides constituted a proportion of more than three-quarters of the total losses by suicide in Canada.

Figure 16.1 presents sex-specific and age-standardized suicide rates for Canada since 1950, spanning more than half a century. The graph for males shows quite clearly the beginning of an incline that we know began on the heels of World War II, ascending quite steeply from the mid-1960s to reach two peaks, a lesser one in 1978 and a slightly higher one in 1983, before sloping downwards towards 2004. In females, we see there is at first no incline but a plateau followed by a shallow trough, until the beginning of the 1960s, when the graph begins to rise into the early 1970s, reaching its peak in 1974 and then beginning a gentle decline that flattens out into a plateau. It is noteworthy that, in both gender groups, the peak that preceded the ultimate decline

Figure 16.1 Age-standardized suicide rates in Canada (1950–2004) shown on a linear scale

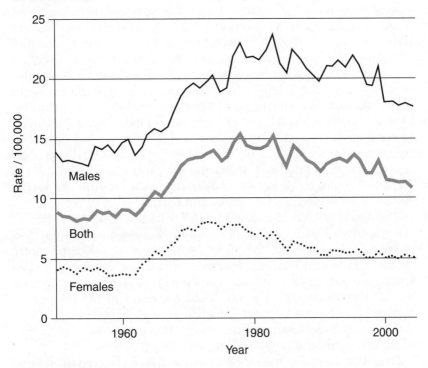

Source: Statistics Canada

clearly anticipated the era of the selective serotonin reuptake inhibitor (SSRI) medications, and the downward gradient shown in the graphs thus appears to have been due to secular causes, probably a reflection of economic and sociocultural changes in society. However, it is impossible to rule out that treatment may have played a role in accelerating the decline.[22]

Canada Compared with the United States

The population of Canada concentrates itself along the border with its much larger neighbour to the south, the United States. Canada's largest trading partner, the United States, along with sending its manufactured goods in exchange for Canadian raw materials, also exports its culture and value systems to Canada through television and the other visual, audio, and print media, as well as through cross-border traffic between the two countries that carries on for tourism or business reasons. It is no secret that Canada is dependent economically on the United States and that economic fluctuations in the latter country have particularly important consequences for the economy north of the border. There is an adage that says that when Uncle Sam sneezes Canada catches a cold. Since both countries are primarily English speaking and share a similar heritage and culture as well, one might anticipate that their suicide rates would be similar, which is, in fact, almost the case. Canada's suicide rates ran behind those of the United States until the early 1970s when they overtook them, and since then have remained the same or slightly higher.[23,24] Figure 16.2 displays the age-standardized rates for Canada and the United States from 1981 to 2004. For comparative age-standardized suicide rates for the earlier period of 1960–1988 see Sakinofsky and Leenaars.[24]

The American and Canadian rates for suicide among males (top of the graph) are closely intertwined, and the Kolmogorov-Smirnov and Kuiper statistics confirm that their distributions are not significantly different from each another. However, this is not the case for rates among women, or for both sexes combined. The significant difference for both sexes combined is no doubt the effect of the divergence between the rates for U.S. and Canadian females. For females, the U.S. rates, while closely approximated to Canadian rates, are distinct, albeit to the eye running at only a slightly lower level.

Overall, a decline in the incidence of suicide can be seen in all three pairs of data series since 1981. However, there appears to be a recent upturn in the rates among U.S. women from 1999 to 2004, and the decline in suicide in American males has plateaued over the same period. The reason for this upturn can only be speculated upon at the present time (perhaps related to firearm availability, for instance,[25] and the greater preference for this method by American women,[26] or maybe even a change in treatment policies after the imposition of Black Box warnings for the use of SSRIs in youth) and it remains to be seen whether the U.S. rates will cross the line for Canadian suicide rates among females.

Canada Compared with the International Community

The magnitude of Canada's suicide problem must also be measured against the backdrop of that of a number of other countries besides the

Figure 16.2 Suicide rates in Canada (1981–2004)

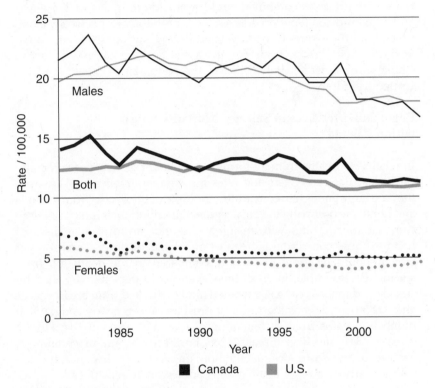

Sources of data: Statistics Canada and WISQARS

United States.[27] Since the fairly recent policies of disclosure to WHO of suicide rates in countries that did not previously submit them, countries of the former USSR have revealed serious suicide problems, for which a high prevalence of alcohol abuse in these societies has been blamed;[28] but it is also likely that rapid social transition[29,30] may be playing a role, although sometimes the relationship between socioeconomic and demographic effects on suicide is not clear-cut.[31] Suicide in the former Soviet Union actually decreased for a while during the period of perestroika, not apparently as a result of political change but because of restrictive measures on alcohol consumption that were introduced by Mr. Gorbachev's government,[32,33] and since then they have been trending upwards. Belarus (with suicide rates of 35.1 per

100,000) and the Russian Federation (34.1) currently report the highest rates for both sexes combined, and for suicide in males they are 63.3 and 61.6, and for females they are 10.3 and 10.7, respectively. Compared with these rates Canada gets off lightly, but not when measured against suicide rates from countries like Argentina, Brazil, urban China, Greece, Israel, Italy, Mexico, the Netherlands, Spain, and the United Kingdom.

Regional Differences in Selected Mortality Rates within Canada

In relation to deaths from all forms of malignant disease or from major cardiovascular causes, suicide rates are comparatively low. However, they are large enough to constitute a multiple of the deaths from assaults and homicide occurring in every regional distribution. It is also unfair to compare suicide rates with malignancies and cardiovascular diseases because these constitute aggregates of related disorders, each one of which should be more reasonably compared to the death toll from suicide. For example, in 2004, there were 3,613 persons who died by suicide and in that year 4,998 women (and men) died from breast cancer and 3,685 men died as the result of prostate cancer, nearly comparable numbers. Deaths from chronic lung disease numbered 10,041, kidney disease 3,541, and liver disease 2,269. Furthermore, among certain age groups suicide is proportionately more important; for instance, it is the second leading cause of death among adolescents aged 10–19.[34]

It is interesting to examine how these selected causes of death are distributed among the regions in Canada and to consider whether the same risk factors might operate between the different causes (see figure 16.3 for males). For example, age-standardized rates for both sexes are very high for suicide in Nunavut and as well for all causes combined, malignancies, accidents, and homicides. By contrast, suicide rates in Ontario are quite low (matching the lower rates for which Newfoundland and Labrador is known)[35,36] and in Ontario rates for deaths from all causes, malignancies, accidents and homicides are also lower. The availability and quality of health care (resulting in early diagnosis and treatment and, in the case of suicide attempts, more timely intervention) could be one reason for the discrepancy between these two areas, but that would be far from the only possible answer.

Among the more populous provinces, Quebec has fairly high suicide rates but relatively low rates for cardiovascular disease, acci-

Figure 16.3 Age-standardized suicide rates in males by region of Canada (2000–4)

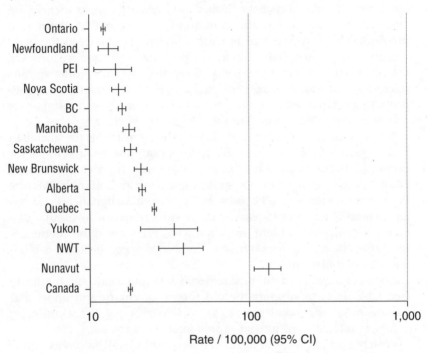

Rate / 100,000 (95% CI)

Source: Statistics Canada

dents, homicides, and malignancies, the finding constituting a dissociation not seen in the previous two examples. Good health care may be operating preventatively for the potential medical causes of mortality in Quebec but clearly the higher suicide rates there are determined by other factors.[37] It is clearly invidious to contrast levels of psychiatric care between the provinces, but it is noteworthy that Langlois and Morrison commented that Quebec paradoxically had the lowest age-standardized hospitalization rates in 1998–99 for suicide attempts among the provinces (49 per 100,000) even though it had the highest suicide rates.[38] The national age-standardized rate for attempted suicide hospitalizations was at that time 89 per 100,000. The highest rates were in Saskatchewan (123) and British Columbia (120), well above the national average.

It is difficult to interpret what such statistics mean. On the one hand it might imply that serious risk of suicide is less often recognized in low hospitalization jurisdictions such as Quebec by gatekeepers in the emergency rooms or in the community, or even that there is a province-wide policy extant to treat psychiatric patients in the community and not hospitalize them, for fiscal or healthcare reasons. On the other hand, it could mean that there are fewer medically serious (including violent) attempts in Quebec; i.e., that a relatively higher proportion than in other regions do not require emergency admissions on physical grounds alone; but this can hardly be the case.

Newfoundland and Labrador, sharing the lowest rates for suicide in both sexes with Ontario over this time-period, also has low rates for homicide and accidents, but its mortality rates from cardiovascular causes and malignancies are quite high. British Columbia has the lowest death rate from all causes and also from malignancies and lies just behind Quebec for the lowest death rates from cardiovascular diseases. Its suicide, accident, and homicide rates are quite moderate. Insofar as the picture for both sexes combined is concerned, it is obviously a good place to live.

There is no evidence from the regional data for suicide and homicide (see table 16.1) to support the old theory of Henry and Short that suicide rates and homicide rates are two sides of the same coin, inversely related as reciprocal expressions of aggression.[39]

With regard to causes of death in males (table 16.1), Nunavut stands out again as the region with the highest death rates for all causes, malignancies, accidents, suicide, and homicide, and has the second highest mortality rate for cardiovascular deaths. Clearly, this calls for urgent attention from federal and provincial policy makers.[40] Among males and for both sexes combined, British Columbia leads the country with its lowest rates for deaths from all causes, malignancies, or cardiovascular disorders, and again returns fairly moderate rates for the other causes of mortality. The dissociation between deaths from major medical causes of death and deaths by suicide emerges again with the high rates for male suicide that are seen in Quebec but the lower rates for other medical causes. The dissociation phenomenon is also seen in Newfoundland and Labrador, which shows relatively low rates for suicide and homicide but high rates for cardiovascular disease and deaths from all causes.

Among females nearly the same picture is present. Death rates are high among Nunavut females for all causes, suicide, and malignan-

Table 16.1
Selected mean mortality rates for Canada and regions (2000–4): Males

	All causes	Malignant	Cardio-vascular	Accidents	Suicide	Homicide
Canada	745.2	219.4	245.6	35.1	17.6	2.2
Newfoundland	894.2	248.9	335.0	34.1	13.2	0.5
PEI	848.5	228.3	321.8	52.8	14.6	0.9
Nova Scotia	812.4	250.1	266.0	36.8	15.3	1.9
New Brunswick	813.0	237.8	268.6	46.2	20.9	1.7
Quebec	782.7	250.0	229.2	32.4	25.2	2.0
Ontario	724.3	212.3	247.4	30.0	12.1	1.8
Manitoba	809.9	221.5	269.1	44.5	17.6	5.1
Saskatchewan	779.4	212.0	262.1	50.0	18.1	4.9
Alberta	727.0	199.3	262.5	40.7	21.3	3.0
BC	673.4	186.7	224.1	40.6	16.0	2.1
Yukon	872.5	271.5	226.2	88.3	33.7	9.8
NWT	951.9	240.2	293.2	67.3	38.8	6.9
Nunavut	1146.1	320.1	301.8	90.8	136.2	10.9

Data Source: Statistics Canada

cies, and are also relatively high for cardiovascular disorders, accidents, and homicide. Suicide rates in women are lowest in Newfoundland and Labrador and Nova Scotia, followed by Ontario. British Columbia reports the lowest rates for deaths from all causes and malignancies and nearly the lowest for cardiovascular disorders and homicides. However, its suicide rates for women are moderately high, which diminishes the relatively benign picture in British Columbia for both sexes combined and for males.

Comparison of Suicide Rates between the Provinces and Regions of Canada

Because of the great variation in population sizes between the regions of Canada, it is essential to validate the apparent differences in their suicide rates by taking into consideration the possibility of statistical error. The base rates for suicide generally are low and in some regions the numbers on which they are based may also be particularly low (e.g., the Yukon and Northwest Territories). Table 16.2 presents mean age-standardized suicide rates (with 95% confidence intervals) for Canada and its regions for 2000–2004. Without doubt, and in spite of

Table 16.2

Age standardized suicide rates (95% confidence intervals) for Canada and regions (2000–4)

	Males 95%CI			Females (95%CI)		
	Rate	Lower	Upper	Rate	Lower	Upper
Canada	17.62	17.33	17.91	5.02	4.87	5.17
Newfoundland	13.16	11.21	15.11	2.62	1.78	3.46
PEI	14.60	10.59	18.61	4.00	1.90	6.10
Nova Scotia	15.28	13.73	16.83	3.34	2.61	4.07
New Brunswick	20.90	18.87	22.93	4.00	3.15	4.85
Quebec	25.24	24.53	25.95	6.82	6.46	7.18
Ontario	12.10	11.71	12.49	3.70	3.49	3.91
Manitoba	17.60	16.07	19.13	6.42	5.48	7.36
Saskatchewan	18.08	16.40	19.76	4.56	3.69	5.43
Alberta	21.30	20.29	22.31	6.42	5.86	6.98
BC	16.04	15.28	16.8	4.88	4.47	5.29
Yukon	33.74	20.51	46.97	4.76	0.10	9.42
NWT	38.82	26.64	51.00	5.06	0.62	9.50
Nunavut	132.14	107.22	157.06	28.72	16.98	40.46

Data source: Statistics Canada

the relatively small numbers of suicide victims, Nunavut has the largest suicide rates of any region in Canada for both sexes. There is no overlap between the 95% confidence intervals for suicide rates in Nunavut and any other province or region for either males or females. Table 16.2 also shows that the suicide rates in both sexes in the Yukon and Northwest Territories are high. Quebec continues to have the highest rates for the more densely inhabited provinces and Ontario and Newfoundland and Labrador the lowest rates for suicide in males.

There is much more overlap to be seen between the regional suicide rates for females, because the numbers of suicides are relatively fewer than those for male suicides and the confidence intervals are therefore considerably wider. In the Yukon, the instability of suicide rates on account of small numbers for suicide in females causes the rates to have such wide confidence intervals that little reliable inference from a statistically significant perspective can be made. Among the more populous regions, regarding suicide in females, Quebec and the western provinces (but not British Columbia) show high rates and Newfoundland and Labrador has the lowest rate. Nunavut's high rates stand out starkly, separating it by a wide margin from all the others.

Figure 16.4a Age-standardized suicide and undetermined rates in males by region of Canada (2000–4)

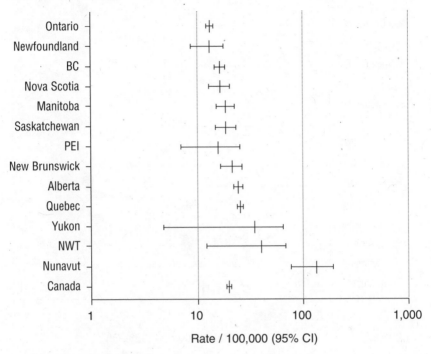

Source of data: Statistics Canada

   There are no recent suicide-related studies from the Yukon or the Northwest Territories. Kehoe[41] attempted to delineate the specific characteristics of suicide in the Yukon, a vast, sparsely populated area with short summers and very long winters, often recording the coldest temperatures to be found in North America. The inimical weather they experience forces the Yukoners to be confined for long periods, resulting in anxiety and depression, which they call 'cabin fever.' Although the particular social stresses of the Gold Rush have passed into history, mining remains the major industry and attracts to the Yukon younger or older migrant workers, single males, who have little to do with their leisure time apart from drinking and who are cut off from their extended families. There is a pervading sense of isolation, and firearms are plentiful.[41]

Figure 16.4b Age-standardized suicide and undetermined rates in females by region of Canada (2000–4)

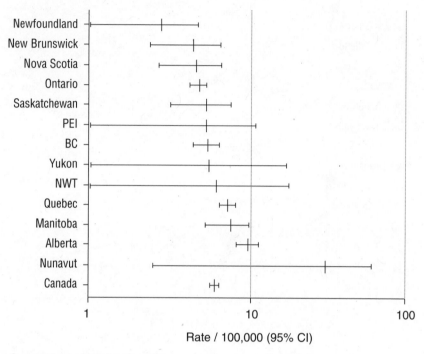

Rate / 100,000 (95% CI)

Source of data: Statistics Canada

What Is the Impact of Possible Errors by Misclassification?

Epidemiologists have long argued over the validity of suicide rates because of alleged errors by understatement (under ascertainment),[22,42,43] especially since the category of deaths from undetermined causes was introduced into the ICD classification in 1969. It is claimed that suicide rates are generally understated in public health data [44, 42] and that non-violent rather than violent deaths permit themselves to be more readily misclassified. Canetto and Sakinofsky[26] calculated the percentages of deaths from each province between 1969 and 1973 that were classified as accidental poisoning or injury undetermined. Since suicide by overdose has been the preferred method chosen by North American women in the past (although U.S. women use firearms more often than do Canadian women), we hypothesized that misclassification of the suicidal motives for overdoses could play a part in the very large differences between the suicide rates of the two sexes. In this context, we found that the proportion of potential under-statement for both sexes by categorization of deaths as accidental poi-sonings or deaths by injury undetermined constituted as much as 15.4% for Newfoundland and Labrador, 12.8% for Nova Scotia, and in excess of 10% each for Alberta and Saskatchewan.[26]

Table 16.3 shows the suicide rates that were presented in table 16.2 combined with the rates for undetermined causes, and including 95% confidence limits (also represented in figures 16.4a and 16.4b). Although the rates for undetermined deaths are quite small they can sometimes make a real difference. Regarding data for suicide in males (table 16.3), the combined rate for Quebec (25.6) is slightly ahead of Alberta's (24.5), but their confidence intervals overlap > 50%, so that the difference is not statistically significant.[45] Nunavut has the highest rates for Canada and Ontario and Newfoundland and Labrador the lowest for suicide in males (13.2), but the overlap of the latter's confidence interval indicates that it is not significantly differ-ent from those of British Columbia and Nova Scotia (see also figure 16.3).

Among the combined rates for females (table 16.3), Newfound-land and Labrador clearly has the lowest rate of 2.8 (95% CI, 0.9–4.7), Ontario's rates for females having expanded to 4.8 (95% CI, 4.2–5.3) after deaths from undetermined causes are included. Alberta has the highest rates among the populous provinces, significantly exceeding those for Quebec. They were not distinct when only the suicide rates were considered, lending force to the possibility that deaths by drug ingestion in women are at greater probability of being classified as undetermined. The rates for Nunavut again tower above the rest and must continue to remain extremely worri-some for Canadians.

Suicide across the Lifespan

During the 1950s and through into the 1970s a strange phenomenon happened to suicide rates in young people. In previous eras, suicide (i.e., completed suicide as opposed to non-fatal suicidality) was con-sidered to be a problem that afflicted the middle-aged and elderly and 'attempts' were more characteristic of young people, particularly

Table 16.3
Mean age-standardized rates (95% CI) for suicide and undetermined causes combined, Canada and its regions (2000–4)

	Males (95%CI)			Females (95%CI)		
	Rate	Lower	Upper	Rate	Lower	Upper
Canada	19.7	19.0	20.4	6.0	5.6	6.4
Newfoundland	13.2	8.8	17.5	2.8	0.9	4.7
PEI	15.9	7.1	24.6	5.3	0.0	10.6
Nova Scotia	16.6	13.0	20.1	4.6	2.7	6.5
New Brunswick	21.3	16.7	25.9	4.4	2.4	6.4
Quebec	25.6	24.0	27.2	7.2	6.4	8.0
Ontario	13.2	12.3	14.1	4.8	4.2	5.3
Manitoba	18.7	15.1	22.2	7.5	5.2	9.7
Saskatchewan	18.8	15.0	22.6	5.3	3.2	7.4
Alberta	24.5	22.0	26.9	9.6	8.1	11.1
BC	16.5	14.8	18.3	5.4	4.4	6.3
Yukon	34.5	4.8	64.2	5.5	−5.3	16.4
NWT	39.8	12.2	67.4	6.1	−4.8	17.0
Nunavut	132.1	76.4	187.9	28.7	2.5	55.0

Data source: Statistics Canada

females.[46,47] The popular myth everyone shared was that young people were supposed to be enjoying their lives protected by freedom from care and responsibility and were not yet expected by society to grapple with the vexatious problems of the adult world. Nevertheless, during the 1950s, suicide rates in young people began to rise quite steeply and in males, in particular, quickly became equal in prevalence to those seen among adults. Figures 16.5a and 16.5b illustrate this development as demonstrated for both sexes, males and females. The line graph shows mean age-specific suicide rates for quadrennia marking the beginning of each decade from 1950–1953 to 2000–2003.

Steele and Doey[34] have discussed the epidemiology of suicide in children and adolescents in Canada and elsewhere. They note the 'precipitous' rise with age group in 1997 in suicide rates from 0.9 per 100,000 for children under the age of 14, to 12.9 in adolescents aged 15–19. Suicide is the second leading cause of death in both sexes for youth aged 10 to 19 in Canada, and in the United States it is the third leading cause of death for children 10–14 years after all accidents and homicides. In Canada, youths use firearms, drugs, carbon monoxide

Figure 16.5a Decennial pattern of suicide in males

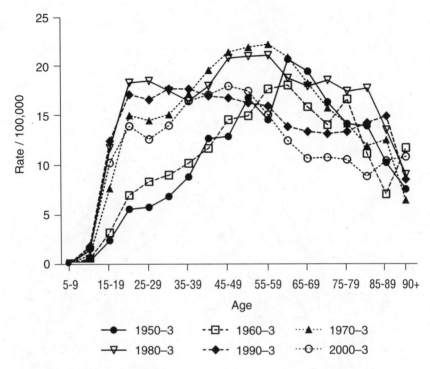

Source of data: Statistics Canada
Reproduced with permission of the *Canadian Journal of Psychiatry* from an article published in June 2007.[27]

poisoning, and hanging for the purpose of suicide but, for non-fatal attempts, overdoses are common. However, firearm use remains lower than that in the United States, while hanging has increased. As always, opportunity selects the method and, even though Canada now has stricter gun control laws (perpetually in danger of being dismantled by changes in government), guns seem to be regularly available, as, of course, they are in indigenous environments as well as in rural populations. Between 1991 and 1997, suicide rates in adolescents aged 15 to 19 decreased in Canada from 13.8 to 12.9 per 100,000. However, the rate was mainly confined to boys; that of girls increasing slightly. Steele and Doey discussed the role that the novel antidepressants (the

Figure 16.5b Decennial pattern of suicide in females

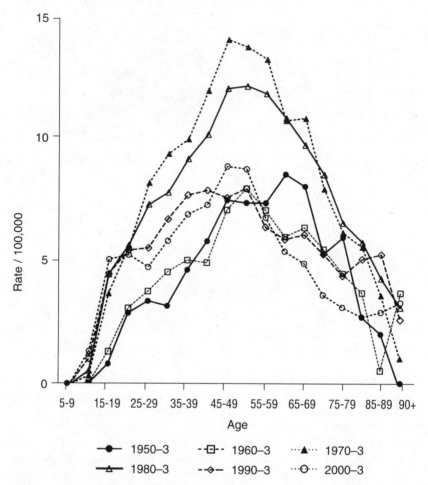

Source of data: Statistics Canada
Reproduced with permission of the *Canadian Journal of Psychiatry* from an article published in June 2007.[27]

SSRIs) may have been playing in the observed downturn of suicide
rates in young people, and at the same time they sound a cautious note
concerning the possibility of emergent suicidality, possibly related to
these antidepressants.

At the other end of the age spectrum the suicide rate in the elderly has also declined, and in 2000 the rate was 10.4 per 100,000 in Canadian residents aged 65 years or older.[48] At one time, suicide rates in Canada were highest in males over the age of 74[49] and social factors, including unemployment, were implicated. Quan et al.[50] undertook a case-control study comparing Albertans over age 55 who completed suicide with those who died as the result of traffic accidents and found that those suicides who were married were more likely to have had cancer (adjusted odds ratio 1.73), chronic pulmonary disease (1.86), prostate disorder other than cancer (1.70), depression (6.70), and other psychiatric illnesses (2.16). Elderly Albertan males were more likely than females to use guns (44%), to come from rural surroundings (47%), and to be single (1 in 8). Physical illness and financial difficulty were more frequent among the men than the women suicides. From Quebec, an observational study reported the characteristics of suicides aged over 60 years in 1998–1999.[51] The prevalence of mental disorders was 43%, mostly depression, but if sub-threshold depressive symptoms could have been included, 65% would have qualified for having had a mental disorder. Fully three-quarters had expressed desires to be dead during the six months prior to their intentional demise. In only 8% could these suicide victims be described as having been physically frail, in contrast to other studies that have reported a high prevalence of physical suffering or impairment.

Suicide among Indigenous Peoples

Although Statistics Canada does not report suicide rates among ethnic, including indigenous, groups separately, it is well known from regional epidemiological studies that the rate among indigenous groups is at least double that found in the general population.[52] Kirmayer noted a marked increase in suicide rates among indigenous populations and that a distinctive feature was that suicide often occurred in clusters.[53] Risk factors included frequent interpersonal conflict, prolonged or unresolved grief, chronic family instability, alcohol or other substance abuse or dependence, and unemployment. Similar factors were implicated as being responsible for the high prevalence of non-fatal suicidality among teenagers on reservations in central Alberta.[13] Compared to other Canadians, substance-abuse levels were high and family pathology was more prevalent. More often than not there was no father in the home and a prior suicide in the household. Aboriginal children were more likely to experience higher rates of school failure, family violence, and substance abuse.[54]

The plight of the Inuit in Canada is particularly deplorable. The suicide rate among them is particularly worrisome. Boothroyd and colleagues carried out a case-controlled study of Inuit people who died by suicide in Nunavik (the vast Arctic region of northern Quebec) between 1982 and 1996. The controls were living persons matched on several variables. Most of the case subjects were single males aged 15 to 24 years and more than half of them died by hanging (55%) and by gunshot in about a third (30%). They were more than four times as likely to have received a lifetime psychiatric diagnosis of depression, personality or conduct disorder, and more than thrice as often to have had a history of solvent sniffing.[55]

The social problems that are uncovered in suicide cases among Canada's native peoples must be viewed as proximate causes only. Group demoralization must somehow have played a role more remotely. Chandler has examined the variation in suicide incidence rates in 200 aboriginal groups in British Columbia and related lower rates to efforts in 196 bands that were engaged in community practices that amount to markers of a collective effort to rehabilitate the cultural continuity of these groups.[56-58] Such efforts at combating anomie are in keeping with the time-worn truths that have been apparent since Durkheim.[23,59,61-62] Recently Hallet, Chandler, and Lalonde[60] added data on mother tongue (specifically Aboriginal language) to their previous indices of cultural continuity and then reanalysed their previous data on youth suicide in 196 First Nations' bands in British Columbia. Remarkably, youth suicide rates were low to absent in bands where the majority spoke their native language but six times as frequent when only the minority of the band were proficient in their native tongue; i.e., there was far less self-destructive behaviour among bands that had been more successful in rehabilitating their native cultures. Hallet et al. warn that many of the Aboriginal languages are in danger of extinction and consequently the persistence of the cultural identities that these languages mediate is also under threat. 'Failures to achieve any viable sense of self or cultural continuity are strongly linked to self-destructive and suicidal behaviours ... Suicide is the "coalminer's canary" of cultural distress.'[60(p394)]

Non-fatal Suicidality

There have been a number of regional community surveys that have included questions about non-fatal suicidality. The oldest emanated from Calgary, Alberta,[63] followed by a survey from Edmonton, Alberta.[64] In Quebec, researchers analysed two waves of data from the Quebec Health Survey (1987 and 1992)[17,65] and in Ontario[66,67] a data analysis of the Ontario Health Survey and its Mental Health Supplement (n = 9,953) was performed. Table 16.4 compares the lifetime prevalences and one-year incidences of non-fatal suicidality (ideation or attempts) between these Canadian surveys as well as two well known ones from the United States, the New Haven[68] and Epidemiologic Catchment Area (ECA)[69] surveys. The agreement between the respective investigations is reasonably close but there are outliers. For lifetime prevalence of ideation and attempts, the figures for New Haven seem low and that for ideation from Quebec is also lowish. The U.S. National Comorbidity Survey (not shown in table) found higher prevalence figures for lifetime ideation (13.5%) and attempts (4.6%).[70] The ECA one-year incidence of suicidal ideation is lowish and the one-year attempt rate in Calgary is high.

Developmental life experiences are clearly important in setting the threshold for suicidality during later life (including during youth) to be triggered then by adverse experiences (consistent with the stress-diathesis theory). These experiences need not appear serious to outsiders, only to the person concerned, who attaches his or her personal meaning and degree of traumatic experience and reacts according to his or her own coping or maladaptive armamentarium. Table 16.5 sets out per cent prevalence figures for a number of the psychosocial risk factors that were analysed in the Ontario Health Supplement.[66] Growing up in a dysfunctional family is clearly a risk factor for non-fatal suicidality. There are significant prevalences and incidences for having parents who were in serious trouble with marital disharmony, whether they separated or stayed together. Parental psychiatric disturbance plays a major role. If the parent attempted suicide, the risk of lifetime and one-year ideation or a lifetime attempt is significantly increased. It is interesting but not surprising that the loss of a parent during childhood per se is not a risk factor for non-fatal suicidality but rather the loss of a close person other than a parent. Loss of continuity of relationships with peers in childhood through domestic dislocation is a potent risk factor.

Table 16.4
Lifetime and one-year prevalence of non-fatal suicidality

Lifetime % prevalence of ideation and attempts	N.Haven ('74)	Calgary ('85)	Edmonton ('88)	ECA ('89)	Que ('93)	OHS ('94)
Ideation	7.4	13.4	11.5	10.7	8	10.7
Attempts	1.1	10.1	3.6	2.9	4	3.3

One-year incidence (%) of ideation and attempts	N.Haven ('74)	Calgary ('85)	Quebec ('87)	ECA ('89)	Que ('93)	OHS ('94)
Ideation	3.8	6.0	3.9	2.6	4	3.4
Attempts	0.6	2.1	0.8	0.3	0.6	0.4

Source: Statistics Canada

Table 16.5

Psychosocial risk factors for non-fatal suicidality

	Ever ideation	1-yr ideation	Ever attempt	1-yr attempt
No parental problem	7.2 (6.3, 8.1)	2.4 (1.9, 2.9)	2 (1.5, 2.5)	0.3 (0.1, 0.5)
Significant parental problem present	17.6 (15.8, 19.4)[b]	5.1 (4.1, 6.1)[b]	6.1 (5.0, 7.2)[b]	0.7 (0.3, 1.1)[a]
Risk of suicidality with parental marital disharmony				
Parents in serious trouble[b]	19.5 (17.3, 21.7)[b]	6.7 (5.3, 8.1)[b]	6.7 (5.3, 8.1)	0.9 (0.4,1.4)[a]
Above not present	8.2 (7.3, 9.1)	2.4 (1.9, 2.9)	2.4 (1.9, 2.9)	0.3 (0.1, 0.5)
Parents separated	21.4 (18.3, 24.5)[a]	7.9 (5.8, 10.0)[a]	6.7 (4.8, 8.6)	1.3*
Parents stayed together but dysfunctional	16.9 (13.7, 20.1)	5.0 (3.1, 6.9)	6.8 (4.7, 8.9)	0.4*
Risk of suicidality with either parent attempting suicide				
History of parent attempting suicide	23.6 (15.6, 31.6)[b]	9.3 (3.8, 14.8)[b]	9.5 (4.0, 15.0)[b]	2.1*
Parent had to seek psychiatric help				
Parent needed help	18.4 (15.9, 20.9)[b]	5.6 (4.1, 7.1)[b]	6.4 (4.8, 8.0)[b]	0.5*
Either parent significantly depressed				
History present	22.9 (19.8, 26.0)[b]	7.1 (5.2, 9.0)[b]	9.2 (7.1, 11.3)[b]	1.4*
Either parent hospitalized or emotionally disabled				
History present	19.8 (16.2, 23.4)[b]	4.7 (2.8, 6.6)[b]	7.6 (5.2, 10.0)[b]	0.5*
Either parent significant alcohol problem				
History present	20.2 (17.5, 22.9)[b]	5.9 (4.3, 7.5)[b]	8.1 (6.2, 10.0)[b]	0.8*
Either parent significant drug abuse problem				
History present	39.2 (27.8, 50.6)[b]	17.6 (8.7, 26.5)[b]	18.2 (9.2, 27.2)[b]	2.2*
Either parent significant personality problems*				
History present	30.5 (22.3, 38.7)[b]	10.0 (4.7, 15.3)[b]	8.1 (3.3, 12.9)[b]	0.1*
Either parent psychotic (hallucinations/delusions =>6m)				
History present	27.8 (20.1, 35.5)[b]	3.0*	12.4 (6.7,18.1)[b]	0.3*
Loss of parent or close person in childhood				
Parental death	8.2 (5.7,10.7)	3.2 (1.6, 4.8)	2.6 (1.2, 4.0)	0.2*
No parental death	10.8 (9.9,11.7)	3.3 (2.8, 3.8)	3.4 (2.9, 3.9)	0.5 (0.3, 0.7)
Death of close person (not parent)	12.5 (11.1,13.9)[a]	4.8 (3.9, 5.7)[b]	4.1 (3.3, 4.9)[a]	0.6 (0.3, 0.9)
No close person death	9.5 (8.5,10.5)	2.4 (1.9, 2.9)	2.8 (2.2, 3.4)	0.3*

Table 16.5 (*continued*)

	Ever ideation	1-yr ideation	Ever attempt	1-yr attempt
Instability while growing up				
Moved twice or more away from friends	14.7 (12.7, 16.7)[b]	4.7 (3.5, 5.9)[b]	4.7 (3.5, 5.9)[b]	0.8*
Home location geographically stable	9.7 (8.8, 10.6)	3.1 (2.6, 3.6)	3.1 (2.6, 3.6)	0.3*
Child welfare services involved	32.3 (25.1, 39.5)[b]	13.1 (7.9, 18.3)[b]	13.1 (7.9, 18.3)[b]	1.7 (0, 3.7)[b]
Above history absent	10.1 (9.3, 10.9)	3.1 (2.6, 3.6)	3.1 (2.6, 3.6)	0.4 (0.2, 0.6)
No confiding relationship with adult	18.9 (16.3, 21.5)[b]	5.7 (4.1, 7.3)±	6.1 (4.5, 7.7)[b]	0.9*
Confiding relationship present	9.2 (8.3, 10.1)	3.0 (2.5, 3.5)	2.8 (2.3, 3.3)	0.3 (0.2, 0.6)
Physical or sexual abuse history in childhood				
Physical abuse history	15.4 (13.2, 17.6)	4.8 (3.5, 6.1)	4.9 (3.6, 6.2)	0.6*
Sexual abuse history present	20.7 (15.2, 26.2)	7.6 (4.0, 11.2)	8.7 (4.9, 12.5)	0.1*
Both forms of abuse present	35.9 (29.7, 42.1)[c]	14.1 (9.6, 18.6)[c]	15.1 (10.5, 19.7)[c]	1.9*

[a] Chi square $p < 0.05$
[b] Chi square $p < 0.01$
[c] Mantel Haenszel test for trend $p < 0.05$
*Unstable numbers
Source: Statistics Canada

If child welfare services were involved, it is clear that there was serious home pathology present that adversely affected the child. There are exceedingly high prevalence rates for non-fatal suicidality with such a history. The presence of physical and sexual abuse in a child growing up is another indicator of extreme family pathology and a powerful risk factor for suicidal ideation and attempts.

Lifetime prevalence and one-year incidence figures for *DSM-III-R* disorders with odds ratios adjusted for age and sex are shown in table 16.6. The risk for non-fatal suicidality is significantly increased with the presence of these psychiatric disorders.

The issue of the ratio of suicide attempts to completed suicides was also examined in the Ontario Health Survey analysis since there is much speculation in the literature but almost no attempts to ground it in actual data, mainly because treated suicide attempts are not notifiable and probably represent the skewed top of the iceberg. Using coroners' data, there were 1,201 deaths on average during 1990 and 1991 (the years when the survey was carried out). Since the estimated weighted one-year frequency of attempted suicides in the household population was over 31,000, then the multiple would be 26:1, a more conservative estimate than the 33:1 derived from Statistics Canada data.[65]

More recently, Rhodes and colleagues analysed data from the Canadian Community Health Survey (cycle 1.2) (N = 36,984 household members aged 15 or more)[71] on prevalence of depression and suicidality (ideation and nonfatal attempts or deliberate self-harm) and their overlap, as well as their utilization of mental health services. In the year prior to the survey, 4.8% reported depression, 4% suicidal ideation, and < 1% reported a suicide attempt, comparable to previous Canadian surveys already mentioned. Of those who reported a one-year history of suicidal ideation, just over one-third had concomitant depressive disorder, but more than half of those with suicide attempt reports had also suffered depression (56%). About 11% of this category reported inpatient care. When respondents reported they had been depressed and suicidal, one-fifth made contact with psychiatric care and one-quarter with a primary care physician. Thereafter the proportions (psychiatric, primary care) declined in the following hierarchy (percentage seeking psychiatric care stated first, followed by primary care): depression, no suicidality – 14%, 26%; suicidality, no depression – 7%, 12%; and neither depression nor suicidality – < 1%, 3%.

Of probably greater significance was the finding that among those who reported being depressed and suicidal, 38% had no contact with

Table 16.6
Lifetime prevalence and one-year incidence of suicidality with *DSM-III-R* disorders

Diagnosis	Ever ideation		1-yr ideation		Ever attempt		1-yr attempt	
	Prevalence(CI)	Adj OR	Incidence(CI)	Adj OR	Prevalence(CI)	Adj OR	Incidence(CI)	Adj OR
No history *DSM-III-R*	7.1 (6.2, 8.0)		2.2 (1.7, 2.7)		1.9 (1.4, 2.4)		0.2 (0.0, 0.4)	
Any history	21.8 (19.7, 23.9)	3.6 (2.8, 4.5)	7.2 (5.9, 8.5)	3.3 (2.2, 4.8)	7.3 (6.0, 8.6)	4.0 (2.7, 6.0)	1.0 (0.5, 1.5)	4.1 (1.3, 12.4)
Any anxiety disorder	24.3 (21.6, 27.0)	3.2 (2.5, 4.0)	8.4 (6.6, 10.2)	2.9 (2.0, 4.3)	8.2 (6.4, 10.0)	3.2 (2.2, 4.7)	1.2 (0.5, 1.9)	3.6 (1.3, 10.1)
Any mood disorder	41.3 (36.8, 45.8)	8.0 (6.1, 10.5)	13.2 (10.1, 16.3)	5.5 (3.6, 8.3)	16.4 (13.0, 19.8)	8.3 (5.6, 12.4)	1.8 (0.6, 3.0)	8.8 (2.2, 20.5)
Dysthymia	48.4 (40.2, 56.6)	9.5 (6.1, 14.6)	11.5 (6.2, 16.8)	4.2 (2.1, 8.3)	21.2 (14.4, 28.0)	9.0 (5.2, 15.5)	1.9 (0.0, 4.2)	8.3 (1.6, 43.4)
Major depression	43.6 (38.6, 48.6)	8.4 (6.3, 11.2)	14.0 (10.5, 17.5)	5.7 (3.7, 8.8)	16.5 (12.8, 20.2)	7.4 (4.9, 11.2)	1.4 (0.2, 2.6)	4.2 (1.2, 14.7)
Excitement >2 weeks	54.8 (38.8, 70.8)	8.6 (3.9, 19.3)	18.8 (6.2, 31.4)	5.1 (1.8, 14.3)	19.8 (7.0, 32.6)	6.1 (2.2, 16.6)	7.8 (0.0, 16.4)	14.5 (2.9, 72.4)
Antisocial disorder	32.8 (24.7, 40.9)	3.4 (1.9, 6.2)	17.7 (11.0, 24.4)	4.8 (2.2, 10.6)	16.6 (10.2, 23.0)	8.4 (4.1, 17.3)	4.5 (0.9, 8.1)	15.8 (3.0, 82.8)
Any substance disorder	22.2 (18.9, 25.5)	2.8 (2.1, 3.7)	6.5 (4.5, 8.5)	2.0 (1.3, 3.3)	8.0 (5.8, 10.2)	3.4 (2.2, 5.4)	1.2 (0.3, 2.1)	4.3 (1.3, 13.6)
Alcohol	20.4 (17.0, 23.8)	2.4 (1.8, 3.2)	6.6 (4.5, 6.7)	2.1 (1.3, 3.4)	7.6 (5.4, 9.8)	3.1 (1.9, 4.9)	1.3 (0.3, 2.3)	4.6 (1.4, 15.0)
Drugs (not cannabis)	35.9 (28.4, 43.4)	6.7 (3.6, 12.5)	11.7 (6.6, 16.8)	7.0 (3.2, 15.1)	14.9 (9.3, 20.5)	10.0 (4.9, 20.7)	3.3 (0.5, 6.1)	20.7 (5.1, 83.5)

*Adjusted for age and sex
Source: Statistics Canada

any care provider. Half of those with depression but no suicidality had no service contact and, worse, of those who reported suicidality without a depressive disorder had no contact at all. In light of the recent audit of 100 New Brunswick suicides[72] which identified short-falls in clinical services that might have prevented a proportion of these deaths, it seems important that more inquiry should be made of the survey respondents who had no contact with health care services in spite of the fact that they were suffering from depressive illness, sui-cidality, or both.

Suicide Methods in Canada

The risk of dying from self-inflicted wounds from firearm use is poten-tially high, whereas if a person who has attempted suicide by other means and is still alive when discovered can be brought to a general hospital emergency department with dispatch, they stand a good chance (less than 2% mortality) of recovery in western societies. How-ever, even speedy emergency care may not save a victim of self-inflicted gunshot. The choice of the method of suicide is considered to depend on its availability.[73–76] Moscicki[76] argued that the choice of lethal versus non-lethal instrument of self-destruction was not one of the factors that could account for the 'gender paradox' of suicide and attempted suicide; i.e., the much higher prevalence of completed suicide in males in contrast with the over representation of females among younger-age suicide attempters. She partly based her argu-ment on the relatively high prevalence of firearm suicide among women in the United States,[77] but this argument could not be extrap-olated to Canada.[26] In 1980–2, 41% of suicides in men in Canada were by firearms and explosives, but in females only 11% of suicide deaths. By 1990–2, the proportion in males had dropped to 31% and in women to 9%. Unlike the United States, Canada, against significant opposition from special interest groups, has enacted a series of legislative acts intended to reduce firearm availability among the public. Following the first of these acts (Bill C-51 in 1978), Carrington and Moyer were able to demonstrate that the reduction in firearm use was associated with a reduction in total rates of suicide without displacement to (sub-stitution by) other methods.[78,79] Leenaars et al.[80] supported this con-clusion even after controlling for the influence of social variables through multiple regression analysis. In 1991, Bill C-17 was enacted to promote firearm registration and safer handling and storage of firearms. Examining trends in suicide rates in youth from 1979–99,

Cheung and Dewa found no changes in the overall rates, but a substantial change in the specific methods used, with suicide by firearms dropping from 60% to 22% with apparent displacement to suicide by hanging or suffocation that increased from 20% to 60% over the same time period.[74]

Tables 16.7 and 16.8 present the data for methods of suicide used by all age groups in Canada from 2000 to 2004.[81] The use of firearms decreased even further in males as compared with 1980–2 and 1990–2 (already mentioned) to a mean of 21% over the five years and in females to less than 4%. However, suicide by hanging and strangulation in men increased to 45% (in 1980–2 it was 25% and in 1990–2 it was 31%). In females it accounted for 36% of suicide deaths in 2000–4, up from 19% in 1980–2 and 22% in 1990–2. Self-poisoning deaths were roughly at the same level (37% in 1990–2 and 35% in 2000–4) and so were deaths from other self-inflicted causes. While this apparent method substitution is disappointing, suicide rates overall and also in youth have been diminishing in Canada and firearm control may be contributing to this decline.

It continues to be necessary for society to reduce the availability of lethal means of suicide that are sometimes used in a sudden fit of rage or depression by youths who, given time to cool down, would not have wished the outcome to have been their own execution. Increasingly in urban Canada, we are also being reminded of the prevalence of gun use by street gangs, often with innocent bystanders as victims, an important reason to reduce the prevalence of firearms in the community and to ensure that those that are available can only be used by law-abiding and responsible adults of sound mental health and personality.

Table 16.7
Methods of suicide for Canadian males, 2000–4

Year	2000		2001		2002		2003		2004		2000–4	
	N	%	N	%	N	%	N	%	N	%	N	%
All intentional self-harm	2,798	100.0	2,869	100.0	2,849	100.0	2,902	100.0	2,734	100.0	14,152	100.0
Self-poisoning	275	9.8	274	9.6	266	9.3	317	10.9	307	11.2	1,439	10.2
Gases, solvents, chemicals	296	10.6	328	11.4	286	10.0	248	8.5	250	9.1	1,408	9.9
Hanging, strangulation	1,229	43.9	1,230	42.9	1,276	44.8	1,341	46.2	1,291	47.2	6,367	45.0
Drowning	68	2.4	73	2.6	73	2.6	53	1.8	57	2.1	324	2.3
Firearms and explosives	649	23.2	617	21.5	615	21.6	585	20.2	543	19.9	3,009	21.3
Jumping from high place	120	4.3	135	4.7	131	4.6	153	5.3	114	4.2	653	4.6
Under moving vehicle	46	1.6	60	2.1	55	1.9	50	1.7	49	1.8	260	1.8
Deliberate collision	25	0.9	26	0.9	25	0.9	28	1.0	17	0.6	121	0.9
Sharp instrument	42	1.5	82	2.9	71	2.5	79	2.7	75	2.7	349	2.5
Other (includes immolation)	48	1.7	44	1.5	51	1.8	48	1.7	31	1.1	222	1.6
Total	2,798	100.0	2,869	100.0	2,849	100.0	2,902	100.0	2,734	100.0	14,152	100.0

Source: Statistics Canada

Table 16.8
Methods of suicide for Canadian females, 2000–4

Year	2000		2001		2002		2003		2004		2000–4	
	N	%	N	%	N	%	N	%	N	%	N	%
All intentional self-harm	807	100.0	819	100.0	799	100.0	862	100.0	879	100.0	4,166	100.0
Self-poisoning	238	29.5	295	36.0	277	34.7	311	36.1	336	38.2	1,457	35.0
Gases, solvents, chemicals	63	7.8	71	8.7	56	7.0	48	5.6	51	5.8	289	6.9
Hanging, strangulation	317	39.3	279	34.1	294	36.8	321	37.2	299	34.0	1,510	36.2
Drowning	26	3.2	33	4.0	33	4.1	39	4.5	49	5.6	180	4.3
Firearms and explosives	37	4.6	35	4.3	18	2.3	34	3.9	27	3.1	151	3.6
Jumping from high place	61	7.6	49	6.0	61	7.6	44	5.1	47	5.3	262	6.3
Under moving vehicle	23	2.9	20	2.4	24	3.0	22	2.6	25	2.8	114	2.7
Deliberate collision	1	0.1	5	0.6	3	0.4	3	0.3	7	0.8	19	0.5
Sharp instrument	12	1.5	12	1.5	18	2.3	19	2.2	21	2.4	82	2.0
Other (includes immolation)	29	3.6	20	2.4	15	1.9	21	2.4	17	1.9	102	2.4
Total	807	100.0	819	100.0	799	100.0	862	100.0	879	100.0	4,166	100.0

Source: Statistics Canada

NOTES AND REFERENCES

1 Sakinofsky I. The epidemiology of suicide in Canada. In: Leenaars AA, Wenckstern S, Sakinofsky I, et al., eds. *Suicide in Canada*. Toronto, University of Toronto Press, 1998:37–66.

2 Solomon MI, Hellon CP. Suicide and age in Alberta, Canada, 1951 to 1977. A cohort analysis. *Arch Gen Psychiatry* 1980;37:511–13.

3 Trovato F. Suicide in Canada: A further look at the effects of age, period and cohort. *Can J Pub Health* 1988;79:37–44.

4 Lester D. An analysis of the suicide rates of birth cohorts in Canada. *Suicide Life Threat Behav* 1988;18:372–8.

5 Barnes RA, Ennis J, Schober R. Cohort analysis of Ontario suicide rates, 1877–1976. *Can J Psychiatry* 1986;31:208–13.

6 Hellon CP, Solomon MI. Suicide and age in Alberta, Canada, 1951 to 1977. The changing profile. *Arch Gen Psychiatry* 1980;37:505–10.

7 Newman SC, Dyck RJ. On the age-period-cohort analysis of suicide rates. *Psychol Med* 1988;18:677–81.

8 Klerman GL. The current age of youthful melancholia. Evidence for increase in depression among adolescents and young adults. *Br J Psychiatry* 1988;152:4–14.

9 Klerman GL, Weissman MM. Increasing rates of depression. *JAMA* 1989;261:2229–35.

10 Sigurdson E, Staley D, Matas M, et al. A five year review of youth suicide in Manitoba. *Can J Psychiatry* 1994;39:397–403.

11 Dhossche DM, Rich CL, Isacsson G. Psychoactive substances in suicides – Comparison of toxicologic findings in two samples. *Am J Forensic Med Pathol* 2001;22:239–43.

12 Kirmayer LJ, Boothroyd LJ, Hodgins S. Attempted suicide among Inuit youth: Psychosocial correlates and implications for prevention. *Can J Psychiatry* 1998;43:816–22.

13 Gartrell JW, Jarvis GK, Derksen L. Suicidality among adolescent Alberta Indians. *Suicide Life Threat Behav* 1993;23:366–73.

14 Sakinofsky I, Roberts R, Van Houten A. *The End of the Journey: A Study of Suicide across Canada and The Social Correlates of Suicide*. Proceedings 8th Annual Meeting International Association of Suicide Prevention (IASP), Jerusalem, 1975

15 Thompson AH, Howard AW, Jin Y. A social problem index for Canada. *Can J Psychiatry* 2001;46:45–51.

16 Thompson AH. Variations in the prevalence of psychiatric disorders and social problems across Canadian provinces. *Can J Psychiatry* 2005;50:637–42.

17 Boyer R, Legare G, St-Laurent D, et al. Epidemiology of suicide, parasui-
    cide, and suicidal ideation in Quebec. In: Leenaars AA, Wenckstern S,
    Sakinofsky I, et al., eds. *Suicide in Canada*. Toronto, University of Toronto
    Press, 1998:67–84.

18 Bland R, Newman SC, Orn H. Help-seeking for psychiatric disorders.
    Can J Psychiatry 1997;42:935–42.

19 Hegerl U. The Nuremberg alliance against depression: Effects of a com-
    munity based intervention progamme for suicidality. *J Affect Disord*
    2004;78:s42.

20 Hegerl U, Althaus D, Stefanek J. Public attitudes towards treatment of
    depression: Effects of an information campaign. *Pharmacopsychiatry*
    2003;36:288–91.

21 Fombonne E. Increased rates of depression: Update of epidemiological
    findings and analytical problems. *Acta Psychiatr Scand* 1994;90:145–56.

22 Sakinofsky I. Treating suicidality in depressive illness. Part 1: Current
    controversies. *Can J Psychiatry* 2007;52(suppl):s71–s84.

23 Sakinofsky I, Roberts R. The ecology of suicide in the provinces of
    Canada, 1969–71 to 1979–81. In: Cooper B, ed. *The Epidemiology of Psychi-
    atric Disorders*. Baltimore, Johns Hopkins University Press, 1987:27–42.

24 Sakinofsky I, Leenaars AA. Suicide in Canada with special reference to
    the difference between Canada and the United States. *Suicide Life Threat
    Behav* 1997;27:112–26.

25 Miller M, Azrael D, Miller M. Firearm availability and suicide, homicide,
    and unintentional firearm deaths among women. *J Urban Health*
    2002;79:26–38.

26 Canetto SS, Sakinofsky I. The gender paradox in suicide. *Suicide Life
    Threaten Behav* 1998;28:1–23.

27 Sakinofsky I. The current evidence base for the clinical care of suicidal
    patients: Strengths and weaknesses. *Can J Psychiatry*
    2007;52(suppl):s7–s20.

28 Wasserman D, Varnik A, Eklund G. Male suicides and alcohol consump-
    tion in the former USSR. *Acta Psychiatr Scand* 1994;89:306–13.

29 Varnik A, Wasserman D. Suicides in the former Soviet republics. *Acta
    Psychiatr Scand* 1992;86:76–8.

30 Pridemore WA, Chamlin MB, Cochran JK. An interrupted time-series
    analysis of Durkheim's social deregulation thesis: The case of the Russian
    federation. *Justice Q* 2007;24:271–90.

31 Rancans E, Renberg ES, Jacobsson L. Major demographic, social and eco-
    nomic factors associated to suicide rates in Latvia 1980–48. *Acta Psychiatr
    Scand* 2001;103:275–81.

32 Wasserman D, Varnik A, Eklund G. Female suicides and alcohol con-

sumption during perestroika in the former USSR. *Acta Psychiatr Scand* 1998;98:26–33.

33 Varnik A, Wasserman D, Dankowicz M, et al. Marked decrease in suicide among men and women in the former USSR during perestroika. *Acta Psychiatr Scand* 1998;98:13–9.

34 Steele MM, Doey T. Suicidal behaviour in children and adolescents. Part 1: Etiology and risk factors. *Can J Psychiatry* 2007;52(suppl):s21–s33.

35 Malla A, Hoenig J. Suicide in Newfoundland and Labrador. *Can J Psychiatry* 1979;24:139–46.

36 Aldridge D, St John K. Adolescent and pre-adolescent suicide in Newfoundland and Labrador. Special Issue: Child and adolescent psychiatry. *Can J Psychiatry* 1991;36:432–6.

37 Krull C, Trovato F. The Quiet Revolution and the sex differential in Quebec's suicide rates: 1931–1986. *Soc Forces* 1994;72:1121–47.

38 Langlois S, Morrison P. Suicide deaths and suicide attempts. *Health Rep* 2002;13:9–22.

39 Lester D. Henry and Short on suicide: A critique. *J Psychol* 1968;70:179–86.

40 Haggarty J, Craven J, Chaudhuri B, et al. A study of multi-media suicide education in Nunavut. *Arch Suicide Res* 2006;10:277–81.

41 Kehoe JP. Suicide and attempted suicide in the Yukon Territory. *Can Psychiatr Assoc J* 1975;20:15–23.

42 Speechley M, Stavraky KM. The adequacy of suicide statistics for use in epidemiology and public health. *Can J Pub Health* 1991;82:38–42.

43 Brown JH. Reporting of suicide: Canadian statistics. *Suicide* 1975;5:21–8.

44 Neeleman J, Wessely S. Changes in classification of suicide in England and Wales: Time trends and associations with coroners' professional backgrounds. *Psychol Med* 1997;27:467–72.

45. Norman, GR, Streiner DL. *Biostatistics: The Bare Essentials.* 3rd ed. Hamilton, ON: BC Decker, 2007.

46 Hawton K, Fagg J, Simkin S, et al. The epidemiology of attempted suicide in the Oxford area, England (1989–1992). *Crisis* 1994;15:123–35.

47 Platt S, Bille-Brahe U, Kerkhof A, et al. Parasuicide in Europe: The WHO/EURO multicentre study on parasuicide. I. Introduction and preliminary analysis for 1989. *Acta Psychiatr Scand* 1992;85:97–104.

48 Grek A. Clinical management of suicidality in the elderly: An opportunity for involvement in the lives of older patients. *Can J Psychiatry* 2007;52(suppl):s47–s57.

49 Agbayewa MO, Marion SA, Wiggins S. Socioeconomic factors associated with suicide in elderly populations in British Columbia: An 11-year review. *Can J Psychiatry* 1998;43:829–36.

50 Quan H, Arboleda-Flórez J, Fick GH, et al. Association between physical

illness and suicide among the elderly. *Soc Psychiatry Psychiatr Epidemiol* 2002;37:190–7.

51 Préville M, Boyer R, Hébert R, et al. Correlates of suicide in the older adult population in Quebec. *Suicide Life Threat Behav* 2005;35:91–105.

52 Malchy B, Enns MW, Young TK, et al. Suicide among Manitoba's Aboriginal people, 1988 to 1994. *Can Med Assoc J* 1997;156:1133–8.

53 Kirmayer LJ. Suicide among Canadian Aboriginal peoples. *Transcultural Psychiatric Research Review* 1994; 31:3–58.

54 Gotowiec A, Beiser M. Aboriginal children's mental health: Unique challenges. *Can Ment Health* 1994;41:7–11.

55 Boothroyd LJ, Kirmayer LJ, Spreng S, et al. Completed suicides among the Inuit of northern Quebec, 1982–1996: A case-control study. *Can Med Assoc J* 2001;165:749–55.

56 Chandler MJ. The problem of self-continuity in the context of rapid personal and cultural change. In: Oosterwegel A, Wicklund, R., eds. *The Self in European and North American Culture: Development and Processes*. The Netherlands: Kluwer, 1995:45–63.

57 Chandler M, Lalonde C. Cultural continuity as a hedge against suicide in Canada's First Nations. *Transcultur Psychiatry* 1998;35:191–219.

58 Chandler MJ. Adolescent suicide and the loss of personal continuity. In: Cicchetti D, Toth SL, eds. *Rochester Symposium on Developmental Psychopathology: Disorders and Dysfunctions of the Self*. Rochester, NY: University of Rochester Press, 1994:371–90.

59 Durkheim E. *Suicide* (Spaulding JA, Simpson G, Trans). New York: The Free Press, 1951.

60 Hallet D, Chandler MJ, Lalonde CE. Aboriginal language knowledge and youth suicide. *Cognitive Development* 2007;22:392–9

61 Lester D. Testing Durkheim's theory of suicide in nineteenth and twentieth century Europe. *Eur Arch Psychiatry Clin Neurosci* 1993;243:54–5.

62 Trovato F. A Durkheimian analysis of youth suicide: Canada, 1971 and 1981. *Suicide Life Threat Behav* 1992;22:413–27.

63 Ramsay R, Bagley, C. The prevalence of suicidal behaviors, attitudes and associated social experiences in an urban population. *Suicide Life Threat Behav* 1985;15(3):151–67.

64 Bland RC, Newman SC, Dyck RJ. The epidemiology of parasuicide in Edmonton. *Can J Psychiatry* 1994;39:391–6.

65 Bellerose C, Lavallée, Camirand J. *Enquête sociale et de santé 1992–1993*. Québec: Santè Québec, 1994.

66 Sakinofsky I, Webster G. *Major Risk Factors for Non-fatal Suicidality in the Community*. XVIII Congress of the International Association for Suicide Prevention, Venice. 1995.

67 Webster G. The epidemiology of attempted suicide and suicidal ideation: An analysis of the Ontario Health Survey and the Ontario Health Supplement [dissertation]. University of Toronto, 1996.

68 Paykel ES, Myers JK, Lindenthal JJ, et al. Suicidal feelings in the general population: A prevalence study. *Br J Psychiatry* 1974;124:460–9.

69 Moscicki EK, O'Carroll P, Rae DS, et al. Suicide attempts in the Epidemiologic Catchment Area Study. *Yale J Biol Med* 1988;61:259–68.

70 Kessler RC, Borges G, Walters EE. Prevalence of and risk factors for lifetime suicide attempts in the national comorbidity survey. *Arch Gen Psychiat* 1999;56:617–26.

71 Rhodes AE, Bethell J, Bondy SJ. Suicidality, depression, and mental health service use in Canada. *Can J Psychiatry* 2006;51:35–41.

72 Seguin M, Lesage AD, Turecki G, et al. Research project on deaths by suicide in New Brunswick between April 2002 and May 2003. 2005. http://gnb.ca/0055/pdf/3182-e.pdf. Accessed January 12, 2007.

73 Brent DA, Perper JA, Moritz G, et al. Firearms and adolescent suicide. A community case-control study. *Am J Dis Child* 1993;147:1066–71.

74 Cheung AH, Dewa CS. Current trends in youth suicide and firearms regulations. *Can J Pub Health* 2005;96:131–5.

75 Miller M, Lippmann SJ, Azrael D, et al. Household firearm ownership and rates of suicide across the 50 United States. *J Trauma* 2007;62:1029–34.

76 Moscicki EK. Gender differences in completed and attempted suicides. *Ann Epidemiol* 1994;4:152–8.

77 Kaplan MS, Adamek ME, Geling O, Calderon A. Firearm suicide among older women in the US. *Soc Sci Med* 1997;44:427–1430.

78 Carrington PJ, Moyer S. Gun control and suicide in Ontario [see comments]. *Am J Psychiatry* 1994;151:606–8.

79 Carrington PJ, Moyer S. Gun availability and suicide in Canada: Testing the displacement hypothesis. *Studies on Crime and Crime Prevention* 1994;3:167–78.

80 Leenaars AA, Moksony F, Lester D, Wenckstern S. The impact of gun control (Bill C-51) on suicide in Canada. *Death Stud* 2003;27:103–24.

81 Statistics Canada. *Deaths by Cause, Chapter XX, External Causes of Morbidity and Mortality.* 2007. http://www.statcan.ca/english/freepub/84-208-XIE/2007001/tb-en.htm#20. Accessed August 12, 2007.

PART FIVE

Mental Health Care Services and Policy

17 Depression and Mental Health Supports and Services in Canada

ANNE RHODES, JULIE THURLOW, NICOLE DONALDSON,
AMANDA T. LO, AND JENNIFER BETHELL

Introduction

The purpose of this chapter is to provide a critical review of the literature on current issues in access and provision of mental health supports and services for those who are living with major depression in Canada. The prevention and control of depression is critical due to its prevalence and the social costs associated with the disability it produces. Effective health promotion programs, prevention, detection, and treatment strategies could, therefore, have a sizeable impact on the health of Canadians. This chapter begins with key findings from the descriptive epidemiology of depression, prevention, and health promotion strategies, screening for depression, and its treatment. It then examines what is known about access and provision of mental health services for those living with major depression in Canada. Last, the implications of this research are discussed.

The Canadian Community Health Survey: Mental Health and Well Being (CCHS 1.2), a nationally representative survey of Canadian residents (see chapter 5), was administered to community-dwelling Canadian residents aged 15 and older in 2002. In the 12 months prior to the survey, 4.8% (95% CI: 4.5–5.1) of respondents experienced a major depressive episode (MDE). The prevalence of MDE was 5.9% (95% CI: 5.4–6.4) among women and 3.7% (95% CI: 3.3–4.1) among men. The prevalence of major depressive disorder (MDD), which excludes those with bipolar disorder, is estimated to be 4.0% (95% CI: 3.7–4.2) in the general population.[1]

These estimates are consistent with, but at the lower end of, prevalence rates reported in other North American and European population surveys.[2–5] With respect to sex differences, findings are consistent with international studies reporting prevalence rates 1.5 to 2.0 times higher for women as compared to men.[3]

While the first episode of major depression can occur at any age, studies report the average or median age at onset is in the mid 20s to early 30s. In Canada, as in a number of other countries, the highest population rates are reported for adolescents and young adults. CCHS 1.2 data estimate annual prevalence of depressive disorders to be 5.3% among those aged 15–24 and 7.6% among those aged 20–24.[1,6] Among those 65 and older, the CCHS 1.2 estimates a prevalence of 1.9% (95% CI: 1.5–2.4) and the Canadian Study of Health and Aging,[7] which includes institutional residents, estimates a prevalence of 2.6% (95% CI: 1.0–4.2).[8] Analysis of CCHS data shows a linear decline in prevalence with age for community dwelling men and women in this age group.[8]

Concurrent medical and psychiatric illness is common among individuals with major depression. In particular, anxiety disorders and dysthymia often co-occur.[9,10] As well, a number of Canadian studies have reported the prevalence of depression to be higher among those with chronic medical conditions and among those reporting chronic pain.[7,11,12]

Studies of incidence are less consistent in their findings. Canadian incidence estimates vary from 2.8% per year, based on data from the Edmonton study[13] to 0.37% per year, using data from the Stirling County study.[14] With respect to age and sex differences, patterns are similar to those reported in studies of prevalence. Higher incidence is found among women and for adolescents and young adults as compared to those in older age groups.[13–15]

Studies of mortality among individuals with major depression suggest an increased risk of death compared to individuals who are not depressed. In particular, major depression is associated with an increased risk of suicide and suicide attempts. A study using CCHS 1.2 data reports that of those respondents with major depression, 28.6% have had thoughts of suicide and 6% have attempted suicide in the prior year.[16] Studies of inpatient and psychiatric samples place estimates of suicide deaths between 12% and 19% for those with major depression.[17,18]

Prevention and Health Promotion Strategies for Depression

There is growing interest in the ways in which major depression or symptoms of depression may be prevented through the modification of the determinants of health by interventions that extend beyond identified clinical populations. Prevention has been defined by the Institute of Medicine[19] as activities that are aimed at reducing the incidence of (new) cases of disorder and can be categorized as: *universal*, where the intervention(s) is delivered to the whole population; *targeted* – selective, where intervention(s) is delivered to those at risk of disorder; and *targeted* – indicated, where intervention(s) is delivered to those with sub-clinical symptoms. A more commonly used typology distinguishes *primary* prevention – which refers to preventing incident cases, from *secondary prevention* – where the target is to lower the rate of prevalent (existing) cases of a disorder/illness in populations, from *tertiary* prevention – where the goal is to reduce the amount of disability associated with disorder/illness.[20]

A helpful model for understanding how modifying determinants of health may affect depression or depressive symptoms is the Population Health Promotion Model, shown in figure 17.1.[21] As the concepts of mental health promotion and population health share many common elements, the Population Health Agency of Canada (PHAC) integrated the core elements together into this model. The model captures how evidence-based decision making can be brought to bear on the determinants of health through comprehensive action strategies at different levels of intervention. Action strategies can be applied in relation to specific determinants of health, health concerns, or groups at risk, such as depression. A full description of the determinants of health is given on the website[21] but include: 1) income and social status, 2) social support networks, 3) education, 4) employment and working conditions, 5) physical environment, 6) biology and genetic endowment, 7) personal health practices and coping skills, 8) healthy child development, and 9) health services.

Accordingly, this model was used to structure a review of prevention and health promotion strategies for depression. More specifically, studies that evaluated promotion and/or prevention interventions *or* directly modified one or more determinants of health with the aim of reducing depressive symptoms and (or) preventing the onset of major depression were identified. (A review of observational studies relating depression or depressive symptoms with each of these determinants of health was considered beyond the scope of this review.) Further, studies that extended beyond clinical samples were emphasized. Based on the literature, the levels of action – i.e., the 'who' – were organized according to specific age/life-stage groups including postpartum women, children and adolescents, adults in the workplace

Figure 17.1 The Population Health Promotion Model

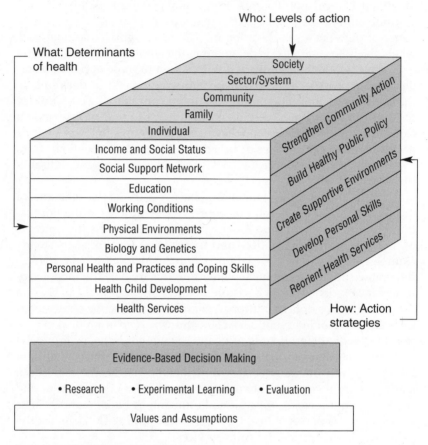

Source: Public Health Agency of Canada

environment, and the elderly. In addition, two systematic reviews that overarch these groupings were examined.[22,23]

Postpartum Women. Several intervention studies and reviews have been conducted on the prevention of postpartum depression.[20,24–27] The available evidence suggests no specific psychosocial or psychological intervention is more effective than another but interventions in the postpartum period and directed to individual mothers may be most effective. Successful uptake of such interventions is likely enhanced if they are inexpensive, simple, and applicable to a large population. As there is uncertainty about an increased risk for depression during the perinatal period,[28] further research comparing potential risk groups and cost-effectiveness can guide future interventions.

Children and Adolescents. Previous meta-analyses and more recent randomized controlled trials directly concerning children and adolescents were recently reviewed by Merry.[29] Psychological interventions have shown a reduction of depressive symptoms in the short term among targeted populations. More evidence on longer-term effects and reduction of the incidence of depression is required. While universal interventions hold appeal, further evidence is needed.[29,30] Interventions with potentially indirect effects on infants, children, and adolescents also merit further attention. For example, an ongoing trial is suggesting that remission of maternal depression is having a beneficial effect on depression in their children.[31]

Adults in the Workplace Environment. Few intervention studies in the workplace have been reported in the literature.[32,33] Organizational level changes as well as more individually tailored practices have great potential; therefore, further research into costs and benefits of specific interventions is desirable. Recently, results from a randomized controlled trial of a screening, outreach, and care management program for workers in a managed behavioural health plan reported significant gains in clinical and work productivity outcomes.[34] Areas needing further research, particularly for the Canadian context, pertain to the nature and effectiveness of privately funded treatment programs in relation to publicly funded care, insurance coverage for treatments, as well as reimbursement for time off work for treatment and for health promotion, prevention, and screening activities.[32,35,36]

Elderly. Systematic reviews of elders have found improvements in depressive symptoms with cognitive-behavioural interventions[37] and programs that include social support.[22] Further study of brief interventions is needed.[38]

   Llopis et al.[22] carried out a meta-analysis of 69 prevention primary programs that focused on reducing depression or symptoms of depression. In this analysis, both targeted and universal programs were equally supported. Overall, an 11% improvement of depressive symptoms was attained through prevention programs, suggesting that a prevention strategy (both universal and targeted) could be cost-effective for the populations. However, information on reducing the incidence of depression was not explored. Although the effect size was small, higher quality studies demonstrated a stronger effect. Assuming that harms associated with the interventions were few, the short- and longer-term benefits may be worth the costs and merits further study. In a systematic review conducted by Cuijpers et al.,[23] the effects of preventative interventions on the incidence of new cases of mental disorders were investigated. Thirteen studies were identified and six studies focused on depression disorders (two being postpartum depression). The studies on depressive disorders resulted in a relative risk of 0.72 (95% CI, 0.54–0.96). Cognitive behavioural and indicated interventions were found most effective.

In reviewing the evidence with respect to the Population Health Promotion Model, it was apparent that the determinants of health most commonly targeted, and apparently most amenable to intervention, were social support networks, and personal health practices and coping skills. From a mental health promotion perspective, it is noteworthy that programs including a competence (but not a behavioural) element were found more effective.[22] Also, the interventions were 'protective' in nature. *Protective factors* refer to circumstances that 'improve people's resistance to risk factors and disorders.'[39]

As found in other reviews, most of the interventions were at the individual level and economic and cost effectiveness data were limited.[35,39] Studies that directly modified determinants of health, such as the physical environment (e.g., housing), access to education, unemployment or low income, or a stressful work environment and then examined the impact on depression or depressive symptoms in exposed/not exposed populations were infrequent. Thus, many questions about their potential impact on depression remain.[40]

The available evidence varied in quality and quantity. For example, few workplace intervention studies were identified.[32,33] On the other hand, while a number of investigations have been conducted with children and adolescents, higher quality studies are needed. For instance, interventions in educational settings have often excluded student absentees and dropouts. Higher quality studies have the potential to demonstrate a stronger effect.[22]

Screening for Depression

Last defines *screening*, described in 1951 by the U.S. Commission on Chronic Illness, as 'the presumptive identification of a disease or defect by the application of tests, examinations or other procedures which can be applied rapidly. Screening tests sort out apparently well persons who probably have the disease from those who do not. A screening test is not intended to be diagnostic. Persons with positive or suspicious findings must be referred to their physician for diagnosis and necessary treatment.'[41(p165)]

The U.S. Preventive Services Task force (USPSTF) conducted a rigorous systematic review based on 14 randomized trials occurring in primary care settings. This review focused on the differences in detection, proportion of patients treated or referred for treatment, and the clinical outcomes of depression. Screening interventions varied in intensity; some trials provided feedback of exclusively screening results, others additionally provided treatment advice (specific or general), and some provided clinicians with advice on developing practices that would augment the quality of treatment and follow-up their patients received. The USPSTF concluded that screening can improve outcomes when compared to usual care, particularly when screening is complemented with effective follow-up and treatment. They recommended that adults be screened for depression 'in clinical practices that have systems in place to assure accurate diagnosis, effective treatment and follow-up.'[42] The evidence on screening adolescents and children was viewed insufficient.[43]

The Canadian Task Force on Preventive Health Care (CTFPHC) later reviewed the same evidence identified by the USPSTF, determined that no new evidence was available, and came to similar conclusions.[44] The CTFPHC endorsed that there is fair evidence (grade B recommendation: there is fair evidence to recommend the clinical preventive action) that screening adults for depression in primary care settings improves health outcomes when coupled with effective treatment and follow-up. As there was not enough evidence to recommend for or against screening adults for depression in primary care settings, when appropriate treatment and follow-up are accessible (grade I recommendation: there is insufficient evidence – in quantity or quality – to make a recommendation, however, other factors may influence decision making), the CTFPHC recommended that physicians endorse screening with integrated treatment and feedback into daily primary care practice. (See 'Implications' section in this chapter regarding chronic disease management models in primary care and adopting shared or collaborative care models).

Overall, the adoption of screening for adults in primary care settings should be supported by clinical evidence and cost-effectiveness. To date, the evidence for screening is not extensive and outstanding issues with regard to cost-effectiveness and feasibility remain. Moreover, there are specific, at-risk populations where the accuracy of screening tools and the effectiveness of subsequent interventions require more research. As there are no clear biomarkers for depression, the identification of depression may vary widely depending on the instrument, subjects, and settings involved. Screening is not indicated when there is no known effective intervention. Also, screening may be considered unethical if such an intervention is known, but cannot be made available to those screening positive.

For example, while depression is common in children and adolescents, little information on the overall effectiveness of screening is available. This may be due, in part, to uncertainties about how to best treat depression in this age group and concerns about potential negative outcomes and costs of false positives. Efforts to accurately identify depression in youths and adolescents in school settings have been made[45] and do not appear to have an immediate distressful effect on those studied.[46] A recent meta-analysis based on eight screening and early psychological intervention studies is promising, but further research is needed.[47] Screening instruments for use among elderly primary care patients are available.[48] Research on screening in work place settings with appropriate treatment management in place would seem a logical next step, given that the evidence for the effective treatment of depression is strongest in adults. (See following section in this chapter and 'Prevention and Health Promotion Strategies for Depression – Adults in the Workplace Environment' section).

Depression and the Use of Mental Health Services in Canada

A consistent finding in Canadian cross-sectional surveys has been that about half of all individuals who meet diagnostic criteria for depression in the past 12 months report a mental health contact during the same time frame. The first major population-based studies of *DSM-III-R* mental disorder and mental health service use in Canada were conducted in Edmonton, Alberta, in the mid to late 1980s[49,50] and then later the MHS-OHS in Ontario in 1990.[51] In the MHS-OHS, of those aged 15–54 years of age with major depression, 48.9% reported use of mental health services in the past 12 months.[52] In the decade after the MHS, the pattern of mental health service use for those with major depression were estimated through a shorter battery of questions in larger national household telephone surveys, the NPHS and in the CCHS 1.1. As the short-form measure of depression is not equivalent to major depression but likely a broader syndrome,[53] it is referred to as 'probable' depression hereafter. In the 1994–5 NPHS, 43% of those with probable depression, age 12 years or more reported having talked to a health professional about their emotional or mental health.[54] More recent estimates of the use of mental health services by persons with *DSM-IV* major depression are now available through the CCHS 1.2 conducted in 2001. The CCHS 1.2, like the earlier studies, conducted structured diagnostic interviews, most often within the respondents' home. Among those with major depression in the past 12 months, contact with a mental health professional was found to be similar to previous estimates, around 50%.[55] This was also the case in the province of Ontario.[56]

While the 50% unmet need estimate has been fairly consistent over time, it is important to recognize there is some 'noise' associated with this estimate. For example, in the CCHS 1.2, homeless persons or those who lived in an institution or on reserves were not included in the sampling frame. Persons who lived at home but were severely depressed may have declined to be interviewed altogether. As well, there is also an ongoing debate as to the reliability and validity of structured diagnostic interviews administered by trained lay interviewers, as opposed to those by clinicians. A more fundamental issue, though, is that the lower prevalence of major depression in the general population mathematically reduces the ability of a diagnostic instrument to accurately predict major depression in an individual.[57] Accordingly, it is not known how many of these people truly suffered from a clinical or major depression that would have benefited from treatment had they accessed it. Tied to this is whether persons who met criteria for major depression in the past but who no longer meet criteria for depression in the present and report current treatment should be counted as having met need.[58]

Further questions pertain to self-reports of mental health service use. For a variety of reasons, people may under-report this use. Two studies that directly compared self-reports of use to administrative claims-based estimates in Ontario suggest that the recall of use is affected by mood states and can be biased when use is self-reported.[58,59] That is, persons with current symptoms may actually recall their use 'better' than those without current symptoms. It is important to note, though, that in both studies, the majority of those with probable depression in the past 12 months had a high level of current distress. Therefore, self-reported estimates of use *among* those with depression may not be biased by current mood state, as most would work equally hard at recalling their use. Indeed, the gap between the prevalence of probable depression and use in these studies and in a later prospective one[60] did not disappear when self-reported data were replaced with administrative records. A more recent study comparing estimates of ambulatory mental health contacts in the CCHS 1.2 with those in administrative records suggests that the elderly are less likely to self-report ambulatory mental health contacts.[61] This may be due to true difficulties in recall coupled with competing mental and physical health concerns addressed in a visit or the ecological nature of the comparisons. Accordingly, more caution should be taken when considering self-reported estimates of service use among the depressed elderly.

The Nature of Care Received

Several researchers have sought to better describe the nature and quantity of mental health contacts received. In particular, the number of mental health contacts reported to a mental health professional and/or the use of antidepressant medications have been examined. While it is unclear exactly what takes place during a contact, in relation to evidence-based treatment guidelines summarized above, ongoing monitoring is viewed necessary for medication monitoring and the provision of evidence-based psychotherapies. In the MHS-OHS, 18% of those with major depression aged 15 to 64 reported antidepressant use in the past 12 months.[62] In depressed persons aged 21 to 54 years of age, 14.9% were defined as having had 'appropriate' management; i.e., self-report of antidepressant use and four or more mental health visits to a health professional in the past 12 months.[54] In the 1994–5 NPHS, 26% of those with probable depression reported four or more contacts in which they talked to a health professional about their emotional or mental health.[54] In Atlantic Canada, of those with probable depression in the CCHS 1.1, 24.4% reported four or more mental health contacts in the previous year.[63] Together, these studies would suggest that about one-quarter of those with major depression in the past 12 months were being actively treated for depression, defined at least in relation to contact and/or medication use.

Again, it should be noted that the same methodological issues above apply to estimates of active treatment for depression. A further consideration is that there is less certainty about how well persons are able to recall the number of contacts they made. Accordingly, estimates of 'active' or 'appropriate use' that are based on self-reports of volume of use may be discordant with administrative records.[58,59] However, it is conceivable that of the 50% who make contact, about half are in the acute treatment phase of depression. Cross-sectional data do not capture these processes well. A prospective study conducted in Ontario followed people sampled in the NPHS 1996/97 with probable depression in the past year and a high level of distress (one month) at baseline. When each individual's medical records were linked to his/her survey response, it was found that 46% made a mental health visit to a physician over the following two years. In terms of the number of visits made, about 25% made two or more mental health visits to a physician in the past year and over the following year, and about 25% made three or more over the following two years.[56,59]

Of greater concern is the potential that antidepressants are being prescribed to more people but the degree of assessment and monitoring has declined over time. There is evidence to suggest that in Canada, more persons with depression are receiving antidepressants than ever before; however, information about the number and nature of the visits in relation to the prescribing of an antidepressant is lacking. An increase in antidepressant two-day use was observed for people with probable depression in the respective NPHS samples: 18.2% in 1994/95 and 32.6% in 1998/99.[64] Most of the increase occurred for newer agents, such as SSRIs.[65] Use of antidepressants over a two-day period was also captured in the CCHS 1.2. Among those with major depression in the past 12 months, 13.5% reported current two-day use of an antidepressant and 10.4% used an SSRI.[66] Self-reported antidepressant use over the past 12 months was also examined in the CCHS 1.2. Among persons with depression in the past year, 40.4% reported taking antidepressants. Overall, 5.8% of Canadians took antidepressants, higher than the annual prevalence of depression (4.8%) in the survey. This difference was explained in part by those with a past history of depression and/or other illnesses measured in the CCHS 1.2. Some of this difference may also be explained by poor recall of a past episode or by use among individuals with subthreshold depression. Without further information, it is difficult to judge whether these patterns of care are appropriate. Of note, depressed women were more likely to report antidepressant use than depressed men. Among the depressed, those over age 25 were more likely than 15–25 year olds to report use of antidepressants.[67]

Differential Patterns of Care

In addition to questions about whether depression is being optimally treated in the population over time are questions related to differential access to quality care over time and the ensuing health care costs and outcomes. This information is necessary for ongoing system evaluation, resource allocation, and training purposes.

Canadian surveys suggest that among persons who were depressed within the past 12 months, indicators of severity such as suicidality,[16,54] level of distress,[59] concurrent anxiety disorders; concurrent physical health problems,[54] and duration of depression[55] are among the strongest predictors of a mental health contact. However, male sex, lower educational attainment,[54,60] younger age (15–25 years),[55] and discomfort with help-seeking[68] may also be deterrents. Due to the large number of subjects required, it has proven difficult to derive estimates of treated prevalence of depression for planning regions[68] or within urban as compared to rural areas.[69,70]

Previously in this chapter it was noted that only about one-half of those with major depression report contact with mental health services over the past 12 months. However, it has been observed that most make contact with a family physician or a general practitioner. For example, in the MHS, 91.5% of those with an affective disorder had contacted a primary care physician for general health reasons.[71] In the 1998–9 NPHS, 90.4% of those with probable depression reported contacting a general practitioner or family physician (GP/FP) for any reason, but only 40.6% reported having received mental health services.[70] A similar proportion (89.1%) was also found in Atlantic Canada, based on the CCHS 1.1.[63] While some of the difference between general use and mental health use may be due to reporting differences, for example in the elderly, it appears there is room for improvement in the detection and treatment of depression in primary care settings. (see under 'Implications') As well, the overall less frequent use of unconventional and self-help services by persons with depression is noteworthy[55] and may be a largely untapped resource worthy of further evaluation.

The size of the CCHS 1.2 provided the opportunity to examine the nature and quality of the care provided at sub-national levels. In Ontario these data were used to describe the care provided to persons with major depression in Ontario during a time when 95% of physicians were reimbursed through the fee-for-service provincial health care plan and prior to the implementation of primary care reforms.[61] Some highlights are:

- Of those with depression who reported a mental health contact, about 91% reported ambulatory mental health contact(s) only. Of this group, almost three-quarters contacted a GP/FP. The next most commonly contacted health professionals were a psychiatrist (41.3%); a social worker, counsellor, or psychotherapist (29.3%), and then a psychologist (15.2%).
- Among those with depression who reported ambulatory mental health contact(s) with a GP/FP, 41.8% contacted a GP/FP 'solo' for their mental health contact(s).
- The median number of contacts made to the 'solo' GP/FP was four and almost three-quarters reported more than one contact with this same GP/FP.
- When more than one provider group was contacted, the median number of visits increased and it became difficult to distinguish one provider group as the most consistent.
- At least 80% of persons with depression who reported contacts with a GP/FP 'solo' or in combination with a psychiatrist or with a social worker/counsellor or psychotherapist reported that they were satisfied or very satisfied with the services or treatments that the GP/FP provided and felt they were helped some or a lot by the GP/FP.

These findings are consistent with the broader literature wherein mental health care is typically provided in ambulatory care settings and GP/FPs are the most commonly contacted providers. Depression is sometimes treated 'solo' by a GP/FP and this may be most appropriate when the depression is not severe in nature. Other specialty groups are frequently involved but how these groups work together over time and with the client is not known. In a similar vein, the extent to which self-help or peer-support groups are integrated into ongoing care is uncertain. The consistency of the care providers and level of satisfaction reported by the clients is encouraging; however, it would be premature to conclude that this translates into better health outcomes.

Implications

Clinical guidelines for the treatment of depression emphasize the importance of education about depression, its diagnosis, and course and treatment options. Monitoring of treatment response is critical, particularly for suicidality when antidepressant therapy is initiated. Recommended treatments for depression are not short term and typically treatment response is not immediate. The acute phase of depression is therefore a key time to educate clients about the illness, its diagnosis, and course and treatment options. Special populations such as children and adolescents, pregnant and breast-feeding women, the elderly, and those with comorbid physical conditions pose more careful consideration given the available and evolving evidence. As depression remits and during the maintenance phase, when individuals are better able to return to regular roles and activities, the ability to monitor oneself and seek help when appropriate becomes essential. This process may take time given denial and feelings of shame about mental illness.[35] Health care providers play an important role in conveying hope and commitment to the treatment process particularly those in ambulatory care settings and general practitioners and family physicians as a first point and possibly only point of contact. At each phase of treatment, other supports and services, such as peer-support and self-help may also contribute. Further research in these areas is desired.[35]

Those who present with mild or sub-threshold depression pose a dilemma, as some may want to be prescribed antidepressants. In the absence of alternatives, it is difficult to deny clients a therapy they may benefit from. Nevertheless, antidepressants are not without systemic effects and some are adverse in nature even if temporary. Others may prefer to pursue psychotherapy; however, this option becomes less feasible given a lack of publicly funded trained psychotherapists. As women in their reproductive years are more likely than men to have depression and tend to access their mental health care from GP/FPs, they stand to benefit the most from known effective treatments delivered in primary care settings. This is also likely true for the elderly. Males may delay seeking help, if it is sought at all and, therefore, be at greater risk for the negative consequences of depression.[72] The finding that among those with depression, males were less likely than females to report taking an antidepressant in the past year[67] may reflect women seeking and getting treatment earlier. However, there is uncertainty about the relative benefits and harms of increased access to antidepressants[73] at unknown levels of medication monitoring. An increase in demand for these medications could affect the quality of care if there has been no change or a reduction in the supply of mental health care providers.[61]

Given that most people with depression access primary care, the potential for improving the detection and treatment of depression in primary care is receiving a great deal of attention. There is a growing interest in applying components of chronic disease management models in primary care and adopting shared or collaborative care models with respect to the detection and treatment of depression in Canada.[74,75] These models have been shown to benefit those with depression in other countries, most frequently in the United States. While the evidence is encouraging, it is not known how much more will be gained through implementation of these models in Canada. The study settings were controlled and the samples select. It is also unclear how control groups (i.e., 'usual care') in these settings compares to that in Canadian jurisdictions. It has been difficult to describe 'usual care' in Canada, given the lack of population-based data on the process and outcomes of care for depression. Previous work has relied heavily on cross-sectional household surveys and self-reports, as opposed to population-based longitudinal studies of depressed people in ambulatory care settings. Successful implementation of new models of care will depend in part on the nature of existing roles and relationships between providers.[76] Adoption of models will also depend upon the existence of trained providers and reimbursement/inclusion of providers not currently publicly funded.[35] Nevertheless, components of these models, such as provider education, client self-management education, care coordination, and pro-active follow-up, may be implemented and evaluated more readily. Some components of these models may already be offered in communities; e.g., through peer-support, and could be better integrated within the existing primary settings. Of note, the provision of education or guidelines alone is not considered effective.

The often early age of onset and high prevalence of depression for those under age 18 coupled with uncertainties about effective treatments make prevention efforts in this age group attractive. For young children, treatment of mental illness in the family members, particularly depression in the mother, may prevent depression in the children.[31] A critical time may be the postpartum period and, therefore, depression prevention and health promotion programs for new mothers in addition to the cost-benefits of screening tied to effective treatment programs merit more research.[25] While the quality of the evidence for universal interventions in preventing depression for children and adolescents in school-based settings is limited, this is also an important area for further research. Screening is less attractive given uncertainties about the effectiveness of treatment, shortages of trained personnel, and inconsistencies in laws concerning consent for screening versus consent for treatment. Carefully constructed and targeted educational programs about mental illness in school settings may help reduce stigma about mental illness and facilitate future help seeking when needed.[35]

For populations in the work force, including men and women who have children or others who depend on them, personal and organizational level changes in the workplace can reach a broad segment of the population. Further research into costs and benefits of specific interventions in Canadian settings is therefore, quite desirable.

REFERENCES

1 Patten SB, Wang J, Williams J, et al. Descriptive epidemiology of major depression in Canada. *Can J Psychiatry* 2006;51:84–90.

2 Hasin DS, Goodwin RD, Stinson FS, et al. Epidemiology of major depressive disorder: Results from the National Epidemiologic Survey on Alcoholism and Related Conditions. *Arch Gen Psychiatry* 2005;62:1097–106.

3 Waraich P, Goldner EM, Somers JM, et al. Prevalence and incidence studies of mood disorders: A systematic review of the literature. *Can J Psychiatry* 2004;49:124–38.

4 Kessler RC, Berglund P, Demler O, et al. The epidemiology of major depressive disorder: Results from the National Comorbidity Survey Replication (NCS-R). *JAMA* 2003;289:3095–105.

5 WHO International Consortium in Psychiatric Epidemiology. Cross-national comparison of the prevalences and correlates of mental disorders. *Bull World Health Organ* 2000;78:413–26.

6 Nguyen CT, Fournier L, Bergeron L, et al. Correlates of depressive and anxiety disorders among young Canadians. *Can J Psychiatry* 2005;50:620–8.

7 Streiner DL, Cairney J, Veldhuizen S. The epidemiology of psychological problems in the elderly. *Can J Psychiatry* 2006;51:185–91.

8 Ostbye T, Kristjansson B, Hill G, et al. Prevalence and predictors of depression in elderly Canadians: The Canadian Study of Health and Aging. *Chronic Dis Can* 2005;26:93–9.

9 Kessler RC, Chiu WT, Demler O, et al. Prevalence, severity, and comorbidity of 12-month DSM-IV disorders in the National Comorbidity Survey Replication. *Arch Gen Psychiatry* 2005;62:617–27.

10 Alonso J, Angermeyer MC, Bernert S, et al. 12-Month comorbidity patterns and associated factors in Europe: Results from the European Study of the Epidemiology of Mental Disorders (ESEMeD) project. *Acta Psychiatr Scand Suppl* 2004;420:28–37.

11 Gagnon LM, Patten SB. Major depression and its association with long-term medical conditions. *Can J Psychiatry* 2002;47:149–52.

12 Beaudet M. Psychological health-depression. *Health Rep* 1999;11:63–75.

13 Newman SC, Bland RC. Incidence of mental disorders in Edmonton: Estimates of rates and methodological issues. *J Psychiatric Res* 1998;32: 273–82.

14 Murphy JM, Laird NM, Monson RR, et al. Incidence of depression in the Stirling County Study: Historical and comparative perspectives. *Psychol Med* 2000;30:505–14.

15 Patten SB. Incidence of major depression in Canada. *CMAJ* 2000;163:714–15.

16 Rhodes A, Bethell J, Bondy S. Suicidality, depression and mental health service use in Canada. *Can J Psychiatry* 2006;51:35–41.

17 Wulsin LR, Vaillant GE, Wells VE. A systematic review of the mortality of depression. *Psychosom Med* 1999;61:6–17.

18 Guze SB, Robins E. Suicide and primary affective disorders. *Br J Psychiatry* 1970;117:437–8.

19 Mrazek P, Haggerty R. *Reducing Risks for Mental Disorders: Frontiers for Preventive Intervention Research*. Washington DC: National Academy Press, 1994.

20 Ogrodniczuk JS, Piper WE. Preventing postnatal depression: A review of research findings. *Harv Rev Psychiatry* 2003;11:291–307.

21 Public Health Agency of Canada. *Population Health Promotion: An Inte-*

grated Model of' Population Health and Health Promotion. Government of Canada 2006. http://www.phac-aspc.gc.ca/ph-sp/php-psp/php3.htm. Accessed August 21, 2007.

22 Jane-Llopis E, Hosman C, Jenkins R, et al. Predictors of efficacy in depression prevention programmes. Meta-analysis. *Br J Psychiatry* 2003;183:384–97.

23 Cuijpers P, Van SA, Smit F. Preventing the incidence of new cases of mental disorders: A meta-analytic review. *J Nerv Ment Dis* 2005;193:119–25.

24 Austin MP. Targeted group antenatal prevention of postnatal depression: A review. *Acta Psychiatr Scand* 2003;107:244–50.

25 Dennis CL, Creedy D. Psychosocial and psychological interventions for preventing postpartum depression. *Cochrane Database Syst Rev* 2004;(4):CD001134.

26 Dennis C, Ross L, Grigoriadis S. Psychosocial and psychological interventions for treating antenatal depression. *Cochrane Database Syst Rev* 2007;(3):CD006309).

27 Ray KL, Hodnett ED. Caregiver support for postpartum depression. *Cochrane Database Syst Rev* 2001;(3):CD000946.

28 Gavin N, Gaynes B, Lohr K, et al. Perinatal depression. A systematic review of prevalence and incidence. *Obstet Gynecol* 2005;5:1071–83.

29 Merry S. Prevention and early intervention for depression in young people – a practical possibility? *Curr Opin Psychiatry* 2007;20:325–9.

30 Larun L, Nordheim L, Ekland E, et al. Exercise in the prevention and treatment of anxiety and depression among children and young people. *Cochrane Database Syst Rev* 2006;3:1–60.

31 Weissman MM, Pilowsky DJ, Wickramaratne PJ, et al. Remissions in maternal depression and child psychopathology: A STAR*D-child report. *JAMA* 2006;295:1389–98.

32 Bilsker D, Gilbert M, Myette L, et al. *Depression and Work Function: Bridging the Gap between Mental Health Care and the Workplace.* 2004. http://www.carmha.ca/ publications/resources/dwf/Work_Depression.pdf. Accessed April 20, 2007.

33 Sanderson K, Andrews G. Common mental disorders in the workforce: Recent findings from descriptive and social epidemiology. *Can J Psychiatry* 2006;51:63–75.

34 Wang PS, Simon GE, Avorn J, et al. Telephone screening, outreach and care management for depressed workers and impact on clinical and work productivity outcomes. A randomized controlled trial. *JAMA* 2007;298:1401–11.

35 The Standing Senate Committee on Social Affairs, Science and Technol-

ogy. Final report on Mental Health, Mental Illness and Addictions. *Out of the Shadows at Last. Transforming Mental Health, Mental Illness and Addiction Services in Canada.* The Honourable Michael J. L. Kirby, Chair. The Honourable Wilbert Joseph Keon, Deputy Chair, May 2006. http://www .parl.gc.ca/39/1/ parlbus/commbus/senate/com-e/soci-e/rep-e/rep02 may06-e.htm. Accessed November 1, 2006.

36 Bilsker D, Wiseman S, Gilbert M. Managing depression-related occupational disability: A pragmatic approach. *Can J Psychiatry* 2006;51:76–83.

37 Pinquart M, Sörensen S. How effective are psychotherapeutic and other psychosocial interventions with older adults? A Meta-analysis. *J Ment Health Aging* 2001;7:207–43.

38 Cole M, Dendukuri N. The feasibility and effectiveness of brief interventions to prevent depression in older adults: A systematic review. *Int J Geriatr Psychiatry* 2004;19:1019–25.

39 World Health Organization. *Prevention of Mental Disorders: Effective Interventions and Policy Options.* 2004.
http://www.who.int/mental_health/evidence/en/prevention_of_ mental_disorders_sr.pdf. Accessed April 20, 2007.

40 Costello E, Compton S, Keeler G, et al. Relationships between poverty and psychopathology: A natural experiment. *JAMA* 2003;290:2023–9.

41 Last M. *A Dictionary of Epidemiology.* 4th ed. Oxford: Oxford University Press, 2001.

42 U.S. Preventive Services Task Force. *Screening for Depression.* Agency for Health Care Research and Quality, 2002. http: //www.ahrq.gov/clinic /uspstf/uspsdepr.htm. Accessed February 2, 2006.

43 Pignone MP, Gaynes BN, Rushton JL, et al. Screening for depression in adults: A summary of the evidence for the U.S. Preventive Services Task Force. *Ann Intern Med* 2002;136:765–76.

44 MacMillan HL, Patterson CJ, Wathen CN, et al. Screening for depression in primary care: Recommendation statement from the Canadian Task Force on Preventive Health Care. *CMAJ* 2005;172:33–5.

45 Shaffer D, Scott M, Wilcox H, et al. The Columbia Suicide Screen: Validity and reliability of a screen for youth suicide and depression. *J Am Acad Child Adolesc Psychiatry* 2004;43:71–9.

46 Gould MS, Marrocco FA, Kleinman M, et al. Evaluating iatrogenic risk of youth suicide screening programs: A randomized controlled trial. *JAMA* 2005;293:1635–43.

47 Cuijpers P, Van SA, Smits N, et al. Screening and early psychological intervention for depression in schools. Systematic review and meta-analysis. *Eur Child Adoles Psychiatry* 2006;15:300–7.

48 Watson L, Pignone MP. Screening accuracy for late-life depression in primary care: A systematic review. *J Fam Pract* 2003;52:956–64.
49 Bland RC, Newman SC, Orn H. Health care utilization for emotional problems: Results from a community survey. *Can J Psychiatry* 1990;35:397–400.
50 Bland RC, Newman SC, Orn H. Help-seeking for psychiatric disorders. *Can J Psychiatry* 1997;42:935–42.
51 Boyle MH, Offord DR, Campbell D, et al. Mental health supplement to the Ontario Health Survey: Methodology. *Can J Psychiatry* 1996;41:549–58
52 Parikh SV, Lesage A, Kennedy S, et al. Depression in Ontario: Under-treatment and factors related to antidepressant use. *J Affect Dis* 1999;52:67–76.
53 Patten S, Wang J, Beck C, et al. Measuring issues related to the evaluation and monitoring of major depression prevalence in Canada. *Chronic Dis Can* 2005;26:100–6.
54 Diverty B, Beaudet M. Depression: An undertreated disorder? *Health Rep* 1997;8:9–18.
55 Wang J, Patten S, Williams J, et al. Help-seeking behaviours of individuals with mood disorders. *Can J Psychiatry* 2005;50:652.
56 Rhodes A, Bondy S, Jaakkimainen L. *Depression – A Grade of Care in an Insured Population.* Poster Presentation, San Francisco, American Public Health Association, 2003.
57 Beck CA, Patten SB. Adjustment to antidepressant utilization rates to account for depression in remission. *Compr Psychiatry* 2007;45:268–74.
58 Rhodes A, Lin E, Mustard C. Self-reported use of mental health services versus administrative records: Should we care? *Int J Methods Psychiatr Res* 2002;11:125–33.
59 Rhodes A, Fung K. Self-reported use of mental health services versus administrative records: Care to recall? *Int J Methods Psychiatr Res* 2004;13:165–75.
60 Rhodes A, Jaakkimainen L, Bondy S, et al. Depression and mental health visits to physicians: A prospective records-based study. *Soc Sci Med* 2006;62:828–34.
61 Rhodes A, Bethell J, Schultz S. *Primary Mental Health Care.* Ontario: Institute for Clinical Evaluative Sciences, Report No. 9, 2006.
62 Katz SJ, Kessler RC, Lin E, Wells K. Medication management of depression in the United States and Ontario. *J Gen Intern Med* 1998;13:77–85.
63 Starkes J, Poulin C, Kisely S. Unmet need for the treatment of depression in Atlantic Canada. *Can J Psychiatry* 2005;50:580–90.
64 Patten S. Progress against major depression in Canada. *Can J Psychiatry* 2002;47:775–80.

65 Patten S. Major depression and mental health care utilization in Canada: 1994 to 2000. *Can J Psychiatry* 2005;49:303–9.

66 Beck C, Williams J, Wang J, et al. Psychotropic medication use in Canada. *Can J Psychiatry* 2006;50:605–13.

67 Beck C, Patten S, Williams J, et al. Antidepressant utilization in Canada. *Soc Psychiatry Psychiatr Epidemiol* 2005;40:799–807.

68 Lin E, Parikh SV. Sociodemographic, clinical and attitudinal characteristics of the untreated depressed in Ontario. *J Affect Dis* 1999;53:153–62.

69 Parikh SV, Wasylenki D, Goering P, et al. Mood disorders: Rural/urban differences in prevalence, health care utilization, and disability in Ontario. *J Affect Dis* 1996;38:57–65.

70 Wang J, Langille D, Patten S. Mental health services received by depressed persons who visited general practitioners and family doctors. *Psychiatr Serv* 2003;54:878–83.

71 Parikh S, Lin E, Lesage A. Mental health treatment in Ontario: Selected comparisons between the primary care and specialty sectors. *Can J Psychiatry* 1997;42:878–83.

72 Rhodes A. Women's need and use of mental health services. In: Romans S, Seeman M, eds. *Women's Mental Health: A Life-cycle Approach.* Baltimore: Lippincott, Williams and Wilkins, 2005:367–75.

73 Hemels M, Koren G, Einarson T. Increased use of antidepressants in Canada: 1981–2000. *Ann Pharmacother* 2002;36:1375–9.

74 Craven M, Bland RC. Better practices in collaborative mental health care: An analysis of the evidence base. *Can J Psychiatry* 2006;51 (Suppl 1):s1–s72.

75 Kates N, Mach M. Chronic disease management for depression in primary care: A summary of the current literature and implications for practice. *Can J Psychiatry* 2007;52:77–85.

76 Gilbody S, Whitty P, Grimshaw J, et al. Educational and organizational interventions to improve the management of depression in primary care: A systematic review. *JAMA* 2003;289:3145–51.

18 Examining the Mental Health of the Working Population: Organizations, Individuals, and Haystacks

CAROLYN S. DEWA, ELIZABETH LIN, MARC CORBIÈRE, AND
MARTIN SHAIN

The purpose of this chapter is to discuss the factors that contribute to the mental health of the working population. In the first section, we consider the salience of this topic and the related economic burden of mental illness in the working population. This is followed by brief reviews of the organizational characteristics that contribute to an unhealthy workplace and individual characteristics that would render a worker susceptible to such an environment. We then look at two examples of how population-based epidemiological surveys have been used to explore the topic. We conclude with a discussion of the strengths and limitations of population-based data for workplace mental health.

Why Is Mental Health in the Working Population Important?

In Canada, there has been growing awareness that mental and emotional health problems are associated with staggering social and economic costs that place a heavy burden on the workplace. In its recent report, the Standing Senate Committee on Social Affairs, Science and Technology[1] raised prevention, promotion, and treatment of mental illness as critical issues to be addressed. The committee went on to identify the workplace as one of the prime areas in which to begin. They state, 'It is in the workplace that the human and economic dimensions of mental health and mental illness come together most evidently.'[1(p171)]

Mental and behavioural disorders account for approximately 12% of all diseases and injuries worldwide.[2] For countries such as Canada, the percentage of all disorders and injuries attributable to mental disorders is closer to 25%, with as much as 13% attributable to depression alone.[3] By the year 2020, it is expected that depression will emerge as one of the leading causes of disability globally, second only to ischaemic heart disease.[2] It is estimated that approximately 5% of the working-aged population suffers from depression during a 12-month period.[4] Moreover, about 10% of the working population has a mental disorder.[5]

In North America, the estimated annual societal costs of mental disorders range from $14.4 billion (CAD) in Canada[6] to $83.1 billion (USD) in the United States.[7] Between 30% and 60% of the societal cost of depression is related to losses associated with work disruptions.[6,7] It has been reported that workplace absenteeism related to mental health problems accounts for about 7% of the total payroll and is one of the principal causes of absences.[8] These estimates provide a strong incentive to promote worker mental health.

Although the effects of mental illness on the labour force are of critical concern, little is known about the causes of mental disorders in the working population. For example, the most advanced etiological models of adult depression include factors related to genetic vulnerability, as well as developmental factors, neurobiological factors, childhood experiences, life events, chronic situations (e.g., a stressful work environment), and the presence of other disorders.[9] It is not yet understood what the due weight of each of these dimensions is and how they fit together.

However, there is awareness that there is a complex relationship among factors that contribute to worker health. Loisel and colleagues[10] conceptualized the contributing factors within systems that include the workplace system, the health care system, the legislative and insurance system, and the personal system/personal coping; all of these exist within an overall societal context. Although they focused on disability management for musculoskeletal pain, there are similarities between worker impairment related to musculoskeletal pain and that related to mental illness.[11] Loisel et al.'s[10] four systems of factors form the broad building blocks contributing to worker mental health.

Workplace stress has been identified as one of the mechanisms through which worker mental health is affected.[12,13] Noblet and LaMontagne[14] reported the conditions under which occupational stress occurs: 'Occupational stress occurs when external demands and conditions do not match a person's needs, expectations or ideas or exceed their physical capacity, skills, or knowledge for comfortably handling a situation.'[14(p346)] This definition suggests that two immediate sources of stress for workers are their working conditions and themselves. But, rather than two distinct entities, Noblet and Lamontagne suggest that stress is also related to the interface between the organization and the individual. This interface involves questions of person-environment fit.

Consequently, it is not surprising that of the four systems identified by Loisel and colleagues,[10] the two that have attracted the greatest research activity are the workplace system and the personal system/personal coping. There is a large and expanding body of research in these two areas examining the relationship between workplace stress, mental illness, and disability.[12,15–17]

The Workplace System:
Overview of Organizational Characteristics
Contributing to Unhealthy Workplaces

Since the seminal work of Karasek and Theorell in the late 1980s and 1990s, research related to the effect of work organization on health has been dominated by the Demand/Control/Social Support Model[18] and more recently by the Effort Reward Imbalance Model.[19] The essence of these models is the proposition that job responsibilities in which a worker perceives s/he is under too much demand, has too little job control, is required to exert too much effort, and is given too little reward are not advantageous to worker health. Together, these job characteristics create unhealthy work situations that contribute to illnesses including depression,[20–24] anxiety,[24–26] and cancer,[27] as well as injury such as repetitive strains and back problems.[28–30]

We know that certain ways of organizing work are more likely than others to increase the risk or probability of harm to the mental or emotional health of workers (for a review, see[31]). This is particularly evident when different organizations in the same geographic area or even departments within a single organization are performing the same type of work, where the same sorts of people are employed to do it, yet the outcomes as measured by worker mental health status or work stress differ. For example, one sawmill was observed to have three times the rate of mental health related absences and accidents as another sawmill owned by the same company in the same valley. Discrepancies of a similar nature were observed between two units in one hospital and two police units in one division.[32]

Essentially the study of such differences allows us to measure at a local level what is referred to at a population level as an *etiologic fraction* (EF). An EF is the proportion of a disease or state that would not have occurred had a risk factor been absent in the population. Based on their studies of countries in the European Union, Levi and Lunde-Jensen[33] estimated that, on average, 10% of the workforce was in a very high stress risk group at any given time due to the effects of adverse but modifiable workplace governance practices. These rates varied across countries between 4% and 23%. Italy, Portugal, and the Netherlands scored low while Germany, Greece, and the United Kingdom scored high based on the 1991–1992 data from the First European Survey of the Working Environment.

Canadian figures derived from Health Canada's Workplace Health System employer surveys are usually in a similar range but with very high stress rates approaching 33% in some instances.[32] The Canadian data, unlike the European Union's,[33] are not population-based but rather are derived from studies of specific workplaces conducted during the implementation of an intervention, namely the Workplace Health System.[32] The Workplace Health System employer database currently is composed of survey information gathered from approximately 650,000 employees from all sectors of the Canadian economy over a 20 year period.

The ability to estimate the EF at a population as well as at a workplace-specific level is of more than academic interest. Indeed, the correct identification of causal sources (etiology) is of practical importance because it contributes to the discussion of how the responsibility might be allocated for reducing the burden of impaired mental health on individuals, families, communities, and society at large. To the extent that the role of the organization of work can be conceptualized and quantified as a cause of, or influence on, mental health problems, we can determine the degree to which this role can be modified and who is responsible for doing this.

The Personal System/Personal Coping: Overview of Individual Worker Characteristics Contributing to Susceptibility

Not only are there data that organizational factors play a significant role in worker mental health, there also is sufficient evidence indicating individual characteristics also make a contribution. In the next section, we consider individual worker factors that could put them at risk to succumbing to the type of unhealthy environmental factors described in the previous section. An important source of information about these factors comes from the work being done to decrease worker disability using cognitive behavourial therapy (CBT). CBT, like other types of psychological interventions, focuses on coping strategies, problem-solving strategies, and belief/attitude adjustments. This is due to observations that the objective criteria regarding work are often less important than subjective perceptions of job-related stress and other psychological hindrances (e.g., perceptions of a demanding job, lack of support from the supervisor; for a review see[34]). That is, an individual's specific misconceptions and maladaptive assumptions can lead to unhealthy behaviours that result in feelings of stress.[35] This suggests that it is not the workplace alone but individual reactions that also contribute to the negative effects of workplace stress. Thus, employees play an active role in their personal recovery and mental health.[36,37] It has been reported that only a few stress-reducing interventions actually focus on the organization while the work environment is involved in almost 90% of the cases linked to work absences due to mental health problems.[38] Part of this may be because there is more evidence for the effectiveness of cognitive behavioural interventions targeting individuals.[39]

Empirical evidence indicates that when cognitive behavioural treatment is used in return-to-work (RTW) interventions, RTW rates are greater than the treatment as usual or control condition.[40] Also, when specific mental health outcomes were evaluated, such as depression and psychological distress, significant results in favour of the CBT were found.[40] However, it is important to highlight that even if CBT can help many injured employees return to work and improve their mental health problems, not everyone improves at the same rate, especially when comorbid depressive symptoms are present. Indeed, Corbière et al.[41] observed that injured employees with chronic pain who also had high depression levels could either deteriorate or improve in terms of depressive symptoms over time. Using an early screening for depressive symptoms, as well as follow-up assessments, could be useful to better understand the processes involved and to intervene more adequately.

Examples Using Population-Based Surveys

From the previous discussion, we see that a variety of factors are significantly associated with work stress and poor worker mental health. One of the advantages of using population-based surveys is that with them, we are able to explore the relationship between organizational factors and individual characteristics on worker disability and stress within the working population. This is useful for the surveillance of the mental health status of workers and their perceptions of their working environments. In this section, we talk about two examples of how a population-based survey, the CCHS 1.2 has been used to explore factors associated with workplace mental health.

Example 1. We used the CCHS 1.2 to explore the relationships among chronic work stress, psychiatric disorders, chronic physical conditions, and disability among workers.[5] We were able to do this because the survey included several questions that asked about employment status, occupation, disability, perception of work organization, and work stress as well as chronic physical conditions and psychiatric disorders.

With the employment status responses, we were able to focus the analyses on the 22,118 CCHS respondents aged 18–64 years old who indicated they were employed during the past year. Using a similar selection process as Kessler and Frank[42] and Dewa and Lin,[43] we were able to exclude respondents who indicated they were a full-time student, permanently unable to work, retired, or currently on maternity leave. In our analyses, we observed that nearly 75% of workers with psychiatric disorder also reported having either a chronic physical condition or chronic work stress or both (table 18.1). Furthermore, 43% of respondents with a psychiatric disorder reported experiencing chronic work stress.

Three disability questions were included in the survey. They asked about the number of days in the past 14 days the respondent had been in bed for all or most of the day (*total disability days*), cut down on their normal activities (*partial disability days*), or were able to complete normal activities only with extreme effort (*extra effort days*). Creating three indicator variables based on the responses to these questions, we examined their associations with combinations of psychiatric disorders, chronic work stress, and chronic physical conditions.

Table 18.1
Prevalence of disorders/conditions in working population, CCHS 1.2

Disorders/conditions	%	95% CI
No disorder/condition	32.80	(31.87, 33.73)
Chronic work stress only	12.25	(11.54, 12.96)
Chronic physical condition only	26.10	(25.30, 26.90)
Psychiatric disorder only	2.69	(2.39, 2.98)
Chronic work stress and chronic physical condition	13.74	(13.08, 14.40)
Psychiatric disorder and chronic physical condition	3.33	(3.04, 3.61)
Psychiatric disorder and chronic work stress	1.62	(1.37, 1.87)
Psychiatric disorder, chronic physical condition, and chronic work stress	2.94	(2.62, 3.27)

We found that the probability of disability related to psychiatric disorders was enhanced in the presence of chronic physical disorders and chronic work stress (figure 18.1). These results corroborated reports indicating comorbid psychiatric disorders and chronic physical conditions are more disabling than either psychiatric disorders or chronic physical conditions.[42-44] In the case of chronic physical conditions, we observed that the presence of chronic work stress along with either a psychiatric disorder or chronic physical condition appeared to increase the probability of disability.

Our findings indicate a more complex disability pattern for the association between psychiatric disorders and disability days in the presence of chronic work stress than previously reported.[43] In the presence of chronic work stress, psychiatric disorders are associated with a greater likelihood of total or partial disability days rather than extra effort days. This suggests that with chronic work stress, workers suffering from mental illness experience more disability days that are debilitating.

Example 2. The results of these analyses raise the question about the factors that are associated with chronic work stress. Using the CCHS 1.2 data, we were able to consider Loisel et al.'s[10] conceptualization of the systems contributing to work health: the workplace system, the health care system, the legislative and insurance system, and the personal system/personal coping.

Figure 18.1 The relationship between different levels of disability days and chronic work stress, chronic physical problems, and psychiatric disorders among workers

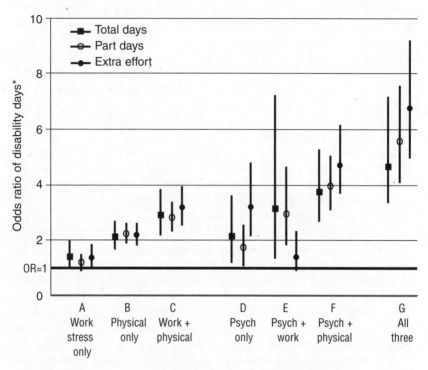

*Comparison group = no chronic work stress *or* chronic illness *or* psychiatric disorder
Source: CCHS 1.2 (Canadian Community Health Survey 1.2, Statistics Canada)

We could observe the associations involving the workplace system because the CCHS 1.2 included 12 items adapted from the Job Content Questionnaire (JCQ) by Karasek et al.[45] The JCQ was developed as an instrument to measure work demands. It has been evaluated cross-nationally in four countries (United States, Japan, Netherlands, and Canada) and has demonstrated good reliability and validity.[45] It is composed of five sub-scales that measure: (1) decision latitude, (2) psychological demands, (3) social support, (4) physical demands, and (5) job security. The 12 CCHS items are from all five sub-scales.[46]

In addition, the provincial/regional indicators available in the CCHS capture several of Loisel et al.'s[10] systems, including the health care system and the legislative and insurance system. With this, we assume that the provincial/regional indicators serve as proxies for unobserved factors that do not change in the short-run, such as the generosity of the province. For example, because the health care system is under provincial jurisdiction, there will be variation among provinces with regard to health care based on variability in provincial culture and values. Furthermore, to an extent, the legislative and insurance factors such as those influencing worker's compensation insurance will also be influenced by provincial culture. We used occupation to adjust for unknown subject and workplace characteristics. Because workers select their occupations to some extent, we assume that the occupation variables reflect individual characteristics.

To examine the factors that are associated with chronic work stress, we used a logistic regression model in which the dependent variable was chronic work stress. The chronic work stress variable was created as a dichotomous one using a single-item question that asked respondents to consider their main job or business and to rate whether they found most days in the past 12 months: (1) not at all stressful, (2) not very stressful, (3) a bit stressful, (4) quite a bit stressful, or (5) extremely stressful. Respondents in the last two categories were identified as experiencing chronic work stress. Thus, in these analyses, rather than a set of symptoms (i.e., psychological distress), chronic work stress indicates the respondent's perceived exposure to stressful stimuli. That is, responses were reflective of how respondents viewed their work environments and job characteristics.

The independent variables included five job characteristic dummy variables. They were created using the five sub-scales from the modified JCQ. The variables indicate whether in their main jobs, respondents experienced: (1) high skill discretion, (2) high job insecurity, (3) high physical exertion, (4) high social support, and (5) higher decision latitude than psychological demand. The high skill discretion, high job insecurity, high physical exertion, and high social support variables were coded a '1' if the respondent's responses on the respective sub-scales was greater than the median and '0' otherwise. The higher decision latitude than psychological demand variable was coded '1' if the value of a respondent's decision latitude sub-scale was larger than his/her psychological demand sub-scale and '0' otherwise. We created nine occupational dummy variables based on the occupational group the respondent endorsed: (1) Managerial, (2) Professional, (3) Technician, (4) Administrative/Financial/Clerical, (5) Sales/Services, (6) Trades/Transport/Equipment Operator, (7) Farming/Fishing/Forestry/Mining, (8) Manufacturing/Processing/Utilities, or (9) Other[47] (see table 18.2).

When professionals are used as the reference group, the results indicated that in comparison, all the other occupation groups had lower odds of reporting chronic work stress. The exceptions were those in management positions; they were 43% more likely to have chronic work stress compared to professionals. This finding is consistent with what has been reported in the literature with a higher rate of stress among managers and professionals.[48]

Considering job characteristics, we observed the odds of experiencing chronic work stress were significantly related to high skill discretion and job insecurity. In contrast, the odds significantly decreased with high social support and greater autonomy than psychological demands.

With regard to provinces, with Ontario as the reference group, workers in all the provinces had comparatively lower odds of reporting chronic work stress. The exception was for workers in Quebec. They were 61% more likely than workers in Ontario to report chronic work stress.

Our findings using the CCHS 1.2 reflect the complexity of the factors contributing to the mental health of the working population. As we would posit based on Loisel et al.'s conceptualization,[10] all the different systems are significantly associated with the average worker's experience of chronic work stress.

As Karasek and Theorell's Demand/Control/Social Support Model[45] and Siegrist's Effort Reward Imbalance Model[19] suggest, we observed job characteristics were related to chronic work stress. Greater autonomy relative to psychological demand, higher job insecurity, and higher skill discretion were related to greater likelihood of reporting chronic work stress. At the same time, greater social support was associated with lower odds of reporting chronic work stress.

But, we also observed that even after controlling for the contributions of job characteristics, certain occupations such as managerial and professional, were also related to chronic job stress. This could indicate two things. First, it may be that the individual characteristics that attract individuals to particular occupations are also associated with perceptions of stress. For example, it could be that people who have

Table 18.2
Association of selected factors with perceived chronic work stress, CCHS 1.2

	OR	95% CI
Job Characteristics		
High skill discretion	1.52[b]	(1.35,1.71)
High job insecurity	1.51[b]	(1.35,1.69)
High physical exertion	1.19	(1.08,1.32)
High social support	0.44[b]	(0.40,0.48)
Autonomy ≥ demand	0.65[b]	(0.58,0.72)
Occupation		
Managerial	1.43[b]	(1.22,1.68)
Technical	0.65[b]	(0.54,0.79)
Administrative/financial/clerical	0.88	(0.73,1.06)
Sales or service	0.65[b]	(0.53,0.76)
Trades/transport/equipment operator	0.53[b]	(0.44,0.64)
Farming, fishing, forestry, or mining	0.40[b]	(0.30,0.54)
Processing, manufacturing or utilities	0.53[b]	(0.42,0.66)
Other	0.54[b]	(0.44,0.65)
Province		
Prairies	0.88[a]	(0.79,0.98)
BC	0.92	(0.80,1.05)
Quebec	1.61[b]	(1.42,1.82)
Maritimes	0.73[b]	(0.64,0.83)
Demographic Characteristics		
Age	1.00	(1.00,1.01)
Male	0.86[a]	(0.77,0.96)
Single	0.83[b]	(0.74,0.93)
Disrupted marriage	1.13	(0.98,1.31)

[a]$p \leq 0.05$
[b]$p \leq 0.001$

tendencies toward being perfectionists and being obsessed with details may be more drawn to becoming professionals – researchers, for example. This drive may also be associated with creating higher expectations of oneself and in turn, greater likelihood of experiencing chronic work stress.

A second interpretation is that different occupations reflect different job characteristics. For instance, professionals may be under different expectations than clerical staff. As a result of the differing job demands, professionals are relatively more likely to experience more chronic work stress than clerical staff.

Interestingly, even after controlling for the contributions of job and individual characteristics, there were significant associations between the province/region in which the respondent resides and chronic work stress. This could reflect a number of things, including differences in the health care systems and the occupational health and safety legislation as well as cultural differences. Because with these data we cannot get any more specific than identifying the existence of provincial/regional differences, we cannot identify the contribution of the specific environmental factors to chronic work stress. We can only say that there is something significant within the different environments associated with chronic work stress.

Role of Population-Based Survey Data to Improve the Mental Health of the Workers

This finding also highlights one of the limitations of population-based surveys. We can collect information about the individual characteristics in terms of their demographics, health status, and their job characteristics, but we are less able to gather information about their environments. Often, individuals will not be fully aware of what is in their environments with regard to government policies regarding workplaces or the healthcare system.

Another limitation is that often population-based surveys are cross-sectional. As a result, we cannot use them to make statements about causality. It is possible that persons experiencing more work stress or persons at risk of having psychiatric disorders may select jobs with more conditions adverse to mental health.

A third limitation of population-based surveys is that the data collected depend on self-report. This is problematic when, for example, respondents are asked to characterize the autonomy that they have in their jobs and to provide a ranking based on their experiences. Because everyone has different experiences and, perhaps, different expectations of autonomy, one person's low autonomy may be another's high autonomy. This leads to imprecision in the measures. This can be problematic if we seek to implement population-wide policies. For example, we know that if you are in a warehouse stacking boxes and one falls on top of you, it is very likely that you will be hurt. We have the physical equations to know at what height and at what mass a falling object will have sufficient force to produce serious injury to a stationary object (i.e., the worker underneath it). Regulations can be set with regard to a height limit up to which boxes can be stacked in warehouses. The limits can be set because there are objective measures for height. In the absence of objective measures for factors such as autonomy, it is difficult to develop population-wide standards to limit hazardous levels of factors that have the potential to produce harm.

On the other hand, it is important to note that the choice of tools/questionnaires used in population-based surveys such as the CCHS have been made according to their psychometric properties and also to reduce the potential imprecision of the measures. Because the imprecision that exists is unlikely to systematically affect the overall patterns in the data, we can obtain valuable information about areas for further investigation. For instance, although we may not be able to distinguish whether stress is related to actual autonomy or perceived autonomy, we know that we need to examine the role of autonomy closer.

The limitations associated with population-based survey data as well as the nature of workplace mental health limit the extent to which they can be used to make policy or to develop interventions. The survey data are important to track trends and changes with regard to health status. The data serve as a screen, calling attention to the working conditions and individual attributes that contribute to the risk of mental illness and those subpopulations that are at risk.

However, after identifying the contributing conditions, we are faced with the question of how to modify their effects within the constraints of the work environment. The challenge is to offer modifications that do not compromise a company's solvency or its ability to compete in a global economy. This means that interventions must not only be effective but cost-effective in terms that are salient from the business perspective such as productivity and decreased disability to the workforce.

This is where population-based survey data has made one of its largest contributions – it has allowed the burden of mental illness in the working population to be quantified. Because of population-based surveys such as the CCHS, we have estimates that indicate we lose about $17.7 billion (CAD) annually in productivity related to mental illness.[49] Figures such as these have raised the awareness of the business community and government to finding solutions.

Another strength of population-based survey data is that it allows us to identify subpopulations who are at risk of mental illness. We can also see for whom chronic work stress is comparatively higher. In terms of prevention and treatment, this is akin to offering us a glimpse into which haystack may contain the needle. But, we are still left to find the needle within the particular haystack. Then again, if there are thousands of haystacks and we are faced with limited resources, that level of direction can be extremely useful.

REFERENCES

1 The Standing Senate Committee on Social Affairs, S. a. T. *Out of the Shadows at Last: Transforming Mental Health, Mental Illness and Addiction Services in Canada*. Ottawa: The Senate, 2006.

2 World Health Organization. *The World Health Report 2001 Mental Health: New Understanding, New Hope*. Geneva: WHO, 2001.

3 Murray CJ, Lopez AD. Alternative projections of mortality and disability by cause 1990–2020: Global Burden of Disease Study. *Lancet* 1997;349(May 24, 9064):1498–504.

4 Sanderson K, Andrews G. Common mental disorders in the workforce: Recent findings from descriptive and social epidemiology. *Can J Psychiatry* 2006;51:63–75.

5 Dewa CS, Lin E, Kooehoorn M, et al. Association of chronic work stress, psychiatric disorders, and chronic physical conditions with disability among workers. *Psychiatr Serv* 2007;58:652–8.

6 Stephens T, Jourbert N. (2001). The economic burden of mental health problems in Canada. *Chronic Dis Can* 2001;22:18–23.

7 Greenberg PE, Kessler R, Birnbaum HG, et al. The economic burden of depression in the United States: How did it change between 1990 and 2000? *J Clin Psychiatry* 2003;64:1465–75.

8 Watson Wyatt Worldwide. *Staying at work 2000/2001 – The Dollars and Sense of Effective Disability Management*. Vancouver, Watson Wyatt Worldwide, 2000.

9 Kendler KS, Gardner CO, Prescott CA. Toward a comprehensive developmental model for major depression in women. *Am J Psychiatry* 2002;159:1133–45.

10 Loisel P, Buchbinder R, Hazard R, et al. Prevention of work disability due to musculoskeletal disorders: the challenge of implementing evidence. *J Occupl Rehabil* 2005;15:507–24.

11 Goldner E, Bilsker D, Gilbert M, et al. Disability management, return to work and treatment. *Healthcare Pap* 2004;5:76–90.

12 Faragher EB, Cass M, Cooper CL. The relationship between job satisfaction and health: A meta-analysis. *Occup Environ Med* 2005;62:105–12.

13 Niedhammer I, Chastang JF, David S, et al. Psychosocial work environment and mental health: Job-strain and effort-reward imbalance models in a context of major organizational changes. *Int J Occup Environ Health* 2006;12:111–19.

14 Noblet A, Lamontagne AD. The role of workplace health promotion in addressing job stress. *Health Promot Int* 2006;21:346–53.

15 D'Souza RM, Strazdins L, Clements MS, et al. The health effects of jobs: Status, working conditions, or both? *Aust N Z J Public Health* 2005;29:222–8.

16 Marchand A, Durand P, Demers A. Work and mental health: The experience of the Quebec workforce between 1987 and 1998. *Work* 2005;25:135–42.

17 Vezina M, Bourbonnais R, Brisson C, Trudel L. Workplace prevention and promotion strategies. *HealthcarePap* 2004;5:32–44.

18 Karasek R, Theorell T. *Healthy work: Stress, Productivity and the Reconstruction of Working Life.* New York: Basic Books, 1990.

19 Siegrist J. Adverse health effects of high effort – low reward conditions at work. *J Occup Health Psychol* 1996;1:27–43.

20 McEwan BS. Protective and damaging effects of stress mediators. *NEJM* 1998;338:171–9.

21 McEwan BS. Stress, adaptation and disease. Allostasis and allostatic load. *Ann N Y Acad Sci* 1998;840:33–44.

22 McEwan BS. Stress and hippocampal plasticity. *Annu Rev Neurosci* 1999;22:105–22.

23 Rick J, Thomson L, Briner RB, et al. *Review of Existing Supporting Knowledge to Underpin Standards of Good Practice for Key Work-related Stressors – Phase 1 Norwich, UK:* Her Majesty's Stationery Office, 2002

24 Melchior M, Caspi A, Milne BJ, et al. Work stress precipitates depression and anxiety in young, working women and men. *Psychol Med* 2007;37:1119–29.

25 Bosma H, Peter R, Siegrist J, et al. Two alternative job stress models and the risk of coronary heart disease. *Am J Pub Health* 1998;88:68–74.

26 Theorell T, Tsutsumi A, Hallquist J, et al. Decision latitude, job strain, and myocardial infarction: A study of working men in Stockholm. The SHEEP Study Group. Stockholm Heart Epidemiology Program. *Am J Pub Health* 1998;88:382–8.

27 Courtney JG, Longnecker MP, Theorell T, et al. Stressful life events and the risk of colorectal cancer. *Epidemiology* 1993;4:407–14.

28 Shannon HS, Mayr J, Haines T. Overview of the relationship between organizational and workplace factors and injury rates. *Saf Sci* 1997;26:201–17.

29 Shannon HS, Walters V, Lewchuck W, et al. Workplace organizational correlates of lost-time accident rates in manufacturing. *Am J Ind Med* 1996;29:258–30.

30 Burton J, Shain M. Psychosocial factors and mental health at work: A Canadian perspective. *World Health Organization GOHNET (Global Occupational Health Network Newsletter)* 2006;10:6–8.

31 Shain M. The duty to prevent emotional harm at work: Arguments from science and law, implications for policy and practice. *Bull Sci Technol Soc* 2004;24:305–15.

32 Health Canada. *Origins and Characteristics of the Workplace Health Needs and Risks Inventory 2001*. Ottawa: Health Canada Policy and Workplace Health Strategies Bureau, Workplace Health and Public Safety Programme, 2004.

33 Levi L, Lunde-Jensen P. *Model for Assessing the Costs of Stressors at the National Level: Socio-economic Costs of Work Stress in Two EU Member States*. Dublin: European Foundation for the Improvement of Living and Working Conditions, 1996.

34 Hildebrandt J, Pfingsten M, Saur P, et al. Prediction of success from a multidisciplinary treatment program for chronic low back pain. *Spine* 1997;22:990–1001.

35 Beck AT, Rush AJ, Shaw BF, et al. *Cognitive Therapy of Depression*. New York: Guilford Press, 1979.

36 Saunders T, Driskell JE, Johnston JH, et al. The effect of stress inoculation training on anxiety and performance. *J Occup Health Psychol* 1996;1:170–86.

37 van der Klink JJ, van Dijk F. Dutch practice guidelines for managing adjustment disorders in occupational and primary health care. *Scand J Work Environ Health* 2003;29:478–87.

38 St-Arnaud L, St-Jean M,. *La réintégration au travail à la suite d'un problème de santé mentale*. Québec: Secrétariat du Conseil du trésor. Centre d'expertise en gestion des ressources humaines, 2004.

39 van der Klink JJ, Blonk RW, Schene AH, et al. The benefits of interventions for work-related stress. *Am J Pub Health* 2001;91:270–6.

40 Corbière M, Shen J. A systematic review of psychological return-to-work interventions for people with mental health problems and/or physical injuries. *Can J Commun Ment Health* 2006;25:261–88.

41 Corbière M, Sullivan M, Stanish W, et al. Pain and depression in injured

430   C.S. Dewa, E. Lin, M. Corbière, and M. Shain

workers and their return to work: A longitudinal study. *Can J Behav Sci* 2007;39:23–31.

42 Kessler RC, Frank RG. The impact of psychiatric disorders on work loss days. *Psychol Med* 1997;27:861–73.

43 Dewa CS, Lin E. Chronic physical illness, psychiatric disorder and disability in the workplace. *Soc Sci Med* 2000;51:41–50.

44 Lim D, Sanderson K, Andrews G. Lost productivity among full-time workers with mental disorders. *J Ment Health Policy Econ* 2000 Sep 1;3:139–46.

45 Karasek R, Brisson C, Kawakami N, et al. The Job Content Questionnaire (JCQ): An instrument for internationally comparative assessments of psychosocial job characteristics. *J Occup Health Psychol* 1998;3:322–55.

46 Wilkins K, Beaudet MP. *Work Stress and Health.* Health reports/Statistics Canada, Canadian Centre for Health Information. 1998 Winter;10:47–62 (ENG);49–66 (FRE).

47 Statistics Canada. *Canadian Community Health Survey (CCHS) Cycle 1.2 Derived Variable (DV) Specifications.* Ottawa: Statistics Canada, 2004.

48 Cherry NM, Chen Y, McDonald JC. Reported incidence and precipitating factors of work-related stress and mental ill-health in the United Kingdom (1996–2001). *Occup Med* 2006;56:414–21

49 Lim KL, Jacobs P, Ohinmaa A, et al. A new population-based measure of the 'economic burden' of mental illness in Canada. *Chronic Dis Can* 2008; 28:92–8.

19 Knowledge Translation in Mental Health: From Epidemiology to Policy

PAULA GOERING AND CHARLOTTE WADDELL

Introduction

In the health field in the last two decades, there has been tremendous international interest in the use of research evidence in public policy making. Compelled by concern about numerous documented research-policy 'gaps,' researchers have called on policy makers to apply more research evidence in the service of improving public policies for health and health care. Many Canadian researchers have been in the forefront of this changing landscape.[1-3] Research funding agencies have had considerable influence. In particular, the Canadian Health Services Research Foundation (CHSRF), led by Jonathan Lomas, has made 'knowledge transfer and exchange' the central aim of a wide scope of activities aimed at both researchers and policy makers.[4,5] The successful articulation and implementation of this direction by the CHSRF has influenced the subsequent development of the Canadian Institutes of Health Research (CIHR), whose mandate now explicitly includes 'knowledge translation' as a key component of all publicly funded research.

Many terms have been used to describe the various activities and structures that aim to increase the use of research evidence in policy making: *knowledge transfer, knowledge utilization, knowledge exchange,* and *evidence-based decision making.* All have somewhat different definitions and connotations. Here, we use the term *knowledge translation* (KT) as defined by the CIHR: 'the exchange, synthesis and ethically-sound application of knowledge – within a complex system of interactions among researchers and users – to accelerate the capture of the benefits of research for Canadians through improved health, more effective services and products, and a strengthened healthcare system.'[6]

Within the broader context of KT discussion and action, increasing attention is being paid to the issue by both policy makers and researchers in the mental health sector in Canada. For example, the recent call for a national mental health commission by Senator Kirby and his committee in their 2006 report, *Out of the Shadows*, includes the development of a knowledge exchange network as a central component.[7] This reflects concerns heard during cross-country consultations with multiple stakeholders about the need to better implement 'best practice' approaches for the benefit of people with mental disorders. Senator Kirby's work complements recent efforts of the CIHR Institute of Neuroscience, Mental Health and Addictions to encourage and support more KT activities by researchers through recent calls for proposals emphasizing KT.[8]

As researchers concerned with public policy and with improving the mental health of adults and children, we have each actively engaged in policy partnerships and in scholarly KT studies.[9–11,12–16] Amid the new directions increasingly placing KT as an integral part of the Canadian research and policy landscapes, it is therefore timely for us to consider to specific role that epidemiology can play as one important form of research evidence to inform public policy making to improve mental health.

We endorse the common definition of epidemiology as the study of the distribution and determinants of health conditions in human populations. Further, we define public policy making as 'making and implementing collective ethical judgments.'[17] In keeping with the CIHR's conceptualization of KT, this definition acknowledges that researchers can be actors in the policy process – together with more traditionally defined players such as politicians, civil servants, journalists, and advocacy groups – influencing ideas, interests, and institutions to bring about social change.[18]

In this chapter, we first summarize salient lessons from KT scholarship, drawing primarily on Canadian research, to address what kind of influence epidemiology researchers can expect to have on policy. We then explore challenges and potential contributions of epidemiology to public mental health policy in Canada, including case examples from our own KT experiences. Finally, we suggest future directions for better connecting epidemiology and policy in mental health.

Lessons from Knowledge Translation Scholarship

Recent interdisciplinary health policy scholarship has emphasized an expanded conceptualization of the use of research evidence in policy making. This scholarship provides solid ground for considering how epidemiology can influence policy. In the health field in Canada, the original impetus for KT arose from concern about increasing the use of research evidence in clinical practice, or decision making about health care for *individuals*. In particular, drawing from the 'evidence-based medicine' movement, randomized controlled trials (RCTs) came to be the standard asserted by researchers to guide practitioner decision making regarding interventions for individual patients.[19] Systematic reviews have been further suggested as an ideal method of conveying *bodies* of such RCT evidence to practitioners (and others).[20]

Concerned with influencing policy making more broadly, KT scholars subsequently turned their attention to administrative and legislative policy making, or decision making about health and health care for *populations*. At this broader level, encouraging interactions between researchers and policy makers and increasing the policy relevance of research both appear to be promising approaches for encouraging research use in policy making.[21] Nevertheless, KT scholars acknowledge that efforts to increase the use of research evidence in policy making have often met with limited results.[22] It has therefore become more evident that the outcomes of interest are not only changes in practice, such as 'instrumental use,' but also changes in awareness and understanding, or 'conceptual or deliberative use'.[23]

Building on this earlier work, an expanded conceptualization of KT has now been developed by scholars who note that research can only ever be a partial influence in the context of much complexity in dynamic policy environments.[24–26] For example, in a survey of Canadian politicians and civil servants, Lavis' group found that the influence of research evidence (of any kind) was overshadowed by the influence of institutional constraints, stakeholder interests, and public beliefs.[1] These findings have been echoed in studies of the policy process in children's mental health specifically; it has been noted, for example, that research contributions *are* valued and used, as one influence among many, but only if researchers appreciate the policy process and actively engage with policy makers.[13] An understanding of these complexities has tempered the thinking of many researchers involved in KT. For example, the CHSRF's recent change of language from 'evidence-based' to 'evidence-*informed*' decision making suggests a more nuanced understanding of the many factors at play.[5]

A related lesson is that much KT research initially focused on policy makers and their presumed need to use more research evidence, from the perspective of researchers. However, factors in the research process too are now being scrutinized more closely. For example, scientific studies are subject to criticisms – that methods (such as RCTs) can be biased or corrupted, that over-reliance on these methods can lead to fragmented knowledge, and that many research studies yield knowledge about efficacy but not the knowledge about effectiveness in 'real world' settings that policy makers require.[22] Meanwhile, KT researchers are documenting the constraints to policy engagement that researchers themselves experience, particularly in conventional academic settings.[15,27] Researchers are recognizing that KT is a 'social process, not a technical task' that will require changes on their part, as well as on the part of policy makers.[3]

In summary, in the health field in Canada, KT scholarship has broadened well beyond its origins in 'evidence-based medicine.' It is now widely acknowledged that KT is a complex and nuanced social process, requiring both researchers and policy makers to make changes. We also better appreciate the specific ways that researchers can have influence and are more humble in our expectations about a direct causal link between data and decisions.

Potential Contributions of Epidemiology to Policy

Taking the complexities of policy making into account, epidemiologic research may occupy a unique position in the KT process. A recent review of KT in public health decision making in Canada defined four different types of research evidence used, the most abundant being basic epidemiologic evidence.[28] Although intervention and implementation research are also needed, program planning in health usually starts with identifying the distribution and determinants of a problem, and with identifying patterns of related service use. Consequently, we focus our discussion primarily on the type of research evidence obtained through community surveys of the distribution (and potentially, determinants) of mental health problems and related service use in the population. Both public health and health care policy makers are potential audiences for this type of research.

This edited collection includes descriptions of many specific community surveys with potential relevance for mental health policy making in Canada. For adult populations, the Canadian Community Health Survey (CCHS) and the Mental Health Supplement to the Ontario Health Survey (the Supplement) are particularly important data sources.[29–31] For children, similarly important data sources include the Ontario Child Health Survey (OCHS), the Quebec Child Mental Health Survey (QCMHS) and the National Longitudinal Survey of Children and Youth (NLSCY).[29,32-34] Ideally, data from these surveys could to be used to:

- estimate needs in order to establish health and health care priorities for the population;
- suggest causal risk and protective factors (if longitudinal surveys) to inform the design of effective prevention and treatment programs; and
- monitor outcomes (such as changes in service utilization, baseline prevalence and causal factors) that are potentially attributable to public programs and services.[35]

A promising recent example of the use of epidemiologic evidence to estimate needs and set priorities comes from Australia. Andrews and colleagues have used prevalence data from their 1997 *National Survey of Mental Health and Well Being* to conduct comparisons of the cost effectiveness of the treatment of 10 mental disorders.[36]

They used their data on the population distribution of illness to address a key policy question: What is the cost of providing optimal care and coverage that approaches that currently being provided for similar physical disorders?[37] These authors have further developed an approach for assessing cost effectiveness that combines technical analysis with policy maker consultation in order to develop policy options and set priorities.[38] Recommendations for change are formulated, taking into account not only the strength of the cost-effectiveness evidence, but also 'second filter criteria' of equity, feasibility, and acceptability. Did this activity work? Andrews thinks it did: 'The costing studies showed that optimal treatment was affordable and that improving access to treatment was practical. In 2006 the Australian Government made reimbursement of some health care costs, previously confined to patients seeing doctors, available to patients referred by doctors to psychologists. This has more than doubled the mental health workforce entitled to reimbursement and has improved access to patients with the common mental disorders' (Andrews, personal communication, May 17, 2007).

Most theories about research used in policy making include the idea that the nature of the evidence and ideas being generated help to determine whether or not there is application. Research evidence generated in partnership with policy makers is considered to be much more likely to be relevant to policy makers and therefore to be applied.[39] The Australian example illustrates that prevalence and cost findings can indeed be generated in collaboration with policy makers, thereby ensuring relevance to policy makers' immediate issues and concerns.

Community survey data regarding prevalence of disorder, disability, and associated costs *are* frequently included in descriptions of needs and priority setting by policy makers and others. In a leading example of this phenomenon, the World Health Organization's (WHO) finding that disability due to depression ranked second in worldwide estimates of the burden of illness is one of the most cited epidemiological findings.[40] This widespread use of this citation reflects the common tactical use of research evidence to support the investment of resources in a particular area (in this particular case, the juxtaposition of depression against other more commonly identified sources of disability such as cardiovascular disease, is a particularly persuasive statement to counter the all too often held belief that mental health problems are not serious disorders in relation to social and economic costs). This same phenomena may also explain the tendency to inflate prevalence estimates of disorder, as documented in a recent systematic review by Waraich and colleagues.[41] Meanwhile, the WHO has gone on to make further use of epidemiologic evidence on the high prevalence of mental disorders to call for new investments in prevention as perhaps the only sustainable strategy for improving mental health population-wide, arguing that treatment services alone will never be able to meet the needs.[42]

In Canada, the influence of the CCHS 1.2 on Senator Kirby's work on mental health is evident in the citations in *Out of the Shadows*, particularly regarding the mental health of adult populations.[7] For example, there are numerous citations regarding work disability findings (described more fully in chapter 18 of this book). *Out of the Shadows* builds on these findings to support a national strategy to address workplace mental health. The CCHS is also cited frequently in the *Overview of Policy and Programs in Canada*, a Standing Senate Committee report that comprehensively reviewed the current state of affairs in adult mental health.[7] The impact of CCHS as a means of raising the profile of mental health at the federal level is fairly clear. As staff from Statistics Canada recently commented, 'The CCHS and the research associated with it have generated additional momentum behind mental health.'[43(p6)] This commentator further points to the follow-up report by the Public Health Agency of Canada[44] and the inclusion of depression in a national surveillance program for chronic conditions as concrete evidence of momentum generated by a community survey. Evidently the CCHS and the epidemiologic data it gathered have been an important source of influence in adult mental health.

For children, Canadian epidemiologic surveys such as OCHS and the QCMHS have provided basic information on prevalence of mental disorders. These same surveys have also provided data on service utilization, indicating that the majority of children with mental disorders do not access the specialized treatment services that have constituted the main public policy investment in children's mental health.[45] However, these surveys do not appear to have the same influence as comparable adult surveys in that children's mental health has never figured highly on the Canadian health policy agenda. As some policy makers have described, if mental health has been one of the 'orphan children' of health and health care,[46] then children's mental health has been the 'orphan's orphan.'[7] Even *Out of the Shadows* focuses most of its attention on issues pertaining to adults.[47] The NLSCY has also made a significant contribution in tracking cohorts of children and taking measures of child development and well-being, including a number pertaining to mental health and disorder. The NLSCY *has* informed the development of early child development programs in Canada and has been used to evaluate the impact of these programs over time,[48,49] even though broader influence on children's mental health policy making has yet to be realized.

Knowledge Translation Examples

In Canada, we have been involved with particular policy partnerships and consultations that help elucidate some of the unique contributions and challenges that are associated with translating epidemiologic research evidence into policy.[11,16,50] We will focus on the use of prevalence and service utilization data to estimate needs and establish priorities, drawing on our experiences in the adult and child mental health sectors.

Adult Mental Health in Ontario

A recurring problem that Paula Goering (one of this chapter's authors) and the Health Systems Research and Consulting Unit (HSRCU) have encountered with regard to documenting prevalence rates is the mismatch between the typical methods of community surveys and the focus of government policy for persons with severe and persistent mental illness. This was evident in the planning of the Supplement in the early 1980s. The research team, headed by Offord, consulted with Ontario Ministry of Health representatives in the design of the study in order to determine their needs for information. Policy makers wanted more information about youth making the transition to adulthood and consequently wanted over-sampling of the 16–21 year age group, a request that was easy to implement. Policy makers also had a number of questions about the population at the centre of mental health reform efforts, namely those with severe and persistent mental illnesses, such as psychotic disorders.

The research team took these policy maker requests seriously and searched for methods of dealing with the low prevalence of psychotic disorders that could be expected using usual conventional, community-based sampling methods. Over-sampling this population required the identification of a two-stage screening method with established psychometric properties. Despite extensive literature reviews and expert consultations, no appropriate method could be found. The decision was made to incorporate the schizophrenia module of the University of Michigan's version of the Composite International Diagnostic Interview (UM-CIDI)[51,52] and to give special attention to training lay interviewers to properly administer the questions. When the Supplement findings were analysed, the measured prevalence of schizophrenia was too low to be accurately reported. Although other data about hospitalization and disability were used to construct an approximate definition of the severe and persistently mentally ill,[53] policy makers were rightfully disappointed with the ability of the study to address their priority concerns.

Other surveys have tackled the problem of low prevalence and hard to measure psychotic disorders by using two-phase survey methods with treated populations in urban areas.[54] But this approach does not mesh well with attempts to get a complete picture of mental disorders. More recently, the psychotic disorder module of the WHO World Mental Health Survey Initiative version of the CIDI[55] was not included in the CCHS, as it did not meet requirements for sample size and methodological rigour applied by the advisory panel. Until more reliable and valid methods of identifying and measuring subpopulations such as those with psychosis are found, large scale community surveys will have limited relevance for planning or evaluating the bulk of specialized services that provincial governments provide. The utility of such community surveys lies much more within the primary care sector. Therefore, a limitation of community surveys is that many of the neediest subpopulations may require specialized studies. For example, while in Canada we have a strong record of immigrant and trans-cultural mental health epidemiology,[56] our coverage of aboriginal populations is seriously deficient as is our knowledge about persons who are homeless.

One of the most common uses of community survey data is to document the 'gap' between need and treatment by identifying the proportion of individuals with disorder who do not report receiving mental health services.[57] The estimates of 'unmet need' produced by this approach are so consistently high as to often engender disbelief on the part of policy makers. One response to this issue has been to include additional measures of disability in the studies so that need is defined in terms of both disorder and disability. Another response is to combine community survey data regarding prevalence with administrative data about use of existing services as a means of assessing unmet needs. Lesage and colleagues have taken this approach in a series of investigations of one catchment area in Montreal.[58,59]

HSRCU researchers have conducted various studies to document both under- and over-utilization of services. Data from the Supplement were used to define rates of 'over-met need' by calculating the proportion of users who had neither disorder nor disability.[31] It is interesting that these findings were frequently challenged or dismissed by mental health colleagues (researchers and clinicians), perhaps because this type of information appears to threaten rather than support advocacy agendas. Uptake and use of findings from a series of level of care surveys in Ontario has been much different.[60] Generating regional estimates of both over and under met service needs, based upon standardized assessments social and behavioural functioning (e.g. self care, social isolation, aggression) has provided information that has been used and cited in mental health reform implementation task forces across the province. It should be noted that there was extensive involvement of local planners and providers in the design and execution of these regional surveys, a factor that likely increased the use of data.

Children's Mental Health in British Columbia

Through a long-term research policy partnership focused on children's mental health in British Columbia, Charlotte Waddell (one of the authors of this chapter) and colleagues have provided regular consultation to policy makers on research findings with potential implications for their decisions. Early on in the partnership, policy makers advised that they were particularly interested in three different kinds of epidemiologic research evidence: (1) the prevalence of a comprehensive range of disorders; (2) the use of existing mental health services; and (3) any data pertaining to implications for redesigning provincial services for children. Funding was provided to the research team to undertake systematic reviews of the existing literature in order to answer these questions.

While conducting systematic searches, the research team quickly learned that the applicability of much of the available epidemiologic research was surprisingly limited. Literature searches yielded high quality community surveys reporting prevalence rates, including OCHS and the QCMHS, as well as British and American surveys. But the diversity of samples and survey methodologies meant that substantial interpretation was required to provide disorder specific prevalence estimates applicable to British Columbia's population of children, particularly given the lack of epidemiologic surveys in British Columbia. For example, surveys that used older diagnostic classifications and groupings had to be translated to be comparable with those using newer classifications. As well, surveys were often difficult to compare due to differences in the particular disorders assessed, or differences in the inclusion (or not) of important measures, such as levels of associated impairment or associated service utilization. Analogous to the Ontario experience, relatively few data were found on low prevalence disorders of considerable interest to policy makers, such as schizophrenia and bipolar disorder.

The research team addressed these challenges in several ways. Special effort was made to conduct a thorough review on the prevalence of children's mental disorders and associated questions, then to interpret findings through a local policy lens.[61] This review yielded estimates that the number of children affected by mental disorders (defined as having both significant symptoms *and* significant impairment) was 14% or one in seven. The same review also produced estimates that 75% of children with mental disorders did not access specialized mental health services (although up to 50% were estimated to access services through primary care and schools). These overall prevalence and need estimates were initially met with strong skepticism by policy makers. Consequently, special effort was also made to convey the findings through a variety of presentations and meetings. The findings became persuasive to policy makers based on the systematic nature of the methods used and were ultimately incorporated into high-level planning documents. These epidemiologic estimates were subsequently quoted by British Columbia's premier as justification for substantial new funding for children's mental health programs and services, including the launching of the first comprehensive plan for children's mental health in Canada.[62]

The question of the implications of the epidemiologic estimates was considerably more complicated. One of the major recommendations stemming from the epidemiologic review was that a new public health strategy was needed, featuring greater investments in prevention in order to extend the reach of mental health services for children.[45] However, the provincial government had competing priorities, including simultaneous reductions in tax revenues and program expenditures. The ensuing climate of fiscal restraint was not conducive to new investments. At the same time, some practitioners and disorder-based advocacy groups were promoting further investment in specialized treatment services, potentially impinging on new funding available for prevention. As a result of these competing influences, new prevention investments were limited to one school-based program for preventing anxiety. Programs for preventing other disorders remain a consideration for the future.

In response to these challenges, the research team sought independent research funding to further investigate prevention, including preparing a systematic review on the prevention of the most common mental disorders in children and a survey of relevant prevention programs across Canada.[63] Researchers continued to encourage prevention initiatives by sharing emerging findings from these independent studies, thereby pursuing an 'evidence-informed' agenda without directly challenging decisions at the political level. This approach in turn assisted amenable policy makers to gradually build support for prevention ideas. As a result, prevention investments grew to comprise 15% of new expenditures through British Columbia's children's mental health plan. This is an incremental but not inconsiderable shift given that, much like other Canadian provinces, British Columbia has typically devoted only 5% of overall health spending to public health including prevention.[64]

Summary

The successes and failures that we have described here suggest that it is possible to integrate epidemiology and policy in mental health. However, our experience also suggests we could do better. The accumulating knowledge about integrating research evidence in health policy making can provide guidance for future efforts.

There is a wealth of experiential and academic knowledge to support an expansion of knowledge transference (KT) activities within epidemiology pertaining to mental health. We have learned to have humble expectations with regard to direct use of research findings, but to nevertheless be mindful of the various other ways in which research evidence (and researchers) can be helpful to policy makers. We know that the nature of research findings will influence their uptake, as will meaningful interaction with policy makers. We can imagine how future research programs can be better designed to increase policy relevance and therefore the likelihood of research use. For example, recent requirements by the CIHR and the CHSRF have mandated that researchers engage with policy makers as collaborators in the design of new studies and in the dissemination of findings, including in mental health.[5,6,8] These initiatives that should encourage greater policy involvement on the part of researchers and greater research receptivity on the part of policy makers.

A scan of the current Canadian mental health landscape suggests that many of the necessary ingredients to realize a new future are also present. There are now programs to better train future researchers to generate research that is relevant to policy in mental health. For example, the Research in Addictions and Mental Health Policy and Services (RAMHPS) program is an innovative initiative spearheaded by mental health researchers with long-term CIHR funding to create links between faculty and trainees in multiple provinces using a curriculum that emphasizes KT.[65] This initiative complements the proposed national knowledge exchange network that should unfold within the coming years, as proposed by Kirby and Keon.[7] There is a thriving association of researchers with an interest in application in the Canadian Academy of Psychiatric Epidemiology. There are also new mental health surveys and surveillance projects on the horizon.

All these developments within mental health are complemented by the generic development of mandates and tools for KT by CHSRF, CIHR, and other funding agencies such as the Social Sciences and Humanities Research Council of Canada. Support is also growing within Canadian universities for researchers to have greater policy involvements. It seems promising that the human and financial resources are increasingly available to realize the vision of establishing model programs for integrating research and policy to better the health of the Canadian population. Epidemiologic research evidence is clearly fundamental to these advances in the mental health sphere.

NOTES AND REFERENCES

Paula Goering thanks Elizabeth Lin and fellow members of the Canadian Academy of Psychiatric Epidemiology for their collegiality and support over the years. Charlotte Waddell thanks Jayne Barker, George McLauchlin, John Lavis, Jonathan Lomas and Cody Shepherd for their contributions to the ideas expressed here.

1 Lavis JN, Ross SE, Hurley JE, et al. Examining the role of health services research in public policymaking. *Milbank Q* 2002;80:25–54.
2 Landry R, Lamari M, Amara N. The extent and determinants of the utilization of university research in government agencies. *Publ Admin Rev* 2003;63:192–205.
3 Lomas J. Postscript: Understanding evidence-based decision-making – or, why keyboards are irrational. In: Lemieux-Charles L, Champagne F, eds. *Using Knowledge and Evidence in Health Care: Multidisciplinary Perspectives.* Toronto: University of Toronto Press, 2004:281–9.
4 Lomas J. Using 'linkage and exchange' to move research into policy at a Canadian foundation. *Health Aff (Millwood)* 2000;19:236–40.
5 *Home Page.* Canadian Health Services Research Foundation (CHSRF), 2007. Available at: http://chsrf.ca/home_e.php
6 *About knowledge translation.* Canadian Institutes of Health Research, 2007. Available at: http://www.cihr-irsc.gc.ca/e/29418.html
7 Kirby MJL, Keon WJ. *Out of the Shadows at Last: Transforming Mental Health, Mental Illness and Addiction Services in Canada.* Ottawa: The Stand-

ing Senate Committee on Social Affairs, Science and Technology, 2006.

8   *Call for proposals.* Canadian Institutes of Health Research, 2007. Available at: http://www.cihr.ca/e/780.html

9   Wasylenki DA, Goering PN. The role of research in systems reform. *Can J Psychiatry* 1995;40:247–51.

10 Goering PN, Wasylenki DA. The use of multiple roles to maximize the utilization of outcome research. *Eval Program Plann* 1993;16:329–34.

11 Goering P, Butterill D, Jacobson N, et al. Linkage and exchange at the organizational level: A model of collaboration between research and policy. *J Health Serv Res Policy* 2003;8(suppl 2):14–19.

12 Jacobson N, Goering P. Credibility and credibility work in knowledge transfer. *Evidence and Policy* 2006;2:151–66.

13 Waddell C, Lavis JN, Abelson J, et al. Research use in children's mental health policy in Canada: Maintaining vigilance amid ambiguity. *Soc Sci Med* 2005;61:1649–57.

14 Waddell C, Lomas J, Lavis JN, et al. Joining the conversation: Newspaper journalists' views on working with researchers. *Healthcare Policy* 2005;1:123–39.

15 Waddell C, Shepherd CA, Lavis JN, et al. Balancing rigour and relevance: Researchers' contributions to children's mental health policy in Canada. *Evidence and Policy* 2005;3(2):181–95.

16 Waddell C, Shepherd CA, Barker J. Developing a research-policy partnership to improve children's mental health in British Columbia. *Canadian Western Geographical Series* 2007;41:183–98.

17 Greenhalgh T, Russell J. Reframing evidence synthesis as rhetorical action in the policy making drama. *Healthcare Policy* 2006;1:34–42.

18 John P. *Analysing Public Safety.* London: Continuum, 1998.

19 Grol R, Grimshaw J. From best evidence to best practice: Effective implementation of change in patients' care. *Lancet* 2003;362:1225–30.

20 Lavis JN, Posada FB, Haines A, et al. Use of research to inform public policymaking. *Lancet* 2004;364:1615–21.

21 Innvaer S, Vist G, Trommald M, et al. Health policy-makers' perceptions of their use of evidence: A systematic review. *J Health Serv Res Policy* 2002;7:239–44.

22 Lewis S. Toward a general theory of indifference to research-based evidence. *J Health Serv Res Policy* 2007;12:166–72.

23 Weiss CH. Many meanings of research utilization. *Public Adm Rev* 1979;39:426–31.

24 Culyer AJ, Lomas J. Deliberative processes and evidence-informed deci-

sion making in healthcare: Do they work and how might we know? *Evidence and Policy* 2006;2:357–71.

25 Oliver TR. The politics of public health policy. *Annu Rev Public Health* 2006;27:195–233.

26 Fox DM. The determinants of policy for population health. *Health Econ Policy Law* 2006;1(4):395–407.

27 Jacobson N, Butterill D, Goering P. Organizational factors that influence university-based researchers' engagement in knowledge transfer activities. *Sci Commun* 2004;25:246–59.

28 Kiefer L, Frank J, Di Ruggiero E, et al. Fostering evidence-based decision-making in Canada: Examining the need for a Canadian population and public health evidence centre and research network. *Can J Public Health* 2005;96:I1–40.

29 Boyle MH, Offord DR, Hofmann HG, et al. Ontario Child Health Study. I. Methodology. *Arch Gen Psychiatry* 1987;44:826–31.

30 Tweed DL, Goering P, Lin E, et al. Psychiatric morbidity and physician visits: Lessons from Ontario. *Med Care* 1998;36:573–85.

31 Lesage AD, Goering P, Lin E. Family physicians and the mental health system. Report from the Mental Health Supplement to the Ontario Health Survey. *Can Fam Physician* 1997;43:251–6.

32 Offord DR, Boyle MH, Fleming JE, et al. Ontario Child Health Study. Summary of selected results. *Can J Psychiatry* 1989;34:483–91.

33 Breton JJ, Bergeron L, Valla JP, et al. Quebec child mental health survey: Prevalence of DSM-III-R mental health disorders. *J Child Psychol Psychiatry* 1999;40:375–84.

34 Willms JD (Ed.). *Vulnerable Children*. Edmonton: University of Alberta Press, 2002.

35 Jenkins, R. Making psychiatric epidemiology useful: the contribution of epidemiology to government policy. *Acta Psychiatr Scand* 2001;103(1):2–14.

36 Andrews G, Issakidis C, Sanderson K, et al. Utilising survey data to inform public policy: Comparison of the cost-effectiveness of treatment of ten mental disorders. *Br J Psychiatry* 2004;184:526–33.

37 Andrews G. It would be cost-effective to treat more people with mental disorders. *Aust N Z J Psychiatry* 2006;40:613–15.

38 Vos T, Haby MM, Magnus A, et al. Assessing cost-effectiveness in mental health: Helping policy-makers prioritize and plan health services. *Aust N Z J Psychiatry* 2005;39:701–12.

39 Denis JL, Lomas J. Convergent evolution: The academic and policy roots of collaborative research. *J Health Serv Res Policy* 2003;8(suppl 2):1–6.

40 Murray CJL, Lopez AD (Eds.). *The Global Burden of Disease.* Vol. 1. Boston: Harvard School of Public Health, WHO, and the World Bank, 1996.

41 Waraich P, Goldner EM, Somers JM, et al. Prevalence and incidence studies of mood disorders: A systematic review of the literature. *Can J Psychiatry* 2004;49:124–38.

42 WHO Department of Mental Health and Substance Abuse. *Prevention of Mental Disorders: Effective Interventions and Policy Options: Summary Report.* Geneva: WHO, 1994.

43 *Research Spotlight.* Institute of Health Services and Policy, 2006. Available at: http://www.cihr-irsc.gc.ca/e/31359.html#6.

44 Public Health Agency of Canada. *The Human Face of Mental Health and Mental Illness in Canada.* Ottawa: Author, 2006.

45 Waddell C, McEwan K, Shepherd CA, et al. A public health strategy to improve the mental health of Canadian children. *Can J Psychiatry* 2005;50:226–33.

46 Romanow RJ. *Building on Values: The Future of Health Care in Canada: Final Report.* Ottawa: Commission on the Future of Health Care in Canada, 2002.

47 McEwan K, Waddell C, Barker J. Bringing children's mental health 'out of the shadows.' *CMAJ* 2007;176:471–2.

48 Boyle MH, Willms JD. Impact of a national community-based program for at-risk children in Canada. *Can Public Policy* 2002;28:461–82.

49 Peters RD, Petrunka K, Arnold R. The Better Beginnings, Better Futures Project: A universal, comprehensive, community-based prevention approach for primary school children and their families. *J Clin Child Adolesc Psychol* 2003;32:215–27.

50 Jacobson N, Butterill D, Goering P. Consulting as a strategy for knowledge transfer. *Milbank Q* 2005;83:299–321.

51 Kessler RC, McGonagle KA, Zhao S, et al. Lifetime and 12-month prevalence of DSM-III-R psychiatric disorders in the United States. Results from the National Comorbidity Survey. *Arch Gen Psychiatry* 1994;51:8–19.

52 Wittchen HU. Reliability and validity studies of the WHO – Composite International Diagnostic Interview (CIDI): A critical review. *J Psychiatr Res* 1994;28:57–84.

53 Premiers Council on Health, Well-Being and Social Justice. *Ontario Health Survey 1990: Mental Health Supplement.* Toronto: Author, 1994.

54 Jablensky A, McGrath J, Herrman H, et al. Psychotic disorders in urban areas: An overview of the Study on Low Prevalence Disorders. *Aust N Z J Psychiatry* 2000;34:221–36.

55 Kessler RC, Ustun TB. The World Mental Health (WMH) Survey Initiative Version of the World Health Organization (WHO) Composite International Diagnostic Interview (CIDI). *Int J Methods Psychiatr Res* 2004. 13:93–121.

56 Beiser,M. *Strangers at the Gate: The Boat People's First Ten Years in Canada.* Toronto: University of Toronto Press, 1999.

57 Kohn R, Saxena S, Levav I, et al. The treatment gap in mental health care. *Bull World Health Organ* 2004;82:858–66.

58 Lesage AD, Clerc D, Uribe I, et al. Estimating local-area needs for psychiatric care: A case study. *Br J Psychiatry* 1996;169:49–57.

59 Lesage AD, Bonsack C, Clerc D, et al. Alternatives to acute hospital psychiatric care in east-end Montreal. *Can J Psychiatry* 2002;47:49–55.

60 Durbin J, Cochrane J, Goering P, et al. Needs-based planning: evaluation of a level-of-care planning model. *J Behav Health Serv Res* 2001;28:67–80.

61 Waddell C, Offord DR, Shepherd CA, et al. Child psychiatric epidemiology and Canadian public policy-making: The state of the science and the art of the possible. *Can J Psychiatry* 2002;47:825–32.

62 Ministry of Children and Family Development. *Child and Youth Mental Health Plan for British Columbia.* Victoria, BC: Author, 2003.

63 Waddell C, McEwan K, Peters RD, et al. Preventing mental disorders in children: A public health priority. *Can J Public Health* 2007;98:174–8.

64 Canadian Institute for Health Information. *National Health Expenditure Trends 1975–2005.* Ottawa: Author, 2005.

65 *Home Page.* Research in Addictions and Mental Health Policy & Service, 2007. Available at: http://www.ramhps-hsr.ca/

PART SIX

Final Thoughts

our opinion, not much. That is not to say that no more surveys are needed. There are many issues that remain unanswered, such as whether the prevalence of mood disorders increases or decreases after age 65;[8,9] and if it declines, whether this is due to age, period, or cohort effects. Other questions arise at the opposite end of the age spectrum. What happens to childhood disorders such as ADHD or phobias when the children and adolescents become adults; do they disappear, remain the same, or presage other problems? Answers to these, and similar, questions cannot come from yet another round of cross-sectional surveys. Rather, what is needed are more focused, longitudinal studies of specific, targeted groups, as was done with the Ontario Child Health Survey.[10]

There are a host of problems associated with longitudinal surveys, especially those begun in childhood. The most obvious is keeping track of the participants over a five- or ten-year time span. In the National Longitudinal Study of Children and Youth (NLSCY),[11] only about 62% of respondents were available for follow-up at wave (cycle) 6. Not only does this affect the sample size (and hence the power) at later times, but it also raises the spectre of differential attrition: that those who drop out are different in some systematic way from those who do not, possibly biasing the results. A thornier problem may be changes in the diagnostic categories and in the scales that are used from one age to another. For example, *DSM-IV* states that for those over 18 years of age, oppositional defiant disorder (ODD; 313.81) must be differentiated from antisocial personality disorder (ASP; 301.7). However, the diagnostic criteria for these two disorders are different, so it is difficult to determine if the natural history of ODD is to become ODD in adulthood (where some of the criteria are inappropriate), morph into ASP, or disappear. Similarly, at earlier ages, questionnaires about children are completed by a surrogate or 'person most knowledgeable of the child,' usually the mother, while they are self-reported at older ages. The literature on the concordance of their judgments is not encouraging. Parents may be adequate reporters of children's overt behaviours, but do poorly when judging covert feelings and beliefs.[12] Hence, changes over time may be due to problems with instrumentation, rather than reflecting the trajectory of the disorder.

Despite these difficulties, we feel it would be more worthwhile to devote resources to smaller, longitudinal studies that better address issues of the natural history of disorders and possible etiology than to broad, less focused studies of prevalence. Indeed, much has been learned already from large, population-based studies of disorder, so the timing is ripe to move from descriptive epidemiology to analytic studies. The emergence of gender differences in depression in adolescence offers one possible take-off point. Large scale, prospective studies clearly indicate age 14 as a critical infliction point where the well-known 'doubling' of risk for depression for girls begins.[13] An inception cohort, possibly of children just entering puberty (likely age 10 or 11), followed over time through the period typically associated with adolescence to early adulthood (say, to age 20), would allow not only for the capture of the critical age period associated with the steep rise in prevalence for girls, but also allow for a more focused array of measures (biological, social, and psychological) to be collected all for one, single analytic purpose – to answer the question, why do rates increase so sharply for girls during this period? We would add to this design (at no additional cost to us) a measure of disorder other than depression, especially one that may be more prevalent in boys (e.g., conduct disorder or substance use), so that gender 'differences' in disorder rather than just gender differences in depression could be explored. It may be the case, for example, that when disorder is defined more broadly than one single clinical entity, apparent gender differences are muted and what we see instead is a critical 'age' period where disorder in general starts to increase in adolescence. The point is, by attempting to dig deeper into associations well documented already by large, descriptive epidemiologic studies, new questions can be posed and, one hopes, new understandings of disorder would ensue.

If Prevalence, Then What Type?

If further prevalence studies are done, such as the more focused ones we just discussed, what type of prevalence should we look at? There are three choices: (a) lifetime – whether a person has had a given disorder at any time in her or his life; (b) period – if the person has had the disorder within a given period of time, usually the past six or 12 months; and (c) point – if the person has the disorder now (or within the past 30 days). Psychiatric epidemiology has traditionally measured the first two, and this is understandable. First, for many disorders, such as depression, anxiety, and schizophrenia, it is notoriously difficult for respondents to state when the onset was. Unlike acute diseases, like cholera or, more recently, Sudden Acute Respiratory

Syndrome, psychiatric disorders often begin insidiously and it may be impossible to say, 'I was well during this week, and became ill the following one.' Second, it was (and is) often believed that many disorders are life-long afflictions – perhaps punctuated by periods of better adaptation due to therapy or medication, but basically chronic conditions.

In an excellent presentation to the Canadian Academy of Psychiatric Epidemiology in 2005, Scott Patten cogently argued that we should dispense with life and period prevalence, and focus on point prevalence.[14] He states that there are two problems with lifetime prevalence. First, citing Andrews et al.[15] and his own work,[16] it's nearly always wrong. People simply cannot recall what happened to them ten, twenty, or more years ago. In fact, in one large-scale survey in the United States, 42% of people did not recall that they had been in hospital for medical reasons one year after the fact![17] Indeed, this may be the reason for the paradoxical finding that lifetime prevalences of anxiety and depression seem to be lower in those over 55 years of age; people simply forget that they had these disorders when they were younger.

The second reason is that, if recall were perfect, then lifetime prevalence becomes extremely insensitive as a measure of mental health status in the population. Even if services were to expand so that all people could be seen, and treatments improved so that all patients got better or remitted entirely, the lifetime prevalence would remain the same, declining only as people died; obviously not the best way to chart improvements in the delivery of mental health services.

Theoretically, period prevalence (often 6 or 12 month estimates in psychiatric epidemiology) is an improvement over lifetime prevalence, because it would be more sensitive to changes in health care delivery and population health. But, Patten argues, it is not sensitive enough, and we should be moving toward point prevalence, which is not only the most sensitive measure, but would also bring psychiatry in line with the rest of medicine with regard to prevalence estimates. Interestingly, in the major instrument now used in psychiatric epidemiology, the CIDI, the emphasis is on lifetime and period prevalence, and point prevalence is added as an 'afterthought.' We would echo Patten's injunctions to focus on point prevalence, as the most realistic assessment of current symptoms and treatment needs.

The immediate problem, however, is that if we consider period prevalence estimates of depression to be small (5% to 6%) for analytic purposes, 30-day or shorter time frames will be even smaller. One potential way around this problem is to use a staged design, where we may first screen for probable disorder using instruments that are quick and easy to administer, then follow-up on a second sample of probable cases with the kinds of methods and measures more commonly used in large-scale epidemiological surveys. Once again, existing data from prevalence studies such as the CCHS 1.2 can be useful to test the feasibility of this strategy. Our research group found, for example, that a 6-item measure of distress, originally developed by Ron Kessler and his colleagues at the University of Michigan, was a reasonably effective screen for 30-day or current depression using the CIDI to generate diagnoses.[18] We will, of course, need to reconsider our current strategy toward sampling. Studies such as the CCHS and the National Co-morbidity Study sample large numbers of people (between 8,000 and 28,000) to ensure adequate numbers of 'cases' can be found. This means that we end up surveying an awful lot of people free from any mental health problems. While this is necessary to estimate prevalence, it is of dubious value when the focus shifts.

How Should We Change the Scales in the Survey?

One of the major hurdles that face all psychiatric surveys is their length. From the researchers' point of view, more information is better. Each variable, though, such as social support, quality of life, or stigma, requires its own questionnaire, leading to an increased burden on the respondent. (One can argue that, after one hour or so, the test battery becomes assault and battery.) However, there have been promising advances on this front, led in part by recent developments in test theory and construction. Until the last decade or so, scale development has been guided by 'classical test theory'(CTT).[19] According to CTT, each question in a scale has some degree of random error associated with it, and the best way to minimize error is to increase the length of the scale, thus giving more opportunity for the random errors to cancel each other out. This resulted in reliable, but lengthy, scales for each construct being measured.

However, item response theory (IRT)[20] has changed the way scales are constructed. Using sophisticated mathematical techniques, instruments can be constructed in such a way that they span the entire range of the attribute with far fewer items, yet retain excellent psychometric properties. While this chapter is being written, various teams around

Canada are looking at the scales used in CCHS 1.2 and seeking better instruments that can be used in the next cycle. Included in this exercise is using IRT to shorten some scales, without losing their discriminating ability.

Should We Change Paradigms?

As we highlighted in the opening chapter in this volume, Klerman[2] stated that of the five major 'schools' of psychiatry (biological, psychodynamic, social, interpersonal, and behavioural) psychiatric epidemiology in North America has been most influenced by the social psychological paradigm, to the almost complete exclusion of the others. As one of us has pointed out in an earlier article,[21] genetic factors have been proposed for various disorders – such as schizophrenia, major depressive disorders, and anxiety – and implicated in such traits as intelligence and extroversion; but with rare exceptions, the stress-diathesis model of psychopathology has rarely been tested. Caspi et al.[22,23] provide a superb example of what can be learned by stretching our conceptual models. They found that abused children whose genotype conferred high levels of monoamine oxidase *A* expression were less likely to develop antisocial problems; and those with long copies of the 5-HTT promoter gene were less likely to become depressed, than adolescents with different alleles.

Such large epidemiological surveys, involving both social and genetic factors, pose considerable challenges. Some biological variables can be gathered using buccal swabs, but others require blood samples. This requires using nurses rather than trained lay people as data gatherers and the need to refrigerate samples. Added costs would come from the cost of the assays themselves. The biological samples could also be subpoenaed, raising the spectre of legal and ethical issues. Finally, the non-participation rate, especially if children are involved, may prove to be prohibitive.

However, the potential rewards of such paradigm-shifting research is extremely exciting. Researchers have long speculated that the determinants of mental disorder include environmental (social and psychological), genetic, and biological risk factors operating synergistically in a complex interactive model of psychopathology. Up until this point, our ability to collect and then analyse the data required to test such models has been severely limited. There has, perhaps, never been a better time to capitalize on methodological and analytic (e.g. multilevel modelling) innovations that now make what once seemed impossible, possible.

REFERENCES

1 Weissman MM. The epidemiology of psychiatric disorders: Past, present, and future generations. *Int J Methods Psychiatr Res* 1995;5:69–78.

2 Klerman GL. Paradigm shifts in USA psychiatric epidemiology since World War II. *Soc Psychiatry Psychiatr Epidemiol* 1990;25:27–32.

3 Gravel R, Béland Y. The Canadian Community Health Survey: Mental Health and Well-Being. *Can J Psychiatry* 2005;50:573–9.

4 Kessler R. The National Comorbidity Survey of the United States. *Int Rev Psychiatry* 1994;6:365–6.

5 Leighton AH. *The Stirling County study of psychiatric disorder and socio-cultural environment. Vol. I: My name is legion.* New York: Basic Books, 1959.

6 Srole L, Langner TS, Michael ST, et al. *Mental health in the metropolis: The Midtown Manhattan study.* New York: McGraw-Hill, 1962.

7 Katz SJ, Kessler RC, Frank RG, et al. The use of outpatient mental health services in the United States and Ontario: the impact of mental morbidity and perceived need for care. *Am J Pub Health* 1997;87:1136–43.

8 Streiner DL, Cairney J, Veldhuizen S. The epidemiology of psychological problems in the elderly. *Can J Psychiatry* 2006;51:185–91.

9 van't Veer-Tazelaar PJ, van Marwijk HWJ, Jansen APD, et al. Depression in old age (75+), the PIKO study. *J Affect Disord* 2008;106:295–9.

10 Boyle MH, Offord DR, Hofmann HG, et al. Ontario Child Health Survey: I. Methodology. *Arch Gen Psychiatry* 1987;44:826–31.

11 Willms JD (2002). A study of vulnerable children in J. Douglas Willms (Editor) Vulnerable Children; Findings from Canada's National Longitudinal Survey of Children and Youth (pp. 3–22). Edmonton: University of Alberta Press

12 Ronen GM, Rosenbaum PL, Law M, Streiner DL. Health-related quality of life (HRQL) in childhood epilepsy: Can parents serve as proxies for their children? *Epilepsia* 1997;38, Suppl. 3:103.

13 Wade DT, Cairney J, Pevalin DJ. Emergence of gender differences in depression during adolescence: National panel results from three countries. *J Am Acad Child Adolesc Psychiatry* 2002; 41: 190–8.

14 Patten S. *Findings from Cycle 1.2 of the Canadian Community Health Survey – What have we learned and where do we go from here?* Paper presented at the

annual meeting of the Canadian Academy of Psychiatric Epidemiology, 2005.

15 Andrews G, Anstey K, Brodaty H, Issakidis C, Luscombe G. Recall of depressive episode 25 years previously. *Psychol Med* 1999;29:787–91.

16 Patten SB. Recall bias and major depression lifetime prevalence. *Soc Psychiatry Psychiatr Epidemiol* 2003;38:290–6.

17 Cannell CF, Fisher G, Bakker T. Reporting on hospitalization in the Health Interview Survey. *Vital and Health Statistics*, Series 3, No. 6. Hyattsville MD: Public Health Service, 1965.

18 Cairney J, Veldhuizen S, Wade TJ, Kurdyak P, Streiner DL. Evaluation of two measures of psychological distress as screeners for depression in the general population. *Can J Psychiatry* 2007; 52: 111–120.

19 Streiner DL, Norman GR. *Health measurement scales: A practical guide to their development and use* (4th ed.). Oxford: Oxford University Press, 2008.

20 Embretson SE. The new rules of measurement. *Psychol Assess* 1996;8:341–9.

21 Streiner DL. L'épidémiologie en santé mentale de l'enfant: Regard sur le passé et perspectives d'avenir. *Prism* 2003;42:16–33.

22 Caspi A., McClay J, Moffitt TE, et al. Role of genotype in the cycle of violence in maltreated children. *Science* 2002;297:851–4.

23 Caspi A, Sugden K, Moffitt TE, et al. Influence of life stress on depression: Moderation by a polymorphism in the 5-HTT gene. *Science* 2003;301:386–9.

Contributors

About the Editors

John Cairney, PhD. At the time of the writing of this book, John was a Canada Research Chair in psychiatric epidemiology in the Health Systems Research and Consulting Unit at the Centre for Addiction and Mental Health, Toronto, and an associate professor in the Department of Psychiatry at the University of Toronto. At the present time, he is the inaugural holder of the McMaster Family Medicine Professorship in Child Health Research, an associate professor in the Department of Psychiatry and Behavioural Neurosciences, and the associate director of research in the Department of Family Medicine at McMaster University. In 2008, he was elected president of the Canadian Academy of Psychiatric Epidemiology. In addition to accruing titles, he spends most of his time researching the social and population determinants of mental health, and has a particular interest in the intersection of physical and mental well-being across the lifecourse, especially in childhood and old age.

David L. Streiner, PhD. David is the director of the Kunin-Lunenfeld Applied Research Unit and assistant vice president, research, at the Baycrest Centre in Toronto, and a professor in the Department of Psychiatry at the University of Toronto. For the previous 30 years, he was a member of the Department of Clinical Epidemiology and Biostatistics and the Department of Psychiatry at McMaster University, and is a professor emeritus in both departments. He is the author of four books on statistics, epidemiology, and measurement theory, and has written a series of twenty-six articles on research methods for the *Canadian Journal of Psychiatry*. His main areas of interest are woodworking, measuring quality of life in various populations, woodworking, the epidemiology of psychological disorders in the elderly, and woodworking.

About the Authors

Tracie O. Afifi, MSc, was a PhD candidate in the Department of Community Health Sciences and a research assistant in the Department of Psychiatry at the University of Manitoba when her contribution was written.

Julio Arboleda-Flórez, MD, PhD, FRCPC, DABFP, is professor emeritus at Queen's University, Kingston, chair of the Forensic Division at the Department of Psychiatry and director of the Queen's/WHO/PAHO Regional Research and Training Unit for Psychiatric and Behavioural Epidemiology.

Diego G. Bassani, MSc, PhD, is a scientist/epidemiologist with the Centre for Global Health Research at the Keenan Research Centre of the Li Ka Shing Knowledge Institute, St. Michael's Hospital, Toronto.

Yves Béland is with Statistics Canada.

Jennifer Bethell, MSc, is pursuing a PhD in epidemiology at the University of Toronto.

Roger C. Bland, MB ChB, MRCS, LRCP, D Obst.RCOG, FRCPC, FRCPsych, is professor emeritus, Department of Psychiatry, University of Alberta, and the executive medical director at the Alberta Mental Health Board.

Michael H. Boyle, MSW, MSc, PhD, is a Canada Research Chair in the Social Determinants of Child Health, and a professor in the Department of Psychiatry and Behavioural Neurosciences at McMaster University.

Augustine Brannigan, PhD, is professor of sociology at the University of Calgary.

Saulo Castel, MD, PhD, FRCPC, is the director of medical education and research at the Whitby Mental Health Centre, a research associate within the Health Systems Research and Consulting Unit at the Centre of Addiction and Mental Health, Toronto, and assistant professor in the Department of Psychiatry, University of Toronto.

Marc Corbière, PhD, is an associate professor at the School of Rehabilitation of the Faculty of Medicine and Health Sciences at the Université de Sherbrooke.

Laurie M. Corna, MSc, PhD, is a doctoral candidate in the Department of Public Health Sciences at the University of Toronto.

Brian J. Cox, PhD, is a professor of psychiatry, psychology, and community health sciences at the University of Manitoba. He also holds a Canada Research Chair in mood and anxiety disorders.

Carolyn S. Dewa, MPH, PhD, is an associate professor in the departments of Psychiatry and Health Policy and Management and Evaluation at the University of Toronto. She is also the program head of the Centre for Addiction and Mental Health's Work and Well-being Research and Evaluation Program and is a senior scientist/health economist in the centre's Health Systems Research and Consulting Unit (HSRCU). She currently holds a Canadian Institutes of Health Research IPPH/PHAC Applied Public Health Chair.

Nicole Donaldson, MHSc, is a recent graduate from the Masters of Epidemiology and Community Health program at the University of Toronto.

Laura Gage, MD, FRCPC, is a geriatric psychiatrist at Whitby Mental Health Centre and a part time assistant professor in the Department of Psychiatry at the University of Toronto.

Katholiki Georgiades, PhD, is an assistant professor in Department of Psychiatry and Behavioural Neurosciences at McMaster University.

Paula Goering, RN, PhD, is section head of the Health Systems Research and Consulting Unit at the Centre of Addiction and Mental Health, Toronto, and professor in the Department of Psychiatry, University of Toronto.

Ronald Gravel is with Statistics Canada.

Brian D. Gushulak, MD. Brian is a consultant in migration health and was the director general of the newly created Medical Services Branch in the Canadian Department of Citizenship and Immigration.

Tara Hanson, BA, was a research program manager with the Alberta Mental Health Board at the time of writing her contribution. She is now director of Operations for the Alberta Centre for Child, Family and Community Research.

Alain D. Lesage, MD, FRCPC, MPhil, is a professor in the Department of Psychiatry at the Université de Montréal. He is also a researcher at the Centre de recherche Fernand-Sequin of Hôpital Louis-H. Lafontaine in Montreal.

Elizabeth Lin, PhD, is a research scientist in the Health Systems Research and Consulting Unit at the Centre for Addiction and Mental Health, Toronto.

Amanda T. Lo, BHSc, is pursuing a Masters degree in health research methodology at McMaster.

Douglas W. MacPherson, MD, MSc(CTM), FRCPC, was the director of Out-patient Infectious Diseases, Tropical Medicine, International Health at Hamilton Health Sciences, director of the Regional Parasitology Laboratory in Hamilton, and a member of the health sciences faculty at McMaster University. He has been a medical consultant and advisor for provincial and federal health departments and the federal immigration department in Canada, as well as several international agencies and foreign governments.

Scott B. Patten, MD, PhD, is a professor in the departments of Community Health Sciences and Psychiatry at the University of Calgary. He is also a Health Scholar with the Alberta Heritage Foundation for Medical Research.

Anne Rhodes, PhD, is a research scientist within the Suicide Studies Unit and the Keenan Research Centre in the Li Ka Shing Knowledge Institute of St. Michael's Hospital, Toronto, and an assistant professor in the departments of Psychiatry and Public Health Sciences at the University of Toronto.

Sarah Romans, MD, is a professor in the Department of Psychiatry at the University of Toronto.

Lori E. Ross, PhD, is a research scientist in the Social Equity and Health Research Section, Centre for Addiction and Mental Health, Toronto, and academic leader, Reproductive Life Stages Program, Women's College Hospital, Toronto.

Brian R. Rush, PhD, is co-director and a senior scientist within the Health Systems Research and Consulting Unit at the Centre of Addiction and Mental Health, Toronto, and is a professor in the Department of Psychiatry at the University of Toronto.

Isaac Sakinofsky, MD, FRCPC, FRCPsych, is professor emeritus of psychiatry and public health sciences in the University of Toronto and director of the High Risk Consultation Clinic at the Centre for Addiction and Mental Health, Toronto.

Jitender Sareen, MD, is an associate professor of psychiatry and community health sciences at the University of Manitoba. He is the director of research and anxiety services in the Department of Psychiatry.

Martin Shain, LLD, is founder of the Neighbour at Work Centre, and also a professor with the Department of Public Health Sciences in the Faculty of Medicine at the University of Toronto.

Heather Stuart, MA, PhD, is a professor in the Department of Community Health and Epidemiology and cross appointed to the departments of Psychiatry and the School of Rehabilitation Therapy at Queen's University, Kingston.

Julie Thurlow, MHSc, has a Masters degree in epidemiology and community health at the University of Toronto. She is a research scientist at the Workplace Safety Insurance Board investigating the association between workplace exposures and occupational diseases.

Karen A. Urbanoski, PhD, is a project scientist with the Health Systems Research and Consulting Unit at the Centre for Addiction and Mental Health, Toronto.

Scott Veldhuizen, BA, is a research analyst at the Centre for Addiction and Mental Health in Toronto and a graduate student in the Department of Applied Health Sciences at Brock University.

Charlotte Waddell, MSc, MD, CCFP, FRCPC, is Canada Research Chair in Children's Health Policy at Simon Fraser University where she is also Children's Health Policy Centre director and associate professor.

Terrance J. Wade, PhD, is Canada Research Chair in youth and wellness and associate professor and vice chair in the Department of Community Health Sciences at Brock University.

Greg Webster, MSc, is the director of research and indicator development at the Canadian Institute for Health Information (CIHI).

T. Cameron Wild, PhD, is an Alberta Heritage Foundation for Medical Research Health Scholar and a professor in the Centre for Health Promotion Studies, School of Public Health, at the University of Alberta. He directs the University of Alberta's Addiction and Mental Health Research Laboratory.